Handbook of
Child and Adolescent
Psychopharmacology

Handbook of
Child and Adolescent
Psychopharmacology

Edited by

Benedetto Vitiello MD

Gabriele Masi MD

Donatella Marazziti MD

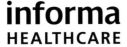

© 2006 Informa Healthcare, an imprint of Informa UK Limited

First published in the United Kingdom in 2006
by Informa Healthcare, an imprint of Informa Limited, 2 Park Square, Milton Park,
Abingdon, Oxon OX14 4RN

Tel: +44 (0)20 7017 6000
Fax: +44 (0)20 7017 6699
Website: http://www.tandf.co.uk/medicine
E-mail: info.medicine@tandf.co.uk

Although every effort has been made to ensure that all owners of copyright material have
been acknowledged in this publication, we would be glad to acknowledge in subsequent
reprints or editions any omissions brought to our attention.

Although every effort has been made to ensure that drug doses and other information are
presented accurately in this publication, the ultimate responsibility rests with the prescribing
physician. Neither the publishers nor the authors can be held responsible for errors or
for any consequences arising from the use of information contained herein. For detailed
prescribing information or instructions on the use of any product or procedure discussed
herein, please consult the prescribing information or instructional material issued by the
manufacturer.

A CIP record for this book is available from the British Library.

Library of Congress Cataloging-in-Publication Data

Data available on application

ISBN-10   1 84184 486 1
ISBN-13   978 1 84184 486 2

Distributed in North and South America by

Taylor & Francis
2000 NW Corporate Blvd
Boca Raton, FL 33431, USA

Within Continental USA
Tel: 800 272 7737; Fax: 800 374 3401
Outside Continental USA
Tel: 561 994 0555; Fax: 561 361 6018
E-mail: orders@crcpress.com

Distributed in the rest of the world by
Thomson Publishing Services
Cheriton House
North Way
Andover, Hampshire SP10 5BE, UK
Tel.:   +44 (0)1264 332424
E-mail: salesorder.tandf@thomsonpublishingservices.co.uk

Composition by C&M Digitals (P) Ltd, Chennai, India
Printed and bound in Great Britain by TJ International, Padstow, Cornwall

Contents

Contributors

Pedro G Alvarenga
Department of Psychiatry
University of São Paulo
  Medical School
São Paulo, SP
Brazil

Cristina Belotto
Department of Psychiatry
University of São Paulo
  Medical School
São Paulo, SP
Brazil

Sonia Borcato
Department of Psychiatry
University of
  São Paulo Medical School
São Paulo, SP
Brazil

Dario Calderoni
Child and Adolescent
  Neurologist and
  Psychiatrist
University of Rome
Rome
Italy

Maura Carvalho
Department of Psychiatry
University of São Paulo
  Medical School
São Paulo, SP
Brazil

Mario Catena
Department of Psychiatry,
  Neurobiology, Pharmacology,
  and Biotechnology
University of Pisa
Pisa
Italy

Priscilla Chacon
Department of Psychiatry
University of São Paulo
  Medical School
São Paulo, SP
Brazil

Maria Alice De Mathis
Department of Psychiatry
University of São Paulo
  Medical School
São Paulo, SP
Brazil

Maria Eugênia De Mathis
Department of Psychiatry
University of São Paulo
    Medical School
São Paulo, SP
Brazil

Juliana B Diniz
Department of Psychiatry
University of São Paulo
    Medical School
São Paulo, SP
Brazil

Ana G Hounie
Department of Psychiatry
University of São Paulo
    Medical School
São Paulo, SP
Brazil

Antonio C Lopes
Department of Psychiatry
University of São Paulo
    Medical School
São Paulo, SP
Brazil

Donatella Marazziti
Professor of Psychiatry
Department of Psychiatry,
    Neurobiology,
    Pharmacology, and
    Biotechnology
University of Pisa
Pisa
Italy

Gabriele Masi
Head of Psychopathology
    and Psychopharmacology
    Research Branch
Stella Maris Scientific Institute
    of Child Neurology and
    Psychiatry
Pisa
Italy

Luigi Mazzone
Division of Child Neurology
    and Psychiatry
Department of Pediatrics
University of Catania
Catania
Italy

Eurípedes C Miguel
Department of Psychiatry
University of São Paulo
    Medical School
São Paulo, SP
Brazil

Márcia Motta
Department of Psychiatry
University of São Paulo
    Medical School
São Paulo, SP
Brazil

Francesco Mungai
Department of Psychiatry,
    Neurobiology, Pharmacology,
    and Biotechnology
University of Pisa
Pisa
Italy

Chiara Pfanner
Division of Child Neurology
  and Psychiatry
IRCCS Stella Maris, Calambrone
University of Pisa
Italy

Adriana Pinto
Department of Psychiatry
University of São Paulo
  Medical School
São Paulo, SP
Brazil

Helena S Prado
Department of Psychiatry
University of São Paulo
  Medical School
São Paulo, SP
Brazil

Silvio Presta
Department of Psychiatry,
  Neurobiology, Pharmacology,
  and Biotechnology
University of Pisa
Pisa
Italy

Lucas Quarantini
Department of
Neuropsychiatry
Federal University of Bahia
Salvador
Brazil

Maria C do Rosário-Campos
Department of Neuropsychiatry
Federal University of Bahia
Salvador
Brazil

Aline S Sampaio
Department of Psychiatry
University of São Paulo
  Medical School
São Paulo, SP
Brazil

André A Seixas
Department of Psychiatry
University of São Paulo
  Medical School
São Paulo, SP
Brazil

Benedetto Vitiello
Chief, Child and Adolescent
  Treatment and Preventative
  Intervention Research Branch
Division of Services and
  Intervention Research
National Institute of Mental
  Health
Bethesda, MD
USA*
and
Adjunct Associate Professor
  of Psychiatry
John Hopkins University
Baltimore, MD
USA

*The opinions and assertions contained in this author's chapters are the private views of the author and are not to be construed as official or as reflecting the views of the National Institute of Mental Health, the National Institute of Health, or the US Department of Health and Human Services

Laura Vivarelli
Department of Psychiatry,
   Neurobiology, Pharmacology,
   and Biotechnology
University of Pisa
Pisa
Italy

Alessandro Zuddas
Child Neuropsychiatry
   Department of
   Neuroscience
University of Cagliari
Cagliari
Italy

Foreword

The purpose of this handbook is to provide clinicians who are directly involved in the care of children and adolescents with mental disorders with updated, practically useful information on how to best use psychotropic medications.

Research in pediatric psychopharmacology has greatly expanded in recent years. This handbook includes the latest research findings with special attention to the clinical context in which care is delivered and treatment decisions are made. To this end, the material has been arranged and presented by disorder rather than by type of medication. Psychopathology is, in fact, the target of treatment and a careful diagnostic evaluation is the foundation of any rational therapy.

Few treatments in medicine can raise more controversy than the use of medications to mange emotional and behavioral disturbances in childhood. Safety concerns should certainly be paramount when considering exposing children to pharmacological agents, and, whenever possible, the possibility of using alternative, psychosocial interventions should be weighed before choosing medications. It remains however that, for many children, a cautions, scientifically informed, and carefully monitored pharmacotherapy can produce major improvements. In this spirit, the handbook is meant to be a contribution towards practicing evidence-based pediatric psychopharmacology.

Benedetto Vitiello, Gabriele Masi,
Donatella Marazziti

chapter 1

Introduction: Psychopharmacotherapy in the developmental age

Benedetto Vitiello, Gabriele Masi, and Donatella Marazziti

Pediatric psychopharmacology informs on how psychotropic medications can be used to treat children with behavioral and emotional disorders. The observation that amphetamine dramatically improved behavior in hyperkinetic children goes back almost 70 years (Bradley, 1937), that is more than 10 years before tranquilizers, lithium, or antidepressants were introduced into the adult pharmacopeia. Still, pediatric psychopharmacology can be considered a relatively new area of inquiry, which only recently has started testing systematically the effects of psychotropics in the developmental age.

The pediatric use of psychotropics has much increased during the last 10 years, especially in the US and with respect to stimulants for the treatment of attention deficit hyperactivity disorder (ADHD) and antidepressants for the treatment of depressive and anxiety disorders (Olfson et al, 2002). Research on the efficacy and safety of psychotropics in children has also dramatically increased over the last few years. Clinical trials have been conducted to test the efficacy of stimulants, antidepressants, mood stabilizers, and antipsychotics in children suffering from a variety of conditions, such as ADHD, depression, obsessive-compulsive disorder, other anxiety disorders, bipolar disorder, autism, and other pervasive developmental disorders.

In spite of, or perhaps because of, this increased utilization and expanding research basis, the pediatric use of psychotropics remains the object of much debate and at times of controversy. While there is minimal resistance to prescribing antibiotics to children for treating infections, bronchodilators for asthma, or anticonvulsants for epilepsy, the notion that psychotropics can be used to treat mental disorders is apparently more difficult to accept. In part, this resistance may be related to the fact that mental disorders still do not have biologic markers that can be used for diagnostic purposes and that the diagnosis is currently based on descriptive phenomenology. Also, common psychiatric disorders, such as ADHD, depression, and anxiety, exist on a continuum with normality, and concerns about medicalization of normal behavior have been raised. To some extent, it may seem arbitrary to diagnose a disorder based on the presence of a certain number of symptoms on a checklist.

Much progress, however, has been made in documenting the negative effects of extreme emotional and behavioral manifestations on the functioning and well-being of children. For most disorders, it is not the symptom that makes the diagnosis, rather the symptom-induced dysfunction that triggers the clinical referral and leads to the diagnosis. Moreover, continuity between "normality" and "psycho-pathology" is not specific to child psychiatry, or even to psychiatry in general. Hypertension and hypercholesterolemia are medical conditions that are on a continuum with normality and are defined by cut-offs based on estimated risk for negative outcomes. The situation of ADHD is not dissimilar since higher rates of hyperactivity have been associated with school failure, social impairment, and underachievement. In parallel, much progress has been made in documenting the neurobiologic bases of psychopathology, even though these advances have not yet translated into diagnostic markers.

A second argument against pharmacologic treatment in children is that childhood psychiatric disorders are "psychologic", with a direct and exclusive connection with negative environmental factors and, consequently, treatable by means of psychologic (i.e., non-pharmacologic) interventions. There is increasing evidence, however, that the traditional dichotomy of psychologic vs biologic factors is not valid, because all psychologic events have underlying biologic substrates and the environment interacts with the genes to determine behavior (Caspi et al, 2002).

Another prominent concern among objectors to pediatric psychophar-macology is that psychotropics may be unsafe for use in children and negatively impact development. This is an important concern that should be taken seriously and lead to careful use and monitoring. It should be noted, however, that drugs that are being used to treat medical conditions can also have safety problems, and some of these drugs, such as corticosteroids, do act on the brain. In fact, we should not assume that any drug is safe per se, rather potential benefits and risks of a drug should be evaluated in the context of the severity of the disorder being treated and the possible alternative approaches (Vitiello et al, 2003). Potential risks of treatment must also be weighed against the possible toxicity of untreated psychopathology.

The issue of whether it is right or wrong to administer psychotropic drugs during the developmental age cannot obviously be oversimplified with a positive or negative answer. In deciding whether psychopharmacologic treatment may be appropriate for an individual child, a number of elements need to be considered, including type, severity, and duration of symptoms, level of functional impairment caused by symptoms, and possibility of treating the condition with psychosocial interventions. Many families and clinicians in the community would prefer to use psychotherapy whenever possible, and leave medications as a second line of treatment. With exceptions, such an approach seems quite sensible. Clearly there are conditions such as schizophrenia and bipolar disorder for which the primary treatment ought to be pharmacologic. However, for most other disorders psychosocial interventions are available and should be used whenever possible and appropriate.

A few studies have directly compared the effectiveness of psychosocial and pharmacologic treatments. Pharmacologic treatment, either alone or in combination with psychotherapy, proved to be more effective than psychotherapy alone for children with ADHD and for adolescents with major depression (MTA Cooperative Group, 1999; TADS Team, 2004). In contrast, cognitive-behavioral therapy, alone or in combination with medication, was superior to medication alone for children and adolescents with obsessive-compulsive disorder (Pediatric OCD Treatment Study Team, 2004). Not enough research, however, has been conducted on the sequential use of psychotherapy and medication. For instance, the current practice guidelines of the American Academy of Pediatrics for the treatment of ADHD indicate either stimulant medication or behavioral therapy as appropriate initial treatment (American Academy of Pediatrics, 2001). Thus, the decision on which treatment should be tried first remains, in most cases, an individual choice, based primarily on personal preferences. It is therefore essential that the expert in pediatric psychopharmacology be familiar not only with potential benefits and risks of medication, but also with available non-pharmacologic interventions, which can be used in lieu of or in combination with medication.

In any case, the critical importance of a careful and comprehensive diagnostic evaluation as the initial step for successful treatment cannot be overstated. Before treatment is started, the type and severity of symptoms must be documented, preferably using a validated rating instrument. This assessment must be periodically repeated during treatment and any adverse events emerging during treatment recorded. Thus, the practice of pediatric psychopharmacology requires multiple skills, among which expertise in developmental psychopathology and pharmacology is just the basic foundation. The ultimate goal is to integrate the current, and ever evolving, scientific knowledge of the efficacy and safety of psychotropics during development with the specific needs of the individual child and family.

References

American Academy of Pediatrics. Clinical practice guideline: treatment of the school-aged child with attention-deficit/hyperactivity disorder. *Pediatrics* 2001; **108**: 1033–44.

Bradley C. The behavior of children receiving benzedrine. *Am J Psychiatry* 1937; **94**: 577–85.

Caspi A, McClay J, Moffitt TE, et al. Role of genotype in the cycle of violence in maltreated children. *Science* 2002; **297**: 851–4.

MTA Cooperative Group. A 14-month randomized clinical trial of treatment strategies for attention-deficit/hyperactivity disorder (ADHD). *Arch Gen Psychiatry* 1999; **56**: 1073–86.

Olfson M, Marcus SC, Weissman MM, Jensen PS. National trends in the use of psychotropic medications by children. *J Am Acad Child Adolesc Psychiatry* 2002; **41**: 514–21.

Pediatric OCD Treatment Study (POTS) Team. Cognitive-behavior therapy, sertraline, and their combination for children and adolescents with obsessive-compulsive disorder: the Pediatric OCD Treatment Study (POTS) randomized controlled trial. *JAMA* 2004; **292**: 1969–76.

TADS Team. The Treatment for Adolescents with Depression Study (TADS): short-term effectiveness and safety outcomes. *JAMA* 2004; **292**: 807–20.

Vitiello B, Riddle MA, Greenhill LL, et al. How can we improve the assessment of safety in child and adolescent psychopharmacology? *J Am Acad Child Adolesc Psychiatry* 2003; **42**: 634–41.

chapter 2

Practicing evidence-based pediatric psychopharmacology: essential concepts

Benedetto Vitiello

The general principle of evidence-based medicine is to make clinical decisions based on the best available evidence of their effectiveness (Gray, 2001). In the same vein, practicing evidence-based psychopharmacology means to hold available evidence of medication effects as the main guiding factor when treating children with psychotropic medications. It has been correctly pointed out that evidence-based medicine and its applications to child psychiatry constitute an ideal toward which one should strive, but which also looks at times elusive or conditioned by economic concerns rather than scientific data (Gray, 2001; Fonagy et al, 2002). Traditionally, these considerations have been especially applicable to pediatric psychopharmacology because of the limited research data supporting treatment decisions.

In fact, most psychotropics have been developed for the treatment of adults and, once marketed, also used for treating children, but without adequate empirical evidence of their efficacy and safety in pediatric subjects (Jensen et al, 1999). In recent years, however, a considerable expansion of research in pediatric psychopharmacology has been providing much needed information on the effects of psychotropics in children, thus allowing truly evidence-based guidelines to be developed (Vitiello et al, 2004).

Treatment decisions, such as whether to treat or which treatment to use, are likely to be influenced by multiple factors and considerations

Table 2.1 Elements likely to influence treatment decisions

Type of symptoms

Severity of symptoms

Severity of impairment associated with symptoms

Evidence for efficacy and safety of treatment

Type of potential side-effects

Clinician's training

Clinician's past clinical experience with specific treatments

Clinician's intuition about individual patients

Family's preference, expectations, and values

Family's past experience with specific treatments

Financial considerations

(Table 2.1). Scientific evidence is only one of these factors, but, according to evidence-based medicine, should be the most influential.

What constitutes evidence of treatment effect

The term "evidence" can have different meanings according to the context in which it is used. Evidence that a treatment produces a certain effect means that a cause–effect relationship has been established between the intervention and the outcome. Causality is generally inferred by comparing a group of patients receiving the treatment in question with another group receiving another treatment and serving as a control. To ensure comparability between groups, treatment assignment is typically randomized and, to avoid biases in assessment, blinded evaluators who are unaware of treatment assignment are employed to measure outcome (Vitiello, 2003). These are the essential features of the randomized controlled clinical trial, which is a true experiment providing the best evidence of treatment effects (Table 2.2).

In the absence of data from controlled clinical trials, however, other, less compelling sources of information can be used to guide treatment decisions. Non-randomized, observational studies and case reports can be suggestive, though not definitive proof, of efficacy. There are numerous examples of medical interventions whose therapeutic benefit had been suggested by non-randomized, observational

Table 2.2   Features of a well-designed controlled clinical trial proving treatment efficacy

Control condition

Randomization

Masking of patient, family, and evaluator (double-blind condition)

Prespecified primary outcome measures

Valid and reliable assessments of variables of interest

Prespecified statistical analyses

Adequate sample to ensure appropriate statistical power to detect differences

Statistically significant difference between study groups

Clinically significant difference between study groups

studies, but then not confirmed by randomized clinical trials. For instance, in pediatric psychopharmacology, tricyclic medications had been used for years in the management of children and adolescents with depression based on clinical experience, but none of the at least 12 randomized trials conducted thus far has been able to demonstrate their advantage over a placebo (Hazell et al, 2002).

It is now generally accepted that evidence for treatment effects in children must come from clinical trials conducted in children and that results of clinical trials conducted in adults, though informative, are insufficient to guide pediatric use. Differences in metabolism, pharmacokinetics, and pharmacodynamics between children and adults have implication for both the efficacy and safety of medications (Riddle et al, 2001; Vitiello and Jensen, 1997). Thus, for instance, young age increases the risk for liver toxicity by valproate or that for skin rash by lamotrigine.

The strength of the evidence supporting treatment effects can be ranked into different levels (Jobson and Potter, 1995; Gray, 2001; GRADE Working Group, 2004). For instance, a five-level strength of evidence ranking is at times used, which includes:

I. Strong evidence from at least one systematic review of multiple, well-designed, randomized controlled trials.
II. Strong evidence from at least one well-designed, randomized controlled trial.

III. Evidence from well-designed, non-randomized trials, such as prepost comparisons, cohort or case-controlled studies.
IV. Evidence from well-designed, non-experimental, observational studies from more than one research group.
 V. Opinion of experts based on descriptive studies or clinical observations (Gray, 2001).

Based on a simpler three-level ranking, if the efficacy of a treatment has been demonstrated by at least two independently conducted, well-designed, randomized clinical trials, this level of evidence is considered to be strong and usually conclusive (level A). If only one well-designed randomized clinical trial supports the treatment effects, the evidence is considered intermediate and usually not conclusive, but in need of replication (level B). Finally, if no randomized controlled trials are available, but only observational studies, case reports, or expert opinion, the data can only be considered as suggestive of an effect (level C) (Table 2.3).

Thus, different levels of evidence currently exist for pharmacologic treatment of major depressive disorder in adolescents (Table 2.4). Clinical guidelines and treatment algorithms integrate available evidence into sequential steps so that the interventions supported by level A evidence are considered first when treating patients, followed, in the order, by level B and level C interventions (Greenhill et al, 2002). As more research data are reported, treatment guidelines and algorithms are to be updated to reflect the most recent level of evidence. In the meantime, the clinician treating conditions for which no intervention with level A evidence of efficacy is available will necessarily have to rely on interventions with less convincing evidence.

Table 2.3 Level of evidence of treatment efficacy

Level A	Efficacy is proven by two or more well-designed, randomized clinical trials
Level B	Efficacy is supported by only one well-designed, randomized clinical trial
Level C	Efficacy is suggested only by observational surveys, uncontrolled studies, or case reports

Table 2.4   Antidepressants for adolescents with major depression: levels of evidence for efficacy

Level A	Fluoxetine
Level B	Sertraline
	Citalopram
Level C	Venlafaxine
	Mirtazapine
	Bupropion
	Tricyclics

Limitations of clinical trials

Clinical trials are the best method for providing evidence of treatment effects. Still, they have limitations. The results of a clinical trial are expressed as group averages, but must be applied to the treatment of individual patients (McAlister et al, 2000). Study participants are not necessarily representative of patients seen in clinical practice. Typically, inclusion and exclusion criteria select study subjects in order to reduce variance and experimental noise, and thus make the experiment more sensitive to detecting treatment effects. This selection process limits the generalizability of the findings. In addition, most efficacy trials are conducted at academic research sites where patients may differ from those usually seen by practitioners in the community.

A distinction has been made between "efficacy," which indicates that a treatment has been shown to be better than a placebo under tightly controlled conditions in research settings, and "effectiveness," which refers to demonstrating that a treatment works under usual clinical practice conditions (Wells, 1999). The use of placebo as a way of detecting treatment effects is, on one hand, experimentally quite advantageous as a difference is more likely to show when an active medication is compared to an inactive compound, but, on the other hand, it decreases the clinical relevance of the study. In fact, placebo is not a realistic treatment choice and it does not equal absence of treatment either. Thus, the ecologic validity of placebo is limited.

Furthermore, "efficacy" refers to effect on symptom reduction, while "effectiveness" refers to improvement in more clinically meaningful outcomes, such as level of functioning or illness recovery. In pediatric psychopharmacology, we currently have good evidence for the efficacy of a number of medications, but the evidence for the effectiveness of pharmacologic interventions is still rather limited. Currently, new models of clinical trials to be conducted in practice settings are being developed and applied to pediatric psychopharmacology (March et al, 2004). It should be pointed out that the terms "efficacy" and "effectiveness" are often used interchangeably in pharmacology, without taking into account this distinction in meaning.

Another limitation has to do with the underreporting of clinical trials that fail to find a treatment difference. These trials, referred to also as "negative trials," tend not to be published, especially when they are funded by industry because marketing considerations discourage the publication of studies that do not support the therapeutic value of a drug (Lexchin et al, 2003). In addition, scientific journals have a publication bias against negative findings. While this situation is being addressed and corrected through a stricter regulation of clinical trials, "consumers" of scientific information should remain aware of this bias.

Importance of systematic reviews and meta-analyses

In most cases, no single clinical trial, no matter how well designed, can conclusively inform on the therapeutic value of a treatment. When multiple trials have been conducted, a systematic and rigorous review of their results yields stronger conclusions than any individual study can provide (Whittington et al, 2004). A review is "systematic" when the specific criteria used to search and select studies are decided a priori. As part of the review, data across studies can be analyzed in order to arrive at an estimate of the overall treatment effect ("meta-analysis").

The value of this approach has been recently shown in the case of the risk/benefit ratio of antidepressants. Anecdotal reports had raised concern about the possibility that use of antidepressants may raise the risk for suicidal behavior in depressed children and adolescents. Because an increased risk for suicidal behavior is intrinsic in the fact of suffering from depression, observational studies cannot be much help and randomized controlled clinical trials are best suited to address this question. However, the rate of suicidal behavior is too low for a single study to have enough statistical power. By analyzing the data of 24 placebo-controlled trials of nine antidepressants involving a total of about 4400 children and adolescents, it was possible to estimate that acute antidepressant treatment for 8–12 weeks is associated with an increased risk for "suicidality" (which includes suicidal attempts and ideation) from about 2% on placebo to about 4% on active medication (Hammad, 2004).

It must be pointed out that this finding does not link antidepressant use to completed suicide, which is too rare of an event to be studied through clinical trials. In fact, no complete suicide occurred among the 4400 subjects included in this meta-analysis. As further discussed in the chapter on the pharmacotherapy of depression, the risk of leaving severe depression untreated likely outweighs potential risks from antidepressant treatment.

Estimating the magnitude of treatment effect

The strength of the evidence for the efficacy of a treatment should not be confused with the magnitude of the treatment effect. For instance, there can be level A evidence, from multiple clinical trials, that a treatment does indeed work, but that its therapeutic benefit is modest. Thus, antidepressants are effective in only about 50–60% of cases, which contrasts with an improvement rate of about 40% on placebo.

From a practical point of view, estimating the strength of a treatment is quite useful as it informs on the likelihood of success of the intervention. To this end, several approaches have been devised. Arguably, the most easily accessible and interpretable are those of the effect size (ES) and the "number needed to treat" (NNT). Both require a comparison condition as a point of reference for estimating treatment effect. The comparison is often a placebo control, which should not, however, be interpreted as absence of treatment. In fact, a placebo is administered in the context of clinical contacts and overall patient management, which, though non-specific, carries considerable therapeutic value.

The ES is the difference in outcome between the group of patients treated with the intervention of interest and the comparison group expressed in standard deviation units. The most commonly used ES (Cohen's d) is the difference between the means of the two groups on the outcome measure at the end of treatment divided by the pooled standard deviation (Cohen, 1998). The greater the d, the larger is the difference between the groups. It is usually accepted that ES values of about 0.2 are "small," 0.5 "moderate," and 0.8 or greater "large." Thus, the effect of stimulants in reducing ADHD symptoms is "large" and that of antidepressants in depression is "small to moderate."

A large effect is easier to demonstrate in a clinical trial, while a smaller effect can escape detection and requires larger sample sizes. This explains why many studies of antidepressants, which tend to have a small to moderate effect size, have failed to detect a difference from placebo. It must be noted that the ES is the result of the therapeutic activity of both the treatment and its control. Antidepressants have a rather small ES also because the placebo effect is quite strong in depression.

The NNT indicates the number of patients that need to be treated in order to add one single improved patient to the number of those who are expected to improve with the control condition (Laupacis et al, 1988). It is computed from the percent response rates in the treatment and control groups, which are provided as part of the results of clinical trials. The ratio between 100 and the mathematical difference between the two rates expressed in percentage units yields the NNT. Thus, in the Treatment for Adolescents with Depression Study (TADS), the response rate on fluoxetine was 61% and that on placebo 35% (TADS Team, 2004). These rates yield a NNT = 100/ (61–35) = 4. This means that one needs to treat four depressed adolescents with fluoxetine in order to add one patient to the three who would improve anyway on placebo. Obviously, the more powerful a treatment is in comparison with placebo, the smaller is the NNT.

Familiarity with the general principles of evidence-based medicine will allow the clinician to better interpret research findings and appreciate both strengths and limitations of practice guidelines and treatment algorithms (Guyatt et al, 2000).

References

Cohen J. *Statistical power analysis for the behavioral sciences*, 2nd edn. Hillsdale, NJ: Erlbaum; 1988.

Fonagy P, Target M, Cottrell D, Phillips J, Kurtz Z. *What works for whom? A critical review of treatments for children and adolescents.* New York: The Guilford Press; 2002.

GRADE Working Group. Grading quality of evidence and strength of recommendations. *BMJ* 2004; **328**: 1490.

Gray JAM. *Evidence-based healthcare*, 2nd edn. London, UK: Churchill Livingstone; 2001.

Greenhill LL, Pliszka S, Dulcan MK, et al. American Academy of Child and Adolescent Psychiatry. Practice parameter for the use of stimulant medications in the treatment of children, adolescents, and adults. *J Am Acad Child Adolesc Psychiatry* 2002; **41**: 26S–49S.

Guyatt GH, Meade MO, Jaeschke RZ, Cook DJ, Haynes RB. Practitioners of evidence based care. Not all clinicians need to appraise evidence from scratch but all need some skills. *BMJ* 2000; **320**: 954–5.

Hammad TA. Results of the analysis of suicidality in pediatric trials of newer antidepressants. Presentation at the Food and Drug Administration, Psychopharmacologic Drugs Advisory Committee and the Pediatric Advisory Committee, 13 September, 2004. Available at website http://www.fda.gov/ohrms/dockets/ac/04/slides/2004-4065S1_08_FDA-Hammad_files/frame.htm.

Hazell P, O'Connell D, Heathcote D, Henry D. Tricyclic drugs for depression in children and adolescents. *Cochrane Database Syst Rev* 2002; **2**: CD002317.

Jensen PS, Bhatara VS, Vitiello B, et al. Psychoactive medication prescribing practices for U.S. children: gaps between research and clinical practice. *J Am Acad Child Adolesc Psychiatry* 1999; **38**: 557–65.

Jobson KO, Potter WZ. International psychopharmacology algorithm project report. *Psychopharmacol Bull* 1995; **31**: 457–9.

Laupacis A, Sackett DL, Roberts RS. An assessment of clinically useful measures of the consequences of treatment. *N Engl J Med* 1988; **318**: 1728–33.

Lexchin J, Bero LA, Djulbegovic B, Clark O. Pharmaceutical industry sponsorship and research outcome and quality: systematic review. *BMJ* 2003; **326**: 1–10.

McAlister FA, Straus SE, Guyatt GH, Haynes RB. Users' guide to the medical literature. XX. Integrating research evidence with the care of the individual patient. *JAMA* 2000; **283**: 2829–36.

March JS, Silva SG, Compton S, et al. The Child and Adolescent Psychiatry Trials Network (CAPTN). *J Am Acad Child Adolesc Psychiatr* 2004; **43**: 515–18.

Riddle MA, Kastelic EA, Frosch E. Pediatric psychopharmacology. *J Child Psychol Psychiatry* 2001; **42**: 73–90.

TADS Team. The Treatment for Adolescents with Depression Study (TADS): short-term effectiveness and safety outcomes. *JAMA* 2004; **292**: 807–20.

Vitiello B. Clinical trials methodology and design issues. In: Martin A, Scahill L, Charney D, Leckman JF, eds. *Child and adolescent psychopharmacology*. New York, NY: Oxford University Press; 2003.

Vitiello B, Heiligenstein JJ, Riddle MA, Greenhill LL, Fegert JM. The interface between publicly funded and industry-funded research in pediatric psychopharmacology: opportunities for integration and collaboration. *Biol Psychiatry* 2004; **56**: 3–9.

Vitiello B, Jensen PS. Medication development and testing in children and adolescents. *Arch Gen Psychiatry* 1997; **54**: 871–6.

Wells KB. Treatment research at the crossroad: the scientific interface of clinical trials and effectiveness research. *Am J Psychiatry* 1999; **156**: 5–10.

Whittington CJ, Kendall T, Fonagy P, et al. Selective serotonin reuptake inhibitors in childhood depression: systematic review of published versus unpublished data. *Lancet* 2004; **363**: 1341–5.

chapter 3

Pharmacotherapy of anxiety disorders in children and adolescents

Gabriele Masi

Clinical features of anxiety disorders

Introduction

Defining boundaries between normal behavior and psychopathology is a frequent dilemma, in children and adolescents even more than in adults. This is particularly true for anxiety symptoms, which are not only extremely frequent, but also may have an organizing effect on normal psychologic and behavioral development. Separation anxieties, simple phobias, and traits of generalized anxiety may have a protective role, and only when they are excessively rigid and severe do they represent a significant pathologic state. The criterion of significant interference with daily life is not easily adaptable to a young child. The severity and stability of anxiety manifestations, as well as an intense subjective distress, irrespective of possible provoking situations, without any possible flexibility in affective modulation, may be considered a possible marker of psychopathology.

Anxiety disorders are among the most common psychiatric disorders affecting pediatric populations, both in the United States (Shaffer et al, 1995) and in Europe (Verhulst et al, 1997), with an estimated prevalence ranging from 6 to 18% of children and adolescents. According to DSM-IV (American Psychiatric Association, 2000) different anxiety disorders can be described, including separation anxiety disorder, panic disorder, social phobia, simple phobias, and generalized anxiety. These disorders often co-occur, and more than 60% of affected children have two or more anxiety disorders. Furthermore, a high comorbidity with affective disorders is reported (Masi et al, 2004). Longitudinal studies suggest that, although most children with anxiety disorders are psychiatrically healthy as adults, childhood anxiety disorders predict adult disorders, and the majority of adult anxiety and depressive disorders is antedated by childhood anxiety (Pine et al, 1998). Finally, social dysfunction may result from the failure to diagnose and treat anxiety disorders during adolescence, increasing rates of use of medical and mental health services (Coyle, 2001).

Anxiety disorders can be managed using non-pharmacologic or pharmacologic options, or a combination thereof. Pharmacotherapy should not be used as the sole intervention, but as an adjunct to psychotherapeutic or behavioral interventions.

Different classes of medications have been used in pediatric anxiety disorders, including benzodiazepines, tricyclic antidepressants, and buspirone. The advent of new antidepressants, selective serotonin reuptake inhibitors (SSRIs) and beyond, has been a major advance in psychiatry, and these drugs have been shown to have fewer side-effects, lower toxicity in overdose, and a potentially broader range of clinical indications. After a brief summary of the clinical features of anxiety disorders in children and adolescents, first- and second-line antianxiety medications will be considered, including newer antidepressants, tricyclics, and benzodiazepines. "Third-line" medications, such as monoamine oxidase inhibitors, antihistamines, and beta-adrenergic antagonists, will not be included in this review. These medications have only case studies or small samples to support their use in anxious youngsters. In addition, there are no recent reports or studies concerning their safety and efficacy in anxiety disorders in children and adolescents.

Categoric and dimensional approach to anxiety disorders

Even though anxiety is a typically dimensional construct, which can be captured prevalently in its quantitative definition (such as fever or blood pressure), all the diagnostic systems have tried to disentangle it into a finite number of specific syndromes, which should represent discrete diagnostic groups. This difficulty is witnessed by the changing structure of chapter of childhood anxiety disorders in the available categoric systems. However, to date, generating syndromes represents a parsimonious approach to estimate pathologic anxiety, which tries to aggregate clusters of anxiety symptoms into more coherent clinical pictures, which will be confirmed or refined with further research.

In this chapter the obsessive-compulsive disorder will not be included in the anxiety disorders; it is considered separately by the International Classification of Diseases 10th edition (ICD-10) (World Health Organization, 1992), but included by the DSM-IV. In contrast, the post-traumatic stress disorder will be included, as proposed by the DSM-IV, but not by the ICD-10.

A brief description of the following anxiety disorders will be provided: separation anxiety disorder, panic disorder, simple phobias (or phobic disorder), social phobia, generalized anxiety disorder, and acute stress disorder/post-traumatic stress disorder.

Separation anxiety disorder

The essential feature of separation anxiety disorder (SAD) is an excessive and developmentally inappropriate anxiety concerning separation from home or attachment figures, with anticipatory anxiety and avoidant behavior (Masi et al, 2001a). Most typical manifestations are:

- excessive distress when separation from home or major attachment figures occurs or is anticipated
- persistent and excessive worry about losing, or possible harm befalling, major attachment figures
- persistent and excessive worry that an untoward event will lead to separation from a major attachment figure (e.g. getting lost or being kidnapped)
- persistent reluctance or refusal to go to school or elsewhere because of fear of separation
- persistent and excessive fearfulness or reluctance to be alone or without major attachment figures at home or without significant adults in other settings
- persistent reluctance to go to sleep without being near a major attachment figure or to sleep away from home
- repeated nightmares involving the theme of separation
- repeated complaints of physical symptoms (such as headaches, stomach aches, nausea, or vomiting) when separation from major attachment figures occurs or is anticipated.

The severity of symptomatology ranges from anticipatory uneasiness to full-blown anxiety about separation, but children are usually brought to the clinician when SAD results in school refusal or somatic symptoms (such as recurrent abdominal pain). Although high rates of comorbidity with anxiety and mood disorders are very common in children with anxiety disorders, children with a primary diagnosis of SAD are the least likely to meet criteria for a concurrent anxiety disorder.

DSM-IV and ICD-10 consider a persistent unwillingness to attend school as one of the possible symptoms of SAD. A prevalence of 1–2% of school refusers in the school-age population is widely reported. The extent to which SAD can account for school refusal is debated. School refusal is reported in about 75% of children with SAD, and SAD is reported to occur in up to 70% of school refusers. Simple and/or social phobia and depression are the other most frequent diagnoses for school refusers, with many of these children having multiple diagnoses.

Different studies have suggested that childhood SAD may be a risk factor for other anxiety disorders, but whether this link is specific, for example to panic disorder and agoraphobia (Silove and Manicavasagar, 1993), or whether SAD represents a general factor of vulnerability for a broad range of anxiety disorders (Silove and Manicavasagar, 1993; Manicavasagar et al, 1998) is still debated. A previous or comorbid SAD has been reported in about 50–75% of children and adolescents with juvenile panic disorder (Biederman et al, 1997; Masi et al, 2001b).

It has been hypothesized that childhood SAD may not transform into panic disorder or other anxiety disorders, but it may simply persist in adulthood, even though with a developmentally modified phenomenology (Manicavasagar and Silove, 1997).

Panic disorder with or without agoraphobia

Panic attack is a discrete period of intense fear and discomfort, with a specific symptomatology, that develops abruptly and reaches a peak in 10 minutes or less. When recurrent and unexpected panic attacks occur, and are followed by a persistent concern of having another panic attack, criteria for panic disorder (PD) are fulfilled. Age of onset of PD is typically early to middle adulthood; nonetheless, in several studies of adults with PD, the subjects retrospectively reported that their panic symptoms began in childhood or adolescence (Weissman et al,

1997). Even though some authors are critical about the validity of retrospective recollections of panic attacks, probably many of the juvenile cases are being misdiagnosed, and/or they do not come to clinical attention. In adults PD is usually a recurrent and disabling condition; an early onset has been widely recognized as a negative predictive factor, associated with high levels of severity and impairment and with a chronic course. According to the available literature, the most common symptoms in younger children are palpitations, shortness of breath, sweating, faintness, and weakness. In adolescence new emerging symptoms become more frequent: chest pain, flushes, trembling, headache, and vertigo. "Cognitive symptoms" appear later: fear of dying is usually the earliest cognitive symptom reported by children and early adolescents; later onset cognitive symptoms are fear of going crazy ("I feel I am losing control") and depersonalization-derealization ("I don't know who I am" or "I don't know where I am").

Agoraphobia usually occurs in the context of a panic disorder, and is characterized by an anxiety about being in places or situations in which a panic attack may occur with a high probability, with a low possibility of help, and in which escape may be difficult or embarrassing. The anticipatory anxiety leads to avoiding a wide variety of situations, mainly including being alone outside home.

The prevalence of PD in adolescents is still under debate, with estimates ranging from 0.6% to 5%, with a mean estimate of 1.6% for PD and 4.3% for panic attacks (Wittchen et al, 1998), and about 10% in clinical settings (Biederman et al, 1997; Masi et al, 2001b), and a clear increment after puberty. Prevalence rates of prepubertal PD are much less clear (Vitiello et al, 1997), because younger children are not able to describe the physiologic or psychologic symptoms of PD, and their descriptions may induce a misinterpretation (e.g. "bad dreams").

Different studies have outlined that a strong familial influence is present in children and adolescents with PD or panic attacks. The presence of a relative with PD, or with anxiety and/or depressive disorders, increases the risk of a PD in the offspring. Other at-risk populations are children with early separation anxiety disorder and/or school refusal, or children with early "behavioral inhibition to the unfamiliar."

Simple phobias

The core feature of the simple phobias is a marked and unreasonable fear of a specific object or situation, lasting at least 6 months. The exposure to the phobic stimulus determines an immediate anxiety response, which may present the characteristics of a panic attack. While adolescents are usually aware that fears are unreasonable, this may not be the case in children. The phobic stimulus is usually avoided, but the anxious anticipation is distressing as well, and it significantly limits daily activities, including social and scholastic performances. The focus of the phobia may be an anticipated harm from the object or situation (e.g. the crash of the plane or the bite of the dog), or the self-reaction in front of the stimulus (e.g. losing control, fainting, panicking). The level of anxiety varies as a function of both the proximity to the stimulus and the possibility of an escape. Sometimes full-blown panic attacks are experienced, especially when escape is limited. Some subtypes of phobia have been delineated: animal type (generally with childhood onset), natural environment (e.g. storms, heights, water), blood injection injury (highly familial and usually associated with strong vasovagal response), and situational type (e.g. tunnels, bridges, elevators, flying, driving). Typical age at onset of specific phobias is during childhood, although the situational type may have a bimodal onset, with a peak in childhood and another peak in the mid-20s. Phobias that persist into adulthood remit only infrequently.

Social phobia

Social phobia (SP) is an anxiety disorder triggered by the exposition or anticipation of social interactions or public performances, and associated with avoidance of feared situations (Beidel et al, 1999). Anticipatory anxiety and avoidance strategies are almost always associated, and they grossly limit performance in everyday life, including social and scholastic interactions. Social phobia is generalized, when most performance and social situations induce a severe anxiety. Specific social phobia is characterized by fear of a single performance, for example eating or writing in front of other people. Social phobia in children and adolescents is usually generalized.

Adolescents may recognize that their fears are unreasonable, while children often do not. Somatic symptoms of anxiety are very frequent (palpitations, tremors, sweating, diarrhea, confusion), and they in turn further increase the anticipatory anxiety. Children with social phobia are usually extremely sensitive to criticism or negative evaluations or rejection, tend to a low assertivity, and have a low self-esteem. Often they have poor social skills (tend to avoid eye-to-eye contact), have no friends or cling to unfulfilling relationships, and have a poorer school performance despite normal or high capacity. In the most severe cases they drop out of school, may stay unemployed, and do not seek work, or seek work without social contacts, and remain with the family of origin.

The prevalence of social phobia is dependent on the selected thresholds, ranging according to the different studies from 3 to 13%. Even though a strong minority of subjects report a childhood onset of social phobia, in continuity with an inhibited temperament, most of the patients have an onset in mid-teens, sometimes insidiously, sometimes abruptly, after a humiliating experience acting on a vulnerable basis, with high rates of persistence in adulthood (Pine et al, 1998), even though it can attenuate during late adolescence or early adulthood. Early detection and treatment of the disorder can reduce the risk of adult mental health difficulties.

Closely related to social phobia is selective mutism, which is considered in DSM-IV as a distinct childhood onset disorder. The essential feature of selective mutism is a persistent failure to speak in social contexts (e.g. school), while in familiar situations there is a normal speaking. Associated features in the non-familiar environment are usually excessive shyness, fear of social embarassment, social isolation, or clinging traits, and, according to some studies, a comorbid social phobia can be diagnosed in about 90% of the subjects. In contrast, mainly in the familial environment, oppositional and controlling behaviors, temper tantrums, and negativism may be prevalent. The onset of the disorder is usually in preschool or early school years and sometimes lasts some months, sometimes several years.

Generalized anxiety disorder

Generalized anxiety disorder (GAD) is characterized by an excessive anxiety of at least 6 months' duration, occurring for most days, hard to control, not focused on a specific situation or objects, and not triggered by recent stressing events (Masi et al, 1999, 2004). Associated symptoms can be restlessness, fatigue, concentration difficulties, irritability, muscle tension, sleep disorders. A forerunner of GAD in children and adolescents, the overanxious disorder (OAD) has been incorporated in GAD after DSM-IV. The diagnostic criteria of GAD have been empirically validated in children and adolescents, and they are sufficiently consistent with the OAD criteria.

The majority of people with GAD experience their first symptoms in their late teenage years, in their twenties, or in their early thirties. However, a bimodal distribution in GAD age of onset has been suggested, with an early-onset GAD, considered a characterologic disturbance and associated with higher degrees of psychopathology, and a later-onset GAD, with a greater role of life events.

Worries in children and adolescents with GAD are mostly related to school performance, but they can apply to social situations, natural phenomena, arriving on time, and are later characterized by continuous self-doubt, high sensitivity to criticism, and need for reassurance. Somatic complaints are frequently reported at all ages.

According to our findings, the great majority of patients with lifetime GAD had another lifetime psychiatric diagnosis. At least another anxiety disorder was present in about half of the patients. More than half of patients with GAD showed a concurrent or lifetime depressive disorder. The high comorbidity between GAD and anxiety and/or depressive disorders has suggested that GAD may be better conceptualized as a prodromal, residual, or severity marker of anxiety and mood disorder. However, comorbidity is a high predictor of help-seeking among people with GAD, thus the frequent comorbidity in clinical samples may be an artifact of sample selection.

Acute stress disorder and post-traumatic stress disorder

Acute stress disorder and post-traumatic stress disorder (PTSD), formally recognized as an adult psychiatric disorder, was initially considered with skepticism in children and adolescents. Since then, many studies considering psychopathologic sequelae in children exposed to acute or chronic traumatic experiences have been published. Unfortunately, developmentally oriented diagnostic criteria are still unsatisfying, although different proposals have been proposed (Scheeringa et al, 1995).

The acute stress disorder is characterized by an acute anxiety lasting at least 2 days but not more than 4 weeks, following the exposure to a traumatic situation which is interpreted by the subjects as threatening life or physical integrity of the self or of significant others, including learning about death, serious harm, or injury of a close associate. The emotional response involves fear, helplessness, horror, and, in children, disorganized or agitated behavior. Subjects tend to re-experience the traumatic event, and avoid the stimuli related to the trauma. A persistent hyperarousal is frequent, mainly in children and adolescents.

When the symptoms last more than 4 weeks, and they become stable and structured, a diagnosis of PTSD is appropriate.

In children the traumatic experience of acute or chronic physical or sexual abuse is most frequent, including a developmentally inappropriate exposure to sexual situations, even without apparent violence. Severe automobile accidents, injuries to or unnatural deaths of close relatives, learning that a friend has a life-threatening disease, and natural disasters are other, not rare traumatic situations.

The re-experiencing of the traumatic experience may occur with recurrent recollections, dreams, or, more rarely, with dissociative states, with psychologic distress and physiologic reactivity. Children often repetitively enact the experience during their games or drawings. Deliberate efforts are made to avoid thought, feelings, conversations about the trauma, as well as persons or situations which may evocate the traumatic experience. A diminished response to the external world, feeling detached from other people, having markedly reduced ability to feel emotions, called "psychic numbing" or "emotional anesthesia", is not rare even in children, and can simulate a depressive anhedonia. Symptoms of increased arousal include difficulty sleeping, hypervigilance, exaggerated startle response, irritability, and outbursts of anger.

Symptoms usually begin within the first 3 months after the trauma, even though more rarely 6 or more months can pass between the experience and the onset of the symptoms. Usually symptoms of acute stress disorder are experienced during the first phase after the trauma, and they resolve within one month. When symptoms persist, the clinical picture fits the diagnostic criteria of the PTSD. The duration of these symptoms can be less than 3 months ("acute" PTSD) or more than 3 months ("chronic" PTSD). The duration and the severity of the symptomatology are affected by the nature of the trauma, the presence of an adequate social and parental support, family history, childhood experiences, personality variables, and pre-existing mental disorders.

Medications for anxiety disorders

Anxiolytic drugs

The concept of anxiolytic, as well as the concept of antidepressant, is misleading, as most of the so-called antidepressants, including

MAOIs, tricyclics, azapyrones (buspirone), SSRIs, serotonergic agents blocking 5HT2A receptors (trazadone, nefazodone), and newer agents acting on both serotonergic and noradrenergic systems (venlafaxine, mirtazapine, duloxetine) have a clear anxiolytic effect, and most of them have also an anti-obsessive-compulsive effect. This clinical observation parallels the psychopathologic observation that boundaries between anxiety disorders and mood disorders have become more and more fluid, with a large comorbidity among these disorders, as well as a continuum between them.

However, there are medications with a specific anxiolytic effect, associated with a sedative-hypnotic effect, without any relevant antidepressant action, such as benzodiazepines (BDZs) and newer non-BDZ anxiolytic agents (zaleplon, zopiclon, zolpidem), and these medications may be considered, strictly speaking, anxiolytic agents.

All the "anxiolytic agents" share a common mechanism of action, that is the modulation of the gamma-aminobutyric acid (GABA) system, through its interaction with the BDZ receptors. A brief summary of the GABAergic neurotransmission will be provided in the next paragraphs and it is more deeply described elsewhere (Stahl, 2000).

GABAergic transmission

Neurotransmitter GABA is a potent inhibitory neurotransmitter, which is synthesized in the GABA neurons from the amino acid (and potent excitatory neurotransmitter) glutamate, through the action of the enzyme glutamic acid decarboxylase. GABA neurons store GABA in vesicles, and then they flow it in the synaptic cleft, where GABA interacts with postsynaptic GABA receptors. Then it is destroyed by an enzyme (GABA transaminase), or captured by presynaptic transporters, which terminate the transmission through the re-uptake inside the GABA neurons for reuse in the following transmission.

Two subtypes of GABA receptors, GABA A, related to the anxiety disorders and to the anxiolytic drugs, and GABA B, are the targets of GABA. GABA A receptors are gatekeepers for a chloride channel, and their activation determines an acute flow of chloride ion from the extracellular to the intracellular environment. The effect of this flow is a decrease of neuron excitability, that is an inhibitory (or anti-excitatory) effect. GABA A receptor is modulated by several nearby receptors, included the BDZ receptor, and the receptors for non-BDZ anxiolytics (zolpidem, zopiclon, zaleplon), for barbiturates, and for alcohol.

The role of GABA B receptors is less well known, as they are not modulated by BDZ receptors, and they are probably not primarily linked to anxiety disorders.

GABA A receptor may be a common final pathway of the anxiolytic and sedative effect of BDZ and non-BDZ medications, as well as of the anticonvulsant effect of some drugs, of the behavioral effects of alcohol, and of several other activities. More specifically, BDZ interaction with its receptor amplifies the effects of the interaction between GABA and its receptor, that is the inhibitory effect deriving from the opening of the chloride channels.

Multiple BDZ receptors are located in different parts of the CNS (cerebellum, striatum, spinal cord) and outside the CNS (i.e. kidney), with different pharmacologic profiles and effects, including the anxiolytic and sedative-hypnotic action, the miorelaxant action, and the anticonvulsant action. Furthermore, they mediate also the negative effects on memory, the adaptive effects after chronic intake, and the dependence and withdrawal phenomena. It is reasonable to hypothesize that the BDZ receptors and the GABA receptors, as well as possible endogenous ligands for BDZ receptors, are closely implicated in a series of emotional and cognitive regulations, and in the pathophysiology of some aspects of the anxiety disorders.

Benzodiazepines

Benzodiazepines were among the first agents used to treat childhood and adolescence anxiety disorders, and have been in use since the early 1960s (chlordiazepoxide). They represented at that time an important step in the treatment of anxiety, replacing previous medications such as barbiturates, which are much more sedative and impairing. Furthermore, they included antianxiety, hypnotic, anticonvulsant and muscle relaxant actions. Finally, they showed a fast onset of action, and were more easily manageable when used to cope with an acute anxiety state, in short-term treatments. Over the last ten years the use of BDZs has decreased, and they have been replaced by safer and at least equally effective agents, such as the so-called antidepressants (in particular the SSRIs). However, they are still the most frequently prescribed psychoactive agents in the world. Because of their ease of use, their low toxicity, and above all their rapidity and effectiveness in alleviating anxiety, they are also the most frequently abused prescription drugs. Currently, they have a specific indication in the initial phase of treatments with medications with slow onset of action. In fact, in short-term treatments with BDZs, the risk of dependence, the negative cognitive effects, and the withdrawal phenomena are much less evident.

The BDZs have an inhibitory effect on CNS activity, through a potentiation of the GABA-ergic neurotransmission. Given the ion-channel-mediated mechanism, all the BDZs share a rapid onset of therapeutic effect. They can be differentiated according to potency, adverse effects, metabolic pathways, and withdrawal phenomena. They may be classified into 2-keto BDZs, 3-hydroxy-BDZs, and triazolo-BDZs, all rapidly absorbed via oral or parenteral routes. The 2-Keto-BDZs (i.e. diazepam, chlordiazepoxide) have a long half-life of 72 hours, which accounts for a long duration of action. The 3-hydroxy-BDZs (i.e. oxazepam, temazepam, lorazepam) have an intermediate half-life of 8–24 hours. The triazolo-BDZs (i.e. alprazolam, triazolam) have a shorter half-life.

Other BDZs cannot be included in these categories, and present specific characteristics. For example, flurazepam and quazepam are considered 2-keto-BDZs, but with a specific metabolic pathway, and a specific active metabolite, desalkyl-flurazepam, with a half-life of 48–120 hours. Clonazepam has also a specific metabolic pathway, but with a half-life similar to diazepam.

In summary, BDZs with faster onset are diazepam, flurazepam, and triazolam; BDZs with an intermediate rapidity of onset are alprazolam, lorazepam, and oxazepam; clonazepam has a (relatively) slower onset of action. BDZs with shorter half-lives are triazolam (1–5 hours), oxazepam (3–24 hours), and lorazepam (8–24 hours), while clonazepam (9–20 hours) and diazepam (20–60 hours) have longer half-lives.

BDZs with rapid onset (e.g. diazepam) more frequently have an initial euphoric-like effect and a higher potential of abuse risk; BDZs with a shorter half-life (e.g. triazolam) have a greater risk for rebound and withdrawal effects; BDZs with a long half-life (e.g. clonazepam) have an increased risk of accumulation during time.

BDZs marketed prevalently as hypnotics have shorter elimination half-lives, and are preferred because they determine less daytime sedation after a bedtime dose. Different BDZs present different patterns of sleep action. For example, alprazolam and diazepam reduce sleep latency and awakenings, but alprazolam is a potent suppressor of REM.

As examples of clinical use, alprazolam can be given at 0.125 mg in children and 0.250 mg in adolescents bid–tid, with a maximum dose of 1–4 mg in children and 8–10 mg in adolescents. Clonazepam can be given at 0.25 mg qid in children and 0.50 mg qid in adolescents with a maximum dose of 0.1–0.2 mg/kg. No specific laboratory evaluation is required at the baseline and as monitoring procedures.

BDZs are contraidicated in the following situations: narrow angle glaucoma, disinhibitory reactions, risk for dependence or abuse, hepatic disorders. The most relevant side-effects of BDZs are sedation, fatigue, drowsiness, slurred speech, and decreased memory and concentration. Behavioral disinhibition is quite frequent in younger patients, and it is manifested by irritability, tantrums, aggression in children, and behavioral outbursts in adolescents. These manifestations are more frequent at higher doses, and in subjects with brain damage and/or personality disorders. Side-effects in children and adolescents receiving BDZs for shorter periods of time are less clear. Cognitive impairment has been documented in adult patients, including visuospatial impairment, memory deficits, and sustained attention problems. Although data on alprazolam use seem to indicate that cognitive symptoms and withdrawal phenomena are less relevant in young patients treated for short periods, these side-effects should be carefully monitored even during short treatments. The slowing of reaction time may interfere with the safe driving of vehicles, and should also be considered in the treatment of adolescents, given that alcohol may further worsen attentional performances. Diplopia, inco-ordination, and tremor have occasionally been reported in adult patients.

Possible development of misuse in adolescents should also be monitored, especially when other addictive behaviors are present, in particular alcohol, hallucinogens, and street drugs. There is a strong association between use by parents and unprescribed use by adolescents, suggesting a modeling effect.

Children usually present an increased rapidity of hepatic metabolism, and this implies more frequent, but not necessarily higher doses. In contrast, lower doses are associated with a good efficacy, whereas higher doses are associated with more frequent side-effects. Tolerance and dependence occur during BDZ treatment in adult patients, but no data are available in children and adolescents. However, given this possible risk of dependence, BDZs should be prescribed only for short periods (weeks).

An important issue is related to the discontinuation of BDZs. A relapse (recurrence of the initial symptoms), a rebound (return of the initial symptoms, with even higher intensity and severity), and a withdrawal (new symptoms resulting from the discontinuation of the medication) can occur at the drug discontinuation. Withdrawal symptoms are severe anxiety, malaise, irritability, headache, sweating, gastrointestinal symptoms, insomnia, and muscle tension. These symptoms are usually more severe after a chronic treatment, or after a fast discontinuation, especially with short or mid half-life BDZs. A gradual tapering of 10% of the total dose every 7 days is recommended, with a further lowering in the presence of withdrawal symptoms. When short half-life BDZs (e.g. alprazolam) are being tapered, a switch to a long half-life BDZ, such as clonazepam, may be considered when withdrawal symptoms are evident.

Overdose of BDZ is relatively safe. Drowsiness, ataxia, confusion, slurred speech, tremor, diplopia are the most frequent manifestations. Respiratory depression, bradycardia and coma can be further increased by adjunctive sedative or hypnotic medications, or alcohol.

In summary, BDZs should be considered for the treatment of anxiety disorders in children and adolescents only when other approaches and medications have failed. Because of the theoretic risk for dependence in children and adolescents they should be prescribed only for weeks rather than months. When titrating BDZ, dosage adjustments should be done gradually, given the more rapid metabolism in children than in adults.

Non-BDZ hypnotics

Newer anxiolytics with prevalent hypnotic action have been more recently marketed, and they are becoming a first-line choice for sleep disorders. Three marketed agents are zaleplon, zopiclone, and zolpidem. Their specificity is that they act less intensively on BDZ receptors involved in cognition, memory, and psychomotor functions. For this reason they may have fewer cognitive side-effects than classic BDZs. Furthermore, all three agents share a rapid onset and a short duration, which reduces both the carryover effect on the next day and accumulated effects after several days of treatment. Finally, the binding of non-BDZs to the receptor is different from that of BDZs, in that they have partial agonist properties. Perhaps for this reason, rebound insomnia, caused by the withdrawal of the drug, dependence and withdrawal phenomena, and loss of efficacy during time seem to be less frequent.

Zaleplon has the most rapid onset (1-hour peak concentration) and short duration (1-hour half-life), with a complete wash-out before arising. For this reason it is more useful for subjects with sleep-onset difficulties, but not in those with problems in the middle of the night or with early awakenings.

Zolpidem has a later peak (2–3 hours) and a longer half-life (1.5–3 hours).

Zopiclone has a peak intermediate between zaleplon and zolpidem, but a significantly longer half-life than either of them (4–6 hours), and it may be more helpful in facilitating sleep continuity.

Antidepressants as antianxiety agents

The role of serotonin and norepinephrine

All the available antidepressant agents act through an enhancing effect on one or more monoamine neurotransmitter systems, including serotonin (5HT), norepinephrine (NE), and, to a lesser degree, dopamine (DA). Several distinct mechanisms can account for this effect: the inhibition of the re-uptake, the blocking of the inhibitory presynaptic autoreceptors (alpha-2 for NE and 5HT, 5HT1A and 5HT1D for 5HT), resulting in a disinhibition of monoamine release, direct action on the postsynaptic receptors, and a gradual change in the receptor's sensitivity to its neurotransmitter (downregulation). These phenomena may represent the first step of this mechanism, as it triggers a sequence of intracellular events in the postsynaptic neuron, which ultimately results in a modulation of the expression of specific genes. This may be the most important effect of the antidepressants, as well as of many other medications, which act through the monoamine system.

The hypothesis of anxiety as an expression of a dysregulation of the serotonergic system has received indirect confirmation by the efficacy of selective serotonergic agents on several anxiety dimensions and syndromes. However, given the high comorbidity between anxiety (namely generalized anxiety disorder) and depression, it is sometimes difficult to disentangle the specific antidepressant and antianxiety effects of these medications, or to attribute the clinical improvement to the antidepressant or to the antianxiety effect of these agents.

An overactivity of the noradrenergic system has been hypothesized in several anxiety disorders, based on the activating effect of the locus coeruleus, in animal models, including somatic symptoms of tachycardia, tremor, and sweating. However, some aspects of anxiety can improve during treatment with medications increasing the noradrenergic neurotransmission, as in antidepressant treatments with tricyclics or venlafaxine.

Alpha-2 agonist agents acting on the inhibitory presynaptic receptors may reduce the norepinephrine release. Clonidine, an alpha-2 agonist, can reduce somatic aspects of anxiety, but is much less effective on emotional aspects. Another point of attack is at the noradrenergic receptors, namely beta receptors, which may be excessively stimulated by a norepinephrine excess release. Beta-blocker medications, such as propanolol, can reduce postsynaptic signaling and improve some autonomic aspects (tremor, sweating, tachycardia) associated with several anxiety disorders, namely social anxiety, without a significant effect on the anxiety symptomatology.

Several categories of antidepressants with potential or putative anti-anxiety action have been marketed, including tricyclic antidepressants, SSRIs, enhancers of both serotonergic and noradrenergic neurotransmission, and blockers of serotonin re-uptake and 5HT2A receptors.

After a brief summary of serotonergic and noradrenergic transmission, these categories of medications will be described.

Serotonergic transmission

Cell bodies of serotonergic neurons are located in an area of the brainstem called the raphe nucleus. In this area 5HT is produced from the amino acid tryptophan, which is converted into 5-hydroxytryptophan by the enzyme tryptophan hydroxylase. Another enzyme, a decarboxylase, converts 5-hydroxytryptophan into 5HT, which is stored in vesicles and then released into the synaptic cleft at the arrival of the neuronal impulse. After its interaction with 5HT receptors, 5HT is terminated by extracellular enzymes (MAO and COMT), or recaptured by a specific presynaptic transporter, and restored in the neuron. The transporter protein is one of the most important targets of the antidepressant agents.

Presynaptic and postsynaptic 5HT receptors are the target of 5HT action. Presynaptic receptors, or autoreceptors, are located on the somatodendritic (5HT1A receptor) or on the axonal part of the neuron (5HT1D receptor), and their interaction with 5HT has an inhibitory effect on further 5HT release. When these autoreceptors are blocked, this can increase the 5HT release.

Two types of noradrenergic receptors, called heteroreceptors, are located on the presynaptic serotonergic neurons, similarly to noradrenergic neurons. The first type, alpha-2, is located on the terminal axon of the serotonergic neuron. Its interaction with NE released by nearby noradrenergic neurons blocks the 5HT release. The second type, alpha-1, is located on the cell body, that is in the raphe, and its interaction with NE has an enhancing effect on the 5HT release. Through these mechanisms the NE system can modulate the 5HT system, and NE agents can affect serotonergic transmission.

Several types of serotonergic receptors are located on the postsynaptic neurons, of which the most important are 5HT1A, 5HT2A, 5HT2C, 5HT3, and 5HT4. Their locations vary in the different projections of the serotonergic neurons from the raphe to other parts of the CNS (mainly frontal cortex, limbic area, basal ganglia and sleep center of brain stem). Other projections descend to the spinal centers and regulate sexual phenomena such as orgasm and ejaculation. Projections to the gastrointestinal tract (5HT3, 5HT4 receptors) regulate appetite and gastrointestinal motility. These projections account for the therapeutic action of serotonergic agents, as well as their side-effects.

Noradrenergic transmission

The cell bodies of the noradrenergic neurons are in the locus coeruleus, an area located in the brainstem. They synthesize their neurotransmitter, NE, from a precursor, tyrosine, through the action of the enzyme tyrosine-hydroxylase, which converts tyrosine in dihydroxyphenylalanine (DOPA). Another enzyme, DOPA decarboxylase, converts DOPA into dopamine. A third enzyme, dopamine-beta-hydroxylase, converts dopamine into NE. At the arrival of the nervous impulse, NE is released in the synaptic cleft and, after interaction with its receptor, it is terminated by two enzymes (MAO, COMT), or by the re-uptake of a specific transporter protein, located in the membrane of the presynaptic neuron.

Several pre- and postsynaptic NE receptors have been found. Presynaptic receptors on the cell body, on the dendrites, and on the terminal axon are alpha-2 autoreceptors, and when they interact with NE, they block the NE release as a brake. Postsynaptic receptors are beta-1, alpha-1, and alpha-2. When NE interacts with those receptors, a sequence of events is triggered, which results in the modulation of gene expression in the postsynaptic neuron.

From the locus coeruleus noradrenergic neurons project into multiple CNS areas, including the frontal and prefrontal cortex, limbic cortex, and cerebellum. Through these projections, noradrenergic neurons control cognition, attention, emotions, and psychomotor functioning, and directly regulate the quality of the relationship with the external world. Other projections in the brainstem, in the heart, and in the urinary tract determine control of blood pressure, heart rate, and bladder emptying. An NE deficiency syndrome includes cognitive effects (impaired attention and difficulty concentrating, memory deficits), depressed mood, loss of energy, fatigue, and psychomotor retardation.

Tricyclic antidepressants

Tricyclic antidepressants (TCAs) have long been the first-line antidepressant in adult patients, even though they have been shown to be much less effective in childhood and adolescent depression, where there is no evidence that TCAs are superior to placebo. The mechanism by which TCAs are effective in mood and anxiety disorders is a block of the 5HT and/or NE pump. Some TCAs are more selective for the NE pump (desipramine, nortriptyline), others for the 5HT pump (clomipramine), and most of them block both pumps. However, TCAs do not exhibit a selective action on the monoamine neurotransmission, as they also block cholinergic, H1 histamine, and alpha-1 adrenergic receptors, and these last actions are responsible for side-effects. Furthermore, TCAs block the sodium channels in the heart and brain, and this may increase the risk for cardiotoxicity and seizures.

Tricyclic antidepressants have a significant hepatic first-pass, and they are more rapidly metabolized in children and adolescents than in adults, given the greater liver mass in relation to body mass. Furthermore, children and adolescents may have 30-fold difference in blood levels at a given dose. About 5% of patients are slow metabolizers, with longer half-lives and higher plasma levels. All these conditions can increase the risk of side-effects, namely CNS and cardiac side-effects.

The most troublesome side-effect in treatment with TCAs is cardiotoxicity. At therapeutic doses and serum levels, TCAs are associated with consistent but mild increases in systolic and diastolic blood pressure, heart rate, and ECG conduction parameters changes, i.e. of PR, QRS, and QTc intervals. Increases in PR and QRS intervals, as well as in pulse rate, are not rare, and when the PR exceeds 0.21 and QRS exceeds 0.12, the cardiac slowing may be dangerous. Cardiotoxicity is of particular concern in children, as they produce higher amounts of toxic hydroxy metabolites, and they are also more sensitive than older adolescents and adults to the cardiac effect of these metabolites. A higher incidence of QTc prolongation may be associated with desipramine. Of note, although the relationship between dosage, serum levels, and the ECG changes is weak, it becomes more robust at relatively high TCA doses or serum levels, being maximum approaching the highest daily dosage of 5 mg/kg per day. Sudden deaths in children treated with TCAs (particularly desipramine) have also been reported.

For these reasons, TCAs are contraindicated in children with cardiac disorders. A baseline ECG must be done in all children and adolescents before starting TCA, and it should be repeated at frequent intervals during the dose increases, when the steady state has been reached, and every 3 months during the maintenance. TCAs should be discontinued when PR > 0.18 and/or QRS > 0.12. Heart rate should be monitored as well, and TCAs should be discontinued with a pulse rate > 110 in children and 100 in adolescents.

Cholinergic blockade may cause dry mouth, urinary retention, constipation, and blurred vision. Histamine blockade may result in sedation and increased appetite with weight gain. Adrenergic blockade may determine orthostatic hypotension and dizziness.

TCAs should be used cautiously in patients with epilepsy, as they can lower the seizure threshold. The risk is higher when cerebral lesions or EEG abnormalities are co-occurring. However, TCAs can be associated with a stable and effective anticonvulsant treatment.

Side-effects can be partly controlled by increasing the dose slowly, starting with 12.5–25 mg/day, with gradual increases, and giving divided doses – bid or tid – whenever possible. Administering the total daily dose at bedtime is not recommended in children, although some clinicians suggest the bedtime dose once the dosage has been stabilized.

Withdrawal symptoms can occur in children more frequently than in adults, given the faster metabolism in younger patients. Withdrawal symptoms include agitation, anxiety, sleep disorder, behavioral activation, and gastrointestinal symptoms. Discontinuation should be gradual, decreasing one quarter of the dose every one or two weeks.

TCA overdose is a potentially lethal condition, and a 15-day supply can result in death, due to heart arrythmias, seizures, hypotension, and coma, developing during the first 24 hours of the overdose.

BDZs, alcohol, and barbiturates further increase CNS toxicity. Close respiratory and cardiac monitoring is needed, as well as serum TCA levels (even though TCA levels do not always reflect the severity of risk). Ventilatory assistance may be indicated when necessary, as well as administration of fluids or pressors (epinephrine) when severe hypotension is present, and anti-arrhythmic medications, or cardioversion. Intravenous BDZs may be necessary in the presence of seizures, with repeated doses until the seizures are controlled.

Given the potential for uncomfortable side-effects, the possibility of cardiac adverse effects, and the need for monitoring by ECG and blood level testing, the TCAs are not a first-line treatment for anxiety disorders.

Selective serotonin re-uptake inhibitors

Six selective serotonin re-uptake inhibitors (SSRIs) are currently marketed: fluoxetine, paroxetine, sertraline, fluvoxamine, citalopram, and escitalopram. Although they differ from each other according to specific pharmacokinetic and pharmacodynamic properties, their similar primary mechanism allows us to consider them as a unique class of medications. All the SSRIs enhance 5HT neurotransmission through a block of the active re-uptake of serotonin by the presynaptic transporter. SSRIs are more selective than TCAs, as they do not have significant anticholinergic, antihistaminergic, and antiadrenergic effects, which account for most of the side-effects. Furthermore, SSRIs do not block the sodium channel, even in overdose, and so they lack danger compared to TCAs.

However, the acute effect on the serotonin transporter of the presynaptic membrane can hardly explain the therapeutic effects which are evident several weeks later. It is likely that neuroadaptative changes in the receptor, involvement of the second messenger system, as well as regulation of the expression of genes in the postsynaptic neuron can account for the therapeutic effect of SSRIs (and other antidepressants) (see Stahl, 2000 for more details).

Recent research has shown that as well as the effect on the serotonin transporter at the axon terminal, the action on the somatodendritic portion of the neuron is also important. After starting SSRI treatment, the block of re-uptake increases serotonin in the synaptic cleft much less than in the somatodendritic portion, at the raphe. While the initial increase in serotonin in the synapse is primarily responsible for the acute side-effects, the therapeutic effect starts at the body cell, in the midbrain. The increased serotonin at the somatodendritic portion of the neuron interacts with inhibitory 5HT1A receptors, resulting in their secondary downregulation and desensitization, through the effect on the genome in the presynaptic neuron's nucleus. This desensitization requires at least 2 or 3 weeks, and it determines a reduction of the inhibiting effect of 5HT1A receptors on serotonin release at the synapse. The interaction between serotonin and postsynaptic receptors determines, in turn, a downregulation of these receptors (through an action on the genome in the postsynaptic neuron's nucleus). This downregulation is responsible for the tolerance to the side-effects. In fact, side-effects are usually acute, and tend to decrease during the first weeks. The acute effect of serotonin on the 5HT2A and 5HT2C postsynaptic receptors at the limbic area is responsible for anxiety, agitation, and even panic attacks. The acute stimulation of 5HT2A in the basal ganglia is responsible for the akathisia, and more rarely for parkinsonism and psychomotor retardation. The effect on the 5HT2A receptors in the sleep centers may determine early-onset sleep disorders and myoclonus during sleep. The effect on the 5HT2A in the spinal cord may interfere with ejaculation or orgasm. The effect on the 5HT3 receptors in the hypothalamus or midbrain may determine nausea or vomiting, while gastrointestinal cramps or diarrhea and bowel effects are related to the interactions with peripheral 5HT3 and 5HT4.

Unfortunately, the serotonergic action is widespread, and agents acting specifically on desired portions of the serotonergic system are not available.

Even though the six available SSRIs share the same basic mechanism, significant pharmacodynamic and pharmacokinetic differences among them partly account for individual responses to one or other agent. For example, citalopram has the most selective serotonergic action, while sertraline is a low blocker of dopamine re-uptake; paroxetine and fluoxetine have low NE re-uptake inhibition, and paroxetine has an additional muscarinic–anticholinergic action. Furthermore, different SSRIs have different profiles of inhibition of the cytocrome P450 liver enzymes (CYP450). Several CYP450 enzymes are involved in the antidepressant metabolism, and different antidepressants differently inhibit specific enzymes, accounting for specific interactions with other co-administered medications. Fluoxetine has a long half-life, 2 days after a single dose and 8 days after repeated dosing, and norfluoxetine, the active metabolite, has a half-life of 7 to 19 days. The half-life of the other SSRIs ranges from 12 to 36 hours. The SSRIs are metabolized in the liver by the cytochrome P450 isoenzyme system.

A withdrawal syndrome can occur when discontinuation is too fast, with a rapid increase in anxiety, irritability, insomnia, and somatic symptoms. Withdrawal symptoms are much more rare with fluoxetine, given its longer half-life.

Formerly proposed as antidepressant agents, SSRIs are extensively used off-label in all the anxiety disorders of children and adolescents. Recent studies from the USA report more than 200 000 mentions of fluoxetine and sertraline in 1994 for children aged 5 to 10 years, suggesting a trend to overprescribing (Emslie et al, 1999). The use of SSRIs as antianxiety medications prevalently rests on studies on adult populations, but a growing evidence supports efficacy and safety in several childhood anxiety disorders (obsessive-compulsive disorder, panic disorder, separation anxiety disorder, generalized anxiety disorder, social phobia, PTSD), without the sedating anticholinergic and cardiotoxic reactions observed with tricyclic antidepressants. However, the incidence of insomnia, nervousness, gastrointestinal complaints, and sexual disorders is high.

Starting doses of SSRIs differ according to the different medications. Fluvoxamine and sertraline should be started at 25 mg in children and 50 mg in adolescents, with slow increases of 25 mg in children and 50 mg in adolescents every 5–7 days, up to a maximum dose of 250 mg for sertraline and 300 mg for fluvoxamine in adolescents. Fluoxetine, paroxetine, and citalopram should start at 5 mg in children and 10 mg in adolescents, with increases of 5 mg in children and 10 mg in adolescents every 5–7 days, up to 20 mg in children and 40 mg in adolescents. Much slower increases should be recommended in patients with panic disorder or panic attacks.

The limited range of action on serotonergic system (without significant implication of the noradrenergic system), as well as possible side effects, partly limits the therapeutic impact of these medications. For these reasons alternative antidepressants have been developed, and those with a higher antianxiety effect will be briefly described in the next paragraphs. These newer, post-SSRI antidepressants have been studied in all the adulthood anxiety disorders, and their efficacy and safety is promising. So far, data on childhood anxiety are still anecdotal.

Serotonin re-uptake inhibitors with 5HT2A antagonism

Some antidepressants have a selective serotonin re-uptake inhibition, even though less potent than that of the SSRIs, but with an additional potent blockade of the 5HT2A receptors. The two antidepressants with this selective action are nefazodone and trazodone. These effects can be evident at the receptor level, decreasing some side-effects resulting from the 5HT2A stimulation, such as anxiety, insomnia, and sexual dysfunction. At the level of the cell nucleus, the decreased stimulation of the 5HT2A receptors can increase the effect of the 5HT1A stimulation on the gene expression.

Given the less activating properties of these compounds, they may be more useful in anxiety than in depressive disorders, namely PTSD, generalized anxiety disorder, and panic disorder.

Trazodone, compared to nefazodone, is a more potent blocker of the histamine receptors, resulting in a sedative effect. For this reason trazodone can be taken when a sleep disorder is co-occurring, primary or secondary to an antidepressant treatment. Orthostatic hypotension is sometimes a side-effect during trazodone treatment. A rare but potentially lethal liver toxicity has been reported during nefazodone treatment.

Dual serotonin and norepinephrine re-uptake inhibitor

A specific antidepressant with a potent antianxiety action, venlafaxine, combines the re-uptake of both 5HT and NE, without blocking cholinergic, histaminergic, and alpha adrenergic transmission. At the lower doses venlafaxine inhibits only 5HT re-uptake, while at higher doses it also blocks NE re-uptake. Finally, at the highest doses it can block, to a lesser extent, the dopamine re-uptake. At the usual dosages, the double action on 5HT and NE has been hypothesized to have a synergistic effect, in terms of amplification of the gene expression. This amplification may have a clinical counterpart in a higher remission rate, and a lower rate of "partial" improvement, with impairing residual symptoms, especially in patients resistant to SSRI treatment. The increase in efficacy with the increase of dosage underlines the importance of the NE involvement in the therapeutic effect. This is particularly true for the anxiolytic effect, which is additional to the antidepressant effect.

Venlafaxine has been approved for the treatment of generalized anxiety disorder in adults. Data on efficacy of venlafaxine as an antianxiety agent in children and adolescents are still lacking. According to available data on controlled studies in children and adolescents with major depression, the relative risk of suicidal behavior or ideation is the highest among antidepressants (see Chapter 4). More recently a newer medication with a relatively balanced inhibition of both serotonin and noradrenaline re-uptake, duloxetine, has been marketed in many countries, but data on children and adolescents are still not available.

Noradrenergic and serotonergic agents

Mirtazapine enhances both serotonergic and noradrenergic transmission, but not via a block of the re-uptake of monoamines from the synaptic cleft. Mirtazapine blocks the alpha-2 receptors, which are presynaptic inhibiting autoreceptors on the noradrenergic and serotonergic neurons. Norepinephrine can inhibit its own release through the interaction with the alpha-2 autoreceptors on the noradrenergic neurons. It can also inhibit the 5HT release through the interaction with the alpha-2 heteroreceptors on the 5HT neurons. Mirtazapine blocks the alpha-2 inhibiting receptors, increasing the release of both NE and 5HT.

Additional effects of mirtazapine are the blockade of 5HT2A, 5HT2C, 5HT3, and histamine receptors. This blockade reduces some side-effects such as anxiety, insomnia, gastrointestinal symptoms, and sexual dysfunction. Furthermore, the 5HT2A and histamine antagonism can increase the anxiolytic and hypnotic effect, while the block of 5HT2C and histamine receptors accounts for the increased appetite and weight gain.

Data on efficacy of mirtazapine as an antianxiety agent in children and adolescents are still lacking.

Buspirone

Efficacy of buspirone as an antianxiety and antidepressant agent in children and adolescents is still debated. It acts as a partial agonist of the 5HT1A presynaptic and postsynaptic receptors, without any interaction with BDZ receptors, and without dependence or withdrawal phenomena in long-term use. It can reduce anxiety symptoms through the interaction with presynaptic (somatodendritic) inhibitory autoreceptors, first resulting in a shutdown of neuronal impulse flow, with 5HT re-accumulation and repletion in the stores, and then in a desensitization of these receptors. This desensitization reduces the limitation of the release of 5HT in the presynaptic neuron. In contrast to BDZ, and similarly to the antidepressants, the onset of action is slow (2–4 weeks). For this reason buspirone may be helpful in chronic anxiety. Data on adults suggest that buspirone may have an effect on depression and on generalized anxiety disorder, but not on obsessive-compulsive disorder and panic disorder. Furthermore, buspirone produces minimal sedation and, therefore, it is not indicated as a hypnotic. Controlled studies in children and adolescents are not available.

Buspirone is started at 5 mg three times a day, gradually increased every 2 weeks to 30, 60, and 90 mg a day, in three divided doses. Side-effects are usually mild and transitory, namely stomach upset, dizziness, sedation, asthenia, and headaches.

More research is needed to confirm efficacy of buspirone in anxious children and adolescents.

Clinical studies on pharmacologic treatments in children and adolescents

Benzodiazepines: available literature

Benzodiazepines have been widely studied in adult patients, but few controlled studies are available in children and adolescents, and they are limited by small sample size, short duration of treatment, and often inadequate dosage.

Bernstein and colleagues (1989) blindly compared for 8 weeks alprazolam (mean 1.4 mg/day), imipramine (mean 135 mg/day), and placebo in 24 anxious and/or depressed children with school refusal, with a trend of efficacy in favor of the medications, even though it was unclear whether the differences in baseline among the groups could affect the results.

In another study Simeon and colleagues (1992) randomized 30 children and adolescents with overanxious and avoidant disorder (the former categorization of childhood social phobia) to alprazolam (0.5–3.5 mg/day, mean 1.6 mg/day) or placebo. After 4 weeks 88% of the completers on alprazolam and 62% of the completers on placebo improved, and the difference between groups was not significant. Another double-blind, cross-over study (Grae et al, 1994) assessed the efficacy of 4-week clonazepam (0.5–2 mg/day) in 15 children with anxiety disorders, prevalently separation anxiety disorder. Outcome differences did not differ between groups.

Finally Kutcher and Reiter (personal communication, cited in Riddle et al, 1999) blindly treated adolescents with panic disorder with clonazepam or placebo. Adolescents on clonazepam had a significant improvement on measures of generalized anxiety disorder, frequency of panic attacks, and school and social measures.

Several open-label studies are also recorded in the literature. Klein (cited in Kutcher et al, 1992) treated 18 children and adolescents with separation anxiety disorder with alprazolam (0.5–6 mg/day), with a significant improvement in 89% of the subjects according to psychiatrists, 82% according to parents, 65% according to self-reports, and 64% according to teachers.

Kutcher and McKenzie (1988) successfully treated four adolescents with panic disorder with clonazepam (0.5 mg twice a day), with a faster improvement of somatic symptoms compared to psychologic symptoms.

Tricyclics: available literature

Most of the available studies have focused on school phobia, which is a non-specific clinical entity, as it may be a consequence of anxiety as well as depressive disorders. Gittelman-Klein and Klein (1971) randomized to placebo or imipramine (100–200 mg/day) 35 children (6–14 years) with school refusal in a 6-week, double-blind, placebo-controlled study. At the end of the study 81% of the group of children on imipramine were attending school regularly versus 47% of the children on placebo. However, the same research group (Klein et al, 1992) did not replicate these findings in another controlled study considering 20 children with separation anxiety disorder.

Berney and colleagues (1981) described a double-blind, placebo-controlled study of low-dose clomipramine (40–75 mg/day) in 46 children and adolescents with school refusal. After 12 weeks of treatment clomipramine was not superior to placebo, but the low dose may have significantly affected the outcome.

Bernstein and colleagues (2000) assessed the efficacy of imipramine in an 8-week, double-blind, placebo-controlled study on 47 subjects with school refusal, who also received a concurrent, cognitive-behavioral, school-reentry treatment. Even though anxiety and depression on clinician rating scales improved significantly for both groups with depression, subjects on medication showed a faster improvement in both depression and school attendance than the placebo group. Posttreatment, the school attendance was significantly higher in the imipramine group (70.7±27.1%) than in the placebo group (29.3±37.7%).

Buspirone: available literature

Kutcher et al (1992) reported on the efficacy of an open treatment with buspirone (15 to 30mg daily for 6 weeks) in a series of adolescents with generalized anxiety disorder/overanxious disorder. Similar findings are reported by Simeon and coworkers (1994) in a 4-week open trial with buspirone in 15 patients (ages 6–14 years) with anxiety disorders.

Pfeffer and colleagues (1997) openly treated with buspirone (10–50 mg/day) 25 inpatient prepubertal children with anxiety and aggressive behavior. After 9 weeks the completers (about 75% of the children) showed a significant improvement in social anxiety, aggressive behavior, and depressive symptoms, but general anxiety did not improve significantly.

SSRIs and beyond: available literature

Separation anxiety disorder/school refusal

Several open-label studies showed efficacy of SSRIs in anxiety disorders in children and adolescents with SAD. Manassis and Bradley (1994) successfully treated with fluoxetine five children (including three with SAD) who had failed to respond to a cognitive behavioral treatment. Improvement started within 6 weeks, according to both subjects' and parents' reports.

Birmaher et al (1994) treated with fluoxetine (mean dosage 25.7 mg/day) 21 children with SAD, overanxious disorder, or social phobia, which was resistant to previous psychotherapeutic and psychopharmacologic treatments. After a 10-week treatment 81% of the subjects showed moderate to marked improvement of anxiety symptoms. Fairbanks et al (1997) examined fluoxetine treatment in 16 outpatients (9–18 years old) with mixed anxiety disorders. Of the ten patients treated for current SAD, four were rated improved and six much improved at the Clinical Global Impression (CGI).

A recent multi-site, double-blind, placebo-controlled study examined the efficacy of fluvoxamine in 128 children and adolescents with SAD and/or generalized anxiety disorder and/or social phobia (Research Unit on Pediatric Psychopharmacology, 2001). The trial used a flexible dosing strategy to a maximum of 300 mg/day for 8 weeks. Psychiatrist-rated clinical responders were 76% in the fluvoxamine group and 29% in the placebo group. Moreover, a significantly greater improvement in anxiety symptoms was found in the fluvoxamine group, compared to the placebo group.

Panic disorder

Very limited published literature is available on pharmacologic treatment of juvenile panic disorder (PD). Previous anecdotal reports (Lepola et al, 1996; Fairbanks et al, 1997) described the efficacy of SSRIs (citalopram, fluoxetine) in young patients (three and five subjects, respectively) with PD and other comorbid anxiety disorders. More recently, two larger open-label studies have explored the efficacy of treatment with SSRIs in children and adolescents with PD. Renaud and coworkers (1999) examined openly effectiveness and safety of different SSRIs (fluoxetine, paroxetine, and sertraline) in 12 children and adolescents with PD, who were followed for about 6 months. Some of these patients assumed BDZs as adjunctive treatment. At the end of the study 75% of patients were much or very much improved at the CGI, without significant side-effects, and 67% no longer fulfilled the criteria for PD. The authors concluded that SSRIs are a safe and promising treatment for juvenile PD.

Masi et al (2001b) have described their clinical experience with paroxetine monotherapy in 18 children and adolescents (7–16 years) with PD followed for about one year. The initial mean dosage of paroxetine was 8.9±2.1 mg/day (range 5–10mg/day), later increased up to 40mg/day, depending on clinical response and occurrence of significant side-effects. The mean dosage at the last observation was 23.9±9.8 mg/day. A significant improvement was evident on the CGI severity scale (*P*<0.0001). Fifteen patients (83.3%) were considered responders at the last evaluation. These patients began to improve after a mean period of 3 weeks. Paroxetine was well tolerated by most patients.

Generalized anxiety disorder

A controlled study that compared the safety and efficacy of sertraline and placebo in the treatment of GAD in children and adolescents was reported by Rynn et al (2001). The study included 22 subjects aged 5 to 17 years with a score of 16 or more on the Hamilton Anxiety Scale. The patients underwent a 9-week, double-blind treatment in which they were randomized to sertraline (up to 50 mg/day) or placebo. The Hamilton Anxiety Scale and CGI (severity and improvement) showed significant differences in favor of sertraline treatment, beginning at week 4.

In the above-mentioned multi-site, double-blind, placebo-controlled study on 128 children and adolescents with anxiety disorders treated with fluvoxamine (up to 300 mg/day), some of the patients had a GAD (Research Unit on Pediatric Psychopharmacology, 2001). A significantly greater improvement in anxiety symptoms was found in the fluvoxamine group, compared to the placebo group.

Two open studies (Birmaher et al, 1994; Fairbanks et al, 1997) have explored the efficacy of fluoxetine in children and adolescents with mixed anxiety disorders, including overanxious disorder, a DSMIII-R diagnostic category which grossly corresponds to GAD according to DSM-IV. According to Birmaher et al's study, about 80% of the patients treated with fluoxetine (mean dosage 25.7 mg/day) had a moderate to marked improvement. In contrast, in Fairbanks et al's study only one of the seven patients treated for current GAD resulted in a responder at the CGI.

Social phobia and social anxiety

There is consensus that treatment of children with SP should begin with a cognitive-behavioral psychotherapy, alone or in conjunction with a pharmacotherapy. Only a few pharmacologic studies have directly addressed SP or selective mutism, which can often be a variant of SP. A 12-week, double-blind, placebo-controlled study of fluoxetine in 15 children with selective mutism showed a significant improvement on parental ratings of anxiety and mutism in the fluoxetine group (Black and Uhde, 1994). Efficacy of fluoxetine in selective mutism is confirmed by a more recent study (Dummit et al, 1996) on 21 children (with other comorbid anxiety disorders), with a significant improvement in 76% of the patients (dose ranging from 10 to 60 mg/day). Another controlled study, mentioned above (Research Unit on Pediatric Psychopharmacology, 2001), included patients with SP successfully treated with fluvoxamine.

Two recent open studies support the efficacy of serotonergic agents in childhood SP. In the first study Mancini et al (1999) reported on a series of seven patients aged 7 to 18 years with generalized social phobia who were treated with paroxetine, sertraline, or nefazodone for up to 7 months. All of the patients appeared to have a very positive clinical response to the serotonergic agents. The second study (Compton et al, 2001) described 14 outpatients with SP treated in an 8-week open trial of sertraline (mean dose 123 ± 37 mg/day). According to CGI (improvement subscale), 36% of subjects were considered responders and 29% (4/14) as partial responders at the end of the 8-week trial. A significant clinical response appeared by week 6.

Post-traumatic stress disorder

Essential components of treatment for children with PTSD are direct exploration of trauma, use of stress management techniques, exploration and correction of inaccurate attributions regarding the trauma, and inclusion of parents in the treatment (Berliner, 1997). Biologic interventions rest on the evidence of the involvement of opioid, glutamatergic, GABAergic, noradrenergic, serotonergic, and neuroendocrine pathways in the pathophysiology of PTSD (Donnelly et al, 1999; Hageman et al, 2001). Few studies indicated that children with PTSD exhibit physiologic abnormalities similar to those seen in adults. Medications shown to be effective in double-blind placebo-controlled trials in adults with PTSD include SSRIs, reversible and irreversible MAO inhibitors, tricyclic antidepressants, and the anticonvulsant lamotrigine (Hageman et al, 2001). Still more agents appear promising in open-label trials.

Few studies have explored the efficacy of medications in childhood PTSD symptoms, such as behavioral dyscontrol (mood stabilizers such as carbamazepine or valproate, adrenergic agents such as clonidine or guanfacine, beta-blockers such as propanolol) or depression and anxiety (newer antidepressants, BDZs).

Data from adult populations suggest the efficacy and safety of newer antidepressants in PTSD patients, SSRIs (Stein et al, 2000), namely paroxetine (Tucker et al, 2001), sertraline (Davidson et al, 2001), and nefazodone (Davis et al, 2000). Even though empirical evidence is lacking, evidence from these studies in adults with PTSD suggests that SSRIs that target broad symptom clusters should be considered initially, especially when anxiety and depressive features are prominent.

Treatment strategy

Separation anxiety disorder – school refusal

Pharmacotherapy should not be used as the primary treatment option in SAD, but as an adjunct to other treatments, in children who failed to respond to previous interventions and who are significantly impaired. Pharmacotherapy of SAD should be considered when it is associated with PD, and/or when it is closely related to school refusal. School refusal can be a symptom of several psychopathologic conditions, including anxiety disorders (mainly SAD, but possibly social phobia, specific phobia), mood disorders (dysthymia, major depressive disorder), and behavioral disorders (oppositional defiant disorder, conduct disorder). Separation anxiety disorder is complicated by a school refusal in at least 70% of cases, and when these situations are severe and chronic, and other behavioral and environmental interventions have failed, a pharmacotherapy may be considered as adjunctive treatment.

Early studies on pharmacotherapy of school refusal explored the efficacy of tricyclics and BDZs, but findings are not consistent and these medications should not be considered as first-line drugs. Short-term treatment with high-potency BDZs (alprazolam, clonazepam) may be of interest in ameliorating acute situational anxiety before entering school, associated with psychologic and environmental interventions. Even though empirical evidence is still scarce, SSRIs should be considered as the first choice at the standard dosages. When effective, the treatment should be continued for at least 4–6 months.

Panic disorder

The first issue in this situation is to suspect the presence of a PD, on the basis of the clinical presentation, a history of separation anxiety disorder and/or school refusal and unexplained somatic complaints, and a positive family history for anxiety disorders and/or panic attacks. The incomplete forms, with few somatic symptoms but no cognitive manifestations, are mostly frequent in childhood, as well as the atypical symptoms ("hyperventilation syndrome"), and the nocturnal occurrence, misdiagnosed as "pavor nocturnus", with related sleep difficulties.

In adolescence the diagnosis is usually easier, given the more "typical" presentation of the disorder, although most of the patients have a history of negative medical consultations and examinations and incorrect medical diagnoses (e.g. asthma).

When a diagnosis of PD is obtained, a careful assessment of possible comorbid conditions, namely other anxiety disorders or mood disorders (both depressive and bipolar), should increase our prognostic abilities, and indicate a more specific treatment. Aims of the treatment are twofold: to control the panic attacks and to limit the consequences of anticipatory anxiety and avoiding strategies. The intervention plan should be considered on the basis of the severity and frequency of the attacks, as well as on the basis of the functional impact of the attacks on daily activities and on the subjective well-being.

A psychoeducational approach, including family environment, is the first step, and it should be considered in all the patients having panic attacks in order to minimize the effects of the episodes. A supportive psychotherapy can further increase the subjects' coping capacities. When severity and frequency of the episodes are clearly exceeding these capacities, anticipatory anxiety and phobic avoidance may rapidly increase. A pharmacologic approach is needed in these cases.

Three possible medications can be used in children and adolescents: SSRIs, BDZs, and tricyclic antidepressants. SSRIs are the most frequently reported medication for PD in the literature, and they should be considered as the first line, on the basis of both efficacy and tolerability. All the SSRIs have been supported by clinical studies on adult populations with PD, whereas no guidelines addressing the choice of a specific SSRI are available for children and adolescents. Sertraline and fluoxetine may be considered on the available experience in mood and anxiety disorders in children and adolescents, with a positive basis of a risk/benefit ratio. Fluoxetine has a long half-life, with once-a-day administration, and plasma levels remain stable even when the intake is not totally regular, because the patient forgets the pill. The long half-life reduces the risk of withdrawal symptoms, even though it implies a longer wash-out period (5 weeks) in the case of a switch to another medication.

Sertraline has a shorter half-life, it has to be taken in two doses, and the intake should be more strictly controlled. Withdrawal symptoms can occur after an abrupt discontinuation, with a rapid increase in anxiety, irritability, insomnia, and somatic symptoms. It is crucial that the titration be extremely slow, given that panic patients are extremely sensitive to the activating effects of antidepressants, and in general of all the stimulants, including caffeine and drugs of abuse. Restlessness, agitation, and worsening of panic attacks can occur in the first days of treatment, and this subjective exacerbation of the anxiety symptoms can induce the patients to discontinue the medication. Fluoxetine treatment should begin at 5 mg/day, with increases of 5 mg every 7 days, up to 10–15 mg in children and 20–30 mg in adolescents. Sertraline treatment should start at 25 mg/day, with weekly increases of 25 mg, up to 100–200 mg/day, according to age and weight.

The onset of a positive response may be not before 4–6 weeks, even though some patients can show some initial improvement after 2 or 3 weeks. This latency period may be too long in patients with an acute and severe symptomatology, who may consider the treatment ineffective after the first 1 or 2 weeks, and interrupt it without contacting the physician. In these cases, a double approach may be needed, with an SSRI for the long-term effect, and with a BDZ for an immediate management of the attacks. Alprazolam may be the first choice, and clonazepam the second, starting with 0.25–0.50 mg bid, with increases every 2 or 3 days, according to the the clinical effectiveness. The BDZ should be gradually and slowly tapered after the SSRI has started its therapeutic effect.

Three different domains should be considered in the assessment of clinical response, that is the number and the intensity of the attacks, the amount of the anticipatory anxiety, and the phobic avoidance (in terms of both number of specific situations avoided and strength of avoidance). The clinical response in the three domains may be different in different subjects.

When an unsatisfactory response is obtained with the SSRI, an alternative is to change the SSRI; the second is to associate an SSRI and a BDZ; the third is to switch from the SSRI to a tricyclic. Further research is needed to explore the efficacy of newer antidepressants (namely venlafaxine and mirtazapine) in treatment-resistant pediatric PD.

When an SSRI treatment is effective, how long should the medication be taken? When the control of panic attacks and anticipatory anxiety has been achieved, the treatment should be maintained at the initial dosage for at least 8 months, then a slow tapering (one quarter of the dose every 4 weeks) may be considered. A persistent anticipatory anxiety with phobic avoidance without persisting panic attacks should be managed with a cognitive-behavioral therapy. A longer treatment period, with higher doses, should be considered after two or three relapses.

Social phobia and selective mutism

First-line treatments for social phobia and selective mutism are psychotherapeutic, including individual and familial approaches. Studies exploring pharmacologic treatment of early-onset social phobia are still few. Even though controlled studies are not available, clinical experience suggests that SSRIs, BDZs and tricyclics are considered the first-line treatment in children and adolescents. In adult social phobia, efficacy of monoamine oxidase inhibitors (MAOIs) is supported by empirical evidence, but these medications are not recommended in young patients because of the risk of a critical increase in blood pressure after intake of tyramine with foods (e.g. cheese, wine, chocolate). A recent controlled study with gabapentin in an adult population (Pande et al, 1999) needs to be confirmed in young patients.

The first-choice medications are SSRIs, namely fluoxetine, sertraline, and fluvoxamine, especially when demoralization, low self-esteem, and helplessness are associated. Fluoxetine is recommended when severe social avoidance and selective mutism are associated. Fluvoxamine and sertraline are recommended when multiple anxiety disorders are comorbid (including separation anxiety disorder, generalized anxiety disorder, obsessive-compulsive disorder). A careful monitoring of behavioral activation in the first weeks of treatment is recommended (Masi et al, 2001c).

Short-acting BDZs can be used in the more acute phases, or before specific phobic situations. No data are available on the long-term treatment of social phobia with BDZ, and this strategy should be avoided in children and adolescents.

Somatic symptoms of social anxiety can often further increase the impairment of affected patients. Beta-blockers have been used to control somatic symptoms of anticipatory social anxiety, including palpitations, tremor, sweating, and dry mouth, but currently they have a limited application in adolescents.

Post-traumatic stress disorder

Pharmacotherapy is not the first-line treatment in children and adolescents with PTSD, and it should be considered as a support to psychotherapeutic approaches, or in acute phases, or when comorbid impairing conditions are associated. Studies on the biologic bases of early-onset PTSD are not so developed to support specific pharmacologic treatments. To date, pharmacotherapy is guided by a symptomatologic evaluation, and the aim of the treatment is to decrease the intensity of specific symptoms, in order to favor psychologic and environmental interventions (Donnelly, 1999).

SSRIs (sertraline) may decrease some depressive and anxiety components of the disorder, related to the avoidance/numbing cluster. They can also be used in obsessive-compulsive or impulsive behaviors. Serotonergic agents blocking the 5HT2A receptors, such as nefazodone, trazodone, and mirtazapine, may improve anxiety, mood, and sleep, with less risk of behavioral activation.

Anticonvulsants can be used when re-experiencing is not well controlled by SSRI antidepressants. When mood fluctuations are more evident, along with impulsivity and irritability, mood stabilizers may be of interest, such as valproic acid (when anxiety is comorbid) or lithium (when impulsivity and aggressiveness are prevalent). Lithium can be used when irritability, impulsivity and aggressiveness are particularly evident.

Acute anxiety symptoms may improve with BDZs (clonzepam, alprazolam), even though they may increase behavioral dyscontrol in some patients during the first period or during the discontinuation.

Beta-blockers, such as propanolol (Famularo et al, 1988), and alpha-adrenergic agents, such as clonidine (Kinzie and Leung, 1989), may reduce the symptoms of hyperarousal, such as impulsivity, startle responses, and insomnia.

Antipyschotic agents (i.e. risperidone, olanzapine, quetiapine) may be useful when psychotic symptoms or flashbacks or severe impulse dyscontrol are present after an acute traumatic experience.

Antagonists of the opiate system (naltrexone) can be used when re-experiencing symptoms do not improve after SSRIs or anticonvulsants.

References

Allen AJ, Leonard H, Swedo SE. Current knowledge of medications for the treatment of childhood anxiety disorders. *J Am Acad Child Adolesc Psychiatry* 1995; **134**: 976–86.

American Psychiatric Association. *Diagnostic and statistical manual of mental disorders.* 4th edn. (revised) Washington, DC: American Psychiatric Association.

Beidel DC, Tuner SM, Marris TL. Psychopathology of childhood social phobia. *J Am Acad Child Adolesc Psychiatry* 1999; **38**: 643–50.

Berliner L. Intervention with children who experienced trauma. In: Cicchetti D, Toth S, eds. *The effects of trauma and the developmental process.* New York: Wiley; 1997: 491–514.

Berney T, Kolvin I, Bhate SR, et al. School phobia: a therapeutic trial with clomipramine and short-term outcome. *Br J Psychiatry* 1981; **138**: 110–118.

Bernstein GA, Garfinkel BD, Borchardt CM. Comparative studies of pharmacotherapy for school refusal. *J Am Acad Child Adolesc Psychiatry* 1989; **29**: 773–81.

Bernstein GA, Borchardt C, Perwien A, et al. Imipramine plus cognitive behavioral therapy in the treatment of school refusal. *J Am Acad Child Adolesc Psychiatry* 2000; **39**: 276–83.

Biederman J, Faraone SV, Marrs A, et al. Panic disorder and agoraphobia in consecutively referred children and adolescents. *J Am Acad Child Adolesc Psychiatry* 1997; **36**: 214–23.

Birmaher B, Waterman GS, Ryan N, et al. Fluoxetine for childhood anxiety disorders. *J Am Acad Child Adolesc Psychiatry* 1994; **33**: 993–9.

Black B, Uhde TW. Treatment of elective mutism with fluoxetine: a double-blind, placebo-controlled study. *J Am Acad Child Adolesc Psychiatry* 1994; **33**: 1000–6.

Compton SN, Grant PJ, Chrisman AK, et al. Sertraline in children and adolescents with social anxiety disorder: an open trial. *J Am Acad Child Adolesc Psychiatry* 2001; **40**: 564–71.

Coyle JT. Drug treatment of anxiety disorders in children. *N Engl J Med* 2001; **344**: 1326–7.

Davidson JR, Rothbaum BO, van der Kolk BA, Sikes CR, Farfel GM. Multicenter, double-blind comparison of sertraline and placebo in the treatment of posttraumatic stress disorder. *Arch Gen Psychiatry* 2001; **58**: 485–92.

Davis LL, Nugent AL, Murray J, Kramer GL, Petty F. Nefazodone treatment for chronic posttraumatic stress disorder: an open trial. *J Clin Psychopharmacol* 2000; **20**: 159–64.

Donnelly CL, Amaya-Jackson L, March JS. Psychopharmacology of pediatric posttraumatic stress disorder. *J Child Adolesc Psychopharmacol* 1999; **9**: 203–20.

Dummit E, Klein R, Tancer N, et al. Fluoxetine treatment of children with selective mutism: an open trial. *J Am Acad Child Adolesc Psychiatry* 1996; **35**: 615–21.

Emslie GJ, Walkup JT, Pliszka SR, Ernst M. Nontryciclic antidepressants: current trends in children and adolescents. *J Am Acad Child Adolesc Psychiatry* 1999; **38**: 517–28.

Fairbanks JM, Pine DS, Tancer NK, et al. Open fluoxetine treatment of mixed anxiety disorders in children and adolescents. *J Child Adolesc Psychopharmacol* 1997; **7**: 17–29.

Famularo R, Kinscherff R, Fenton T. Propanolol treatment of childhood posttraumatic stress disorder, acute type: a pilot study. *Am J Dis Child* 1988; **142**: 1244–7.

Gittelman-Klein R, Klein DF. School phobia: diagnostic considerations in the light of imipramine effects. *J Nerv Ment Dis* 1973; **156**: 199–215.

Grae F, Milner J, Rizzotto L, Klein RG. Clonazepam in childhood anxiety disorders. *J Am Acad Child Adolesc Psychiatry* 1994; **33**: 372–6.

Hageman I, Andersen HL, Jorgensen MB. Post-traumatic stress disorder: a review of psychobiology and pharmacotherapy. *Acta Psychiatr Scand* 2001; **104**: 411–22.

Kinzie JD, Leung P. Clonidine in Cambodian patients with post-traumatic stress disorder. *J Nerv Ment Dis* 1989; **177**: 546–50.

Klein RG, Koplewicz HS, Kanner A. Imipramine treatment of children with separation anxiety disorder. *J Am Acad Child Adolesc Psychiatry* 1992; **31**: 21–28.

Kutcher SP, MacKenzie S. Successful clonazepam treatment of adolescents with panic disorder. *J Clin Psychopharmacol* 1988; **8**: 299–301.

Kutcher SP, Reiter S, Gardner DM, Klein RG. Pharmacotherapy of anxiety disorders in children and adolescents. *Psychiatr Clin North Am* 1992; **15**: 41–67.

Last CG, Perrin S, Hersen M, et al. DSM-III-R anxiety disorders in children: sociodemographic and clinical characteristics. *J Am Acad Child Adolesc Psychiatry* 1992; **31**: 1070–6.

Lepola U, Leinonen E, Koponen H. Citalopram in the treatment of early-onset panic disorder and school-phobia. *Pharmacopsychiatry* 1996; **29**: 30–2.

Manassis K, Bradley S. Fluoxetine in anxiety disorders. *J Am Acad Child Adolesc Psychiatry* 1994; **33**: 761–2.

Mancini C, van Ameringen M, Oakman J, Farvolden P. Serotonergic agents in the treatment of social phobia in children and adolescents. *Depress Anxiety* 1999; **10**: 33–9.

Manicavasagar V, Silove D. Is there an adult form of separation anxiety disorder? A brief clinical report. *Aust NZ J Psychiatry* 1999; **31**: 299–303.

Manicavasagar V, Silove D, Hadzi-Pavlovic D. Subpopulations of early separation anxiety: relevance to risk of adult anxiety disorder. *J Affect Disord* 1998; **48**: 181–90.

Masi G, Mucci M, Favilla L, Romano R, Poli P. Symptomatology and comorbidity of generalized anxiety disorder. *Comprehen Psychiatry* 1999; **40**: 210–15.

Masi G, Mucci M, Millepiedi S. Separation anxiety disorder in children and adolescents: epidemiology, diagnosis and management. *CNS Drugs* 2001a; **15**: 93–104.

Masi G, Toni C, Mucci M, et al. Paroxetine in child and adolescent outpatients with panic disorder. *J Child Adolesc Psychopharmacol* 2001b; **11**: 151–7.

Masi G, Toni C, Perugi G, et al. Anxiety comorbidity in consecutively referred children and adolescents with bipolar disorder: a neglected comorbidity. *Can J Psychiatry* 2001c; **46**: 766–71.

Masi G, Millepiedi S, Mucci M, et al. Generalized anxiety disorder in children and adolescents. *J Am Acad Child Adolesc Psychiatry* 2004; **43**: 752–800.

Pande AC, Davidson JR, Jefferson JW, et al. Treatment of social phobia with gabapentin: a placebo-controlled study. *J Clin Psychopharmacol* 1999; **19**: 341–8.

Pfeffer CR, Jiang H, Domeshek LJ. Buspirone treatment of psychiatrically hospitalized prepubertal children with symptoms of anxiety and moderately severe aggression. *J Child Adolesc Psychopharmacol* 1997; **7**: 145–155.

Pine DS, Cohen P, Gurley D, Brook J, Ma Y. The risk of early adulthood anxiety and depressive disorders in adolescent with anxiety and depressive disorders. *Arch Gen Psychiatry* 1998; **55**: 123–9.

Renaud J, Birmaher B, Wassick SC, Bridge J. Use of selective serotonin reuptake inhibitors for the treatment of childhood panic disorder: a pilot study. *J Child Adolesc Psychopharmacol* 1999; **9**: 73–83.

Research Unit on Pediatric Psychopharmacology. Fluvoxamine for the treatment of anxiety disorders in children and adolescents. The Research Unit on Pediatric Psychopharmacology Anxiety Study Group. *N Engl J Med* 2001; **344**: 1279–85.

Riddle MA, Bernstein GA, Cook EH, et al. Anxiolytics, adrenergic agents, and naltrexone. *J Am Acad Child Adolesc Psychiatry* 1999; **38**: 546–56.

Rynn MA, Siqueland L, Rickels K. Placebo-controlled trial of sertraline in the treatment of children with generalized anxiety disorder. *Am J Psychiatry* 2001; **158**: 2008–214.

Scheeringa MS, Zeanah CH, Drell MJ, Larrieu JA. Two approaches to diagnosing post-traumatic stress disorder in infancy and early childhood. *J Am Acad Child Adolesc Psychiatry* 1995; **34**: 191–200.

Shaffer D, Fisher P, Dulcan MK, et al. The NIMH Diagnostic Interview for Children Version 2.3 (DISC 2.3) Description, acceptability, prevalence rates, and performance in the MECA study. *J Am Acad Child Adolesc Psychiatry* 1995; **35**: 865–77.

Silove D, Manicavasagar V. Adults who feared school: is early separation anxiety specific to the pathogenesis of panic disorder? *Acta Psychiatr Scand* 1993; **88**: 385–90.

Simeon JG, Ferguson HB, Knott V, et al. Clinical, cognitive, and neurophyiological effects of alprazolam in children and adolescents with overanxious and avoidant disorder. *J Am Acad Child Adolesc Psychiatry* 1992; **31**: 29–33.

Simeon JG, Knott VJ, Dubois C, et al. Buspirone therapy of mixed anxiety disorders in childhood and adolescence: a pilot study. *J Child Adolesc Psychopharmacol* 1994; **4**: 159.

Stahl SM. *Essential psychopharmacology*, 2nd edn. New York: Cambridge University Press; 2000.

Stein DJ, Seedat S, van der Linden GJ, Zungu-Dirwayi N. Selective serotonin reuptake inhibitors in the treatment of post-traumatic stress disorder: a meta-analysis of randomized controlled trials. *Int Clin Psychopharmacol* 2000; **15**: S31–S39.

Tucker P, Zaninelli R, Yehuda R, et al. Paroxetine in the treatment of chronic post-traumatic stress disorder: results of a placebo-controlled, flexible-dosage trial. *J Clin Psychiatry* 2001; **62**: 860–8.

Verhulst FC, van der Ende J, Ferdinand RF, Kasius MC. The prevalence of DSM-III-R diagnoses in a normal sample of Dutch adolescents. *Arch Gen Psychiatry* 1997; **54**: 329–36.

Vitiello B, Behar D, Wolfson S, McLeer SV. Diagnosis of panic disorder in prepubertal children. *J Am Acad Child Adolesc Psychiatry* 1997; **29**: 782–4.

Weissmann MM, Bland RC, Canino GJ, et al. The cross-national epidemiology of panic disorder. *Arch Gen Psychiatry* 1997; **54**: 305–9.

Wittchen HU, Reed V, Kessler RC. The relationship of agoraphobia and panic in a community sample of adolescents and young adults. *Arch Gen Psychiatry* 1998; **55**: 1017–24.

World Health Organization. *International classification of diseases*, 10th edn. Geneva. World Health Organization.

chapter 4

Pharmacologic treatment of children and adolescents with major depressive disorder

Benedetto Vitiello, Dario Calderoni, and Luigi Mazzone

Depressive disorders are mood disturbances characterized by persistent and pervasive depression, irritability, or loss of interest or pleasure in all, or almost all, activities, and accompanied by other symptoms such as disruption in appetite, sleep, energy, and ability to concentrate, and feelings of worthlessness, excessive guilt, or recurrent thoughts of death (American Psychiatric Association, 1994). The category of depressive disorders includes major depressive disorder (MDD), dysthymic disorder, and depressive disorder not otherwise specified.

MDD is defined by the presence of at least five depressive symptoms that persist for at least 2 weeks and cause clinically significant distress and/or functional impairment. MDD often has a profound negative impact on the ability of the youth to function interpersonally and academically. Dysthymic disorder has fewer and less severe symptoms lasting at least 1 year and causing significant distress and/or functional impairment. Depressive disorders not otherwise specified constitute a heterogeneous group of conditions, such as minor depressive disorder (episodes of depression that are less severe than MDD and are not chronic like dysthymic disorder) and other disturbances where depressed mood is prominent but without meeting full criteria for better defined disorders. Almost all research in child and adolescent depression has focused on MDD as the most clinically important and best characterized condition. The treatment considerations in this chapter refer to MDD.

MDD is an episodic condition that tends to recur. It is estimated to affect at any time about 1–2% of children 6–12 years old and 4–6% of adolescents 13–17 years old (Lewinsohn et al, 1993; Kessler et al, 2001). By age 18, about 25% of individuals have experienced at least one episode of MDD. MDD improves with time and eventually, usually after many months, remits in the large majority of cases (Birmaher et al, 1996). Occurrence of a second episode, however, is common and about 40% of youths who have recovered from an episode of MDD have another episode within a 1-year period (Emslie et al, 1998). MDD can be associated with psychotic symptoms, such as delusion and hallucinations, and is often comorbid with other psychiatric conditions, such as anxiety, attention deficit hyperactivity disorder (ADHD), conduct disorder, eating disorder, or substance abuse. MDD is a major risk factor for future psychopathology, suicidal attempts, and completed suicide (Weissman et al, 1999; Fombonne et al, 2001). Suicide is the third leading cause of death in the USA and the second in most European countries (National Center for Injury Prevention and Control, 2002).

A high rate (33%) of later emergence of mania has been reported among adolescents with major depression, suggesting that a major depressive episode can be the first manifestation of a bipolar disorder in youth (Geller et al, 2001). The possible development into a bipolar illness has implications for treatment because antidepressants can worsen mania, unless administered together with mood stabilizers.

No diagnostic laboratory tests are currently available. MDD remains an entirely descriptive and clinical diagnosis requiring a comprehensive evaluation and integration of information about symptoms, interpersonal and social context, personal and family history of psychiatric disorders, and medical history.

Approach to treatment

Once a comprehensive evaluation has concluded that the youth suffers from MDD, treatment is usually indicated. In fact, even though untreated MDD eventually remits, remission may take many months to achieve and the depression-associated functional impairment may become in the meantime more difficult to reverse. In some cases, when depressive symptoms are mild and of recent onset, watchful waiting may be initially acceptable, but, if there is no substantial improvement within 3–4 weeks, specific treatment should be initiated.

The goals of treatment are to achieve complete remission and then recovery of the depressive episode and to minimize the risk of relapse and recurrence. Remission is not just symptomatic improvement, rather complete normalization of mood for at least 2 consecutive weeks, so that the patient no longer meets criteria for MDD (Frank et al, 1991). If this state of normal mood persists beyond 2 months, recovery has been achieved. Depression may return during the period of remission (relapse) or after recovery (recurrence).

Accordingly, treatment consists of an initial acute phase (2–3 months) to improve mood, followed by a consolidation phase (1–2 months) to achieve remission, and a maintenance phase (6–9 months) to reach recovery and prevent relapse and recurrence. Continuation of treatment beyond 9–12 months depends on the characteristics and needs of the individual patient. For instance, if the youth has a history of recurrent depressive episode, continuous treatment is indicated.

Both psychotherapeutic and psychopharmacologic interventions have been found to be of benefit in the treatment of children and adolescents with major depression. Cognitive-behavioral therapy (CBT) and interpersonal psychotherapy have been shown to be superior to supportive or family therapy in controlled clinical trials (Brent et al, 1997; Harrington et al, 1998; Mufson et al, 2004). The evidence for supportive therapy, or other psychotherapies such as family therapy, is weaker as it comes from anecdotal clinical experience, and not from controlled studies. Among the medications, only fluoxetine has been shown superior to placebo in more than one controlled study (Emslie et al, 1997, 2002) and is currently approved by the Food and Drug Administration (FDA) for the treatment of depression in subjects age 8 years and above.

In the only direct controlled comparison between fluoxetine and CBT, either alone or in combination, medication was found to be superior to psychotherapy after 3 months of treatment, and especially when used in combination with CBT, for adolescents with moderate to severe MDD (TADS Team, 2004). No study has yet systematically examined possible advantages and disadvantages of starting treatment with either modality. In usual practice, the choice between the two may be influenced by several factors, such as age of the child, severity of depressive symptoms, presence of psychosis or comorbid conditions, and the family's characteristics and preference (Table 4.1).

Table 4.1 Pharmacotherapy or psychotherapy as the first-step treatment?

To consider	Approach
Age of the patient	Under 7 years: use support therapy for child and psychoeducation for family, as there is currently no evidence from controlled studies to support efficacy and safety of antidepressant medication or specific psychotherapies
	7–12 years: consider support therapy, cognitive-behavioral therapy, or medication
	13–17 years: consider support therapy, cognitive-behavioral therapy, interpersonal therapy, or medication
Severity	If symptoms are moderate to severe, medication has a higher rate of success than psychotherapy
Presence of psychosis	Antidepressant and antipsychotic medications are usually indicated
Treatment history	Give preference to interventions that have been effective during previous treatments, and avoid interventions that were not effective or caused adverse effects in the individual patient
Presence of stressors	Psychotherapy may be indicated for improving coping skills
Patient's and family's preference	Youths and parents tend to prefer non-pharmacologic interventions
Services availability	Cognitive-behavioral therapy and interpersonal therapy require trained therapists experienced in these treatment modalities
Family availability to monitor medication effects	Pharmacotherapy requires frequent contacts with the prescribing physician and monitoring by parents at home for mood changes, irritability, insomnia, agitation as possible precursors of suicidal behavior
Cost	Pharmacotherapy is usually less expensive than intensive cognitive-behavioral therapy

Before prescribing antidepressant medication, it is necessary to ensure that a number of previous steps have been accomplished, such as a comprehensive diagnostic evaluation and a discussion of possible treatment approaches with the patient and family (Table 4.2). This is especially important for monitoring the possible emergence of

Table 4.2   Checklist of what to do prior to prescribing an antidepressant medication for major depressive disorder (MDD)

Valid diagnosis of MDD?	If no, antidepressant medication may not be appropriate treatment; in particular, if there is a history of mania, the diagnosis should be bipolar disorder, a condition that requires treatment with a mood stabilizer with or without antidepressant
History of hypomania?	If so, antidepressant treatment can still be used but requires special monitoring for possible emergence of hypomania and mania
Family history of mania?	If so, carefully weigh possible advantages and risks of medication and discuss with parents; plan for close monitoring of mood during treatment for possible emergence of mania
Presence of psychotic symptoms?	Concomitant treatment with an antipsychotic should be considered
Presence of comorbidities?	To be taken into account during treatment
Previous antidepressant treatment?	If so, obtain information about response and adverse events
Informed family of possible adverse events and risks?	Family must be aware of potential risks, and agree to watch for possible emergence of adverse events
Discussed alternative treatments to medication?	Effective psychotherapy exists
Quantify the severity of MDD	This can be accomplished with symptom rating scale. This baseline information is necessary for evaluating treatment effects
Assess and document pretreatment levels of key symptoms such as suicidal ideation, irritability, anxiety, agitation, and insomnia	This baseline information is necessary for assessing possible treatment-associated adverse events
Establish a medication management plan	Patient and parents are given schedule of visits and phone contacts to ensure proper and safe use of medication

adverse events during antidepressant treatment, as further discussed in the safety section of this chapter.

Quantification of the severity of depressive symptoms using a validated rating scale before and during treatment is extremely useful for assessing improvement and estimating treatment effects.

Clinician-administered scales, such as the Child Depression Rating Scale–Revised (Poznanski and Mokros, 1996), or patient self-administered scales, such as the Child Depression Inventory for children (Kovacs et al, 1985), and the Beck Depression Inventory (Beck et al, 1996) for adolescents, can be used for this purpose.

Psychopharmacologic treatment of depression is a multi-component intervention. A medication management plan should be developed and shared with patient and family when medication is first prescribed. The plan should outline the frequency of follow-up visits and instructions for parents' monitoring for possible adverse events. Under usual conditions, weekly contacts between the prescribing clinician and the family and patient are recommended during the first 4 weeks of treatment. Later, if there is satisfactory improvement and no significant adverse effects, contacts can become biweekly or monthly. Finally, once recovery has been reached, a visit every 2–3 months can be sufficient.

An adequate trial of antidepressant medication can be expected to result in clinically significant improvement in about 50–60% of cases. An adequate trial is defined as treatment at full dosage for at least 6 weeks. Thus, treatment non-response is a common occurrence and, by necessity, pharmacotherapy of depression is often a multi-step approach. Treatment planning must take into account the need to ensure an adequate trial of the chosen medication with the understanding that one may need to move to a second-step medication should the first fail.

Even a successful trial of antidepressant will leave most patients still symptomatic, although improved, at the end of the first 8–12 weeks of treatment. Thus, treatment must be continued at least for an additional 4–6 months with the aim of achieving full remission and preventing relapse. Early discontinuation of antidepressant medication entails a substantial risk of relapse. After about 5 months of fluoxetine treatment, relapse occurred in about 60% of children and adolescents who were switched to placebo, as compared with 34% who continued fluoxetine (Emslie et al, 2004). Thus, continuous antidepressant treatment significantly reduces, but does not eliminate, the risk of relapse. If possible, discontinuation of antidepressant medication should occur gradually, for instance by decreasing the daily dosage by 25% every week. This tapering decreases the chance of withdrawal symptoms, which are especially likely in the case of medications with a short elimination half-life.

An integral part of treatment is educating patient and family about depression and its treatment. A better understanding of the illness and of the treatment potential benefits and drawbacks is likely to increase adherence to pharmacotherapy and safety procedures, and thus improve outcome. Moreover, if there are environmental stressors or family conflicts, targeted psychotherapy is indicated.

Depression, antidepressants, and risk of suicide and suicidal behavior

Depression is a major risk factor for suicide. Other risk factors are being male, abusing alcohol or drugs, having conduct disorder, and easy access to potentially lethal weapons. The parents of a depressed youth should be informed of the risk of suicide and instructed to impede access to firearms or dangerous substances.

Antidepressants are expected to reduce depressive symptoms and thus also the risk of suicide. In fact, epidemiologic and observational studies have found an inverse correlation between the extent of use of selective serotonin re-uptake inhibitor (SSRI) antidepressants and rate of suicide in the community (Gibbons et al, 2005). In the US, the increased use of SSRIs in adolescents has been accompanied by a decrease in suicide rate in the 1990s (Olfson et al, 2003). Although association studies cannot prove causality, these data suggest that pharmacologic treatment of depression has a favorable impact in protecting from death from suicide.

It is therefore somewhat paradoxical that the use of antidepressants has been recently found to increase the risk for "suicidality," a category which includes suicidal attempts, suicidal threats, and persistent suicidal ideation. Suicidality and suicide are not synonymous, although they are linked. In fact, based on data in adults, most subjects who attempt suicide do not eventually commit suicide, and most subjects who commit suicide do not have a history of previous attempts. Still, having attempted suicide increases the risk for further attempts and ultimately for suicide.

This link between antidepressants and "suicidality" was established through a meta-analysis conducted by the US Food and Drug Administration (FDA) on the data from 24 separate placebo-controlled clinical trials of antidepressants, most of which were SSRIs, conducted between 1983 and 2004 (Hammad, 2004). Of the 24 studies, 15 were in

Table 4.3 Relative risk (RR) of suicidal behavior and ideation during treatment with antidepressants versus placebo, overall and for selected medications (Hammad, 2004)

	RR	95% CI
Fluoxetine (4 studies in MDD[a] and 1 study in OCD)	1.52	0.75–3.09
Sertraline (2 studies in MDD and 1 study in OCD)	1.48	0.42–5.24
Paroxetine (3 studies in MDD and 1 study in SAD)	2.65	1.00–7.02
Citalopram (2 studies in MDD)	1.37	0.53–3.50
Venlafaxine (2 studies in MDD and 1 study in GAD)	4.97	1.09–22.72
Overall[b] (15 studies in MDD 5 in OCD, 2 in GAD, and 2 in SAD)	1.95	1.28–2.98

[a]MDD: major depressive disorder; OCD: obsessive-compulsive disorder; SAD: social anxiety disorder; GAD: generalized anxiety disorder.

[b]Including all data from 25 pediatric studies across 9 different antidepressants.

CI: confidence interval.

MDD and the remainder were in obsessive-compulsive disorder or other anxiety disorders (Table 4.3). A total of about 4400 children and adolescents took part in these studies. Of these, about half were randomized to receive active medication and half placebo for about 2 months under double-blind conditions. No completed suicide occurred among these subjects, but the rate of "suicidality" was about 4% among the subjects on antidepressants and about 2% among those on placebo (Hammad, 2004). The overall relative risk (risk on active medication divided by risk on placebo) was 1.95 (95% CI 1.28–2.98) (Table 4.3).

Based on the available data, this increased risk for "suicidality" cannot be restricted to a particular drug or group of antidepressants. Thus, in the US, the labeling information of all antidepressants currently carries the same warning that the use of the medication increases the risk of "suicidality." In 2003, the UK Committee on

Safety of Medicines warned against the use of SSRIs or the serotonin/ norepinephrine re-uptake inhibitor (SNRI) venlafaxine in the treatment of depression in children and adolescents, with the only exception of fluoxetine, whose risk/benefit ratio was deemed to be favorable (Whittington et al, 2004). In 2005, the European Medicines Agency concluded that SSRIs and SNRIs should not be used in children and adolescents except for their approved indication, which in Europe does not include depression under age 18 (European Medicines Agency, 2005).

These warnings are likely to restrict the use of pharmacotherapy for depressed youths, especially in Europe where no antidepressant has an officially approved indication for the treatment of depression under age 18 years. The risk for adverse effects, however, must be weighed against the risk of untreated depression unresponsive to non-pharmacologic interventions. In fact, medication treatment with fluoxetine was shown to be superior to psychotherapy for adolescents with moderate to severe depression (TADS Team, 2004).

The mechanism through which antidepressants may cause "suicidality" is not known. Some patients may be "negatively activated" by antidepressant treatment, with agitation, akathisia, and anxiety, and it is possible that these symptoms increase the risk of suicidal behavior. It has also long been observed that depressed patients are paradoxically at higher risk for suicide when depressive symptoms seem to improve.

The important practical implication of the increased risk for suicidality during antidepressant treatment is that antidepressants must be used carefully and only in the context of a comprehensive treatment plan that includes monitoring for possible adverse effects by both family and clinicians.

Selective serotonin re-uptake inhibitors

SSRIs constitute the primary line of pharmacologic treatment of depression in children and adolescents (Table 4.4). Currently available SSRIs include: fluoxetine, sertraline, paroxetine, citalopram, escitalopram, and fluvoxamine. These medications are marketed for the treatment of depression, obsessive-compulsive disorder, or social phobia in adults, and also used, often off-label, in children and adolescents with depression, obsessive-compulsive disorder, or anxiety disorders. In the US, fluoxetine is approved by the FDA for the treatment of depression in children aged 8 and above. Fluoxetine, sertraline, and fluvoxamine

Table 4.4   Pharmacotherapy for children and adolescents (age 6–18 years) with major depressive disorder: lines of treatment to consider sequentially based on evidence of efficacy and safety

First-line	Fluoxetine
Second-line	Another SSRI such as sertraline, citalopram, or escitalopram
Third–fifth-line	Bupropion, venlafaxine, or mirtazapine
Sixth-line	Tricyclics

are FDA-approved for the treatment of obsessive-compulsive disorder in children 7 years and older.

All SSRIs share the same basic pharmacologic action by selectively blocking the re-uptake of serotonin into the pre-synaptic nerve terminal, thus increasing the synaptic availability of this neurotransmitter. The side-effect profile is also similar across SSRIs. Nausea, vomiting, headache, agitation, nervousness, and insomnia are adverse events that have been found to be more common during SSRI treatment than on placebo. SSRIs cause sexual dysfunction, such as anorgasmia, delayed ejaculation, and impotence, in about 5–15% of treated adults and similar problems can occur in adolescents.

Symptoms of hypomania and mania can emerge during SSRI antidepressant treatment, with a highly variable rate ranging between 1 and 6% during a period of 8–12 weeks. A switch to mania can occur during the natural course of depression in adolescence regardless of antidepressant treatment. Thus, it is difficult to determine at the individual patient level if the mania was drug-induced or part of the course of illness. In any case, the presence of mania is a reason for discontinuing antidepressant treatment. Overall, the tolerability of these drugs in children and adolescents is good. In clinical trials, less than 10% of patients discontinued treatment because of side-effects and, for most trials, the rate was not different from that observed on placebo.

SSRIs can be considered relatively safe drugs, especially if compared with the "old" antidepressants, such as the tricyclics or monoamine oxidase inhibitors. Overdose of SSRIs is seldom life-threatening. However, at least one case of death has been reported that was associated with unusually high plasma levels of fluoxetine in a 9-year-old child who had a genetic deficiency of P-450 2D6 enzymes and was consequently unable to metabolize the drug properly (Sallee et al, 2000).

This child, who was also taking methylphenidate and clonidine in addition to fluoxetine 100 mg/day, for 6 months, presented with gastrointestinal symptoms, fever, inco-ordination, and disorientation, which were followed by seizures, status epilepticus, and death.

As previously described, the administration of SSRIs carries a risk for "suicidality", which includes suicidal attempts, suicidal threats, or intense and recurrent suicidal ideation. Because of this risk, it is necessary to carefully weigh potential benefits and harms of SSRI treatment and monitor for possible emergence of adverse events, especially during the first 4–6 weeks of treatment (Tables 4.5 and 4.6).

Table 4.5   Advantages and disadvantages of SSRI medications

Advantages	Disadvantages
Effective in about 50–60% of patients	Non-effective in 40–50% of patients
Easy dose titration	Take several weeks to produce an improvement
Safe in overdose	Can increase risk for suicidal behavior Require monitoring for possible emergence of irritability, agitation, insomnia, suicidal behavior
More effective than psychotherapy for moderate to severe depression	Less accepted than psychotherapy by patients and families

Table 4.6   What to monitor during treatment with antidepressant medication

Depressive symptom severity	Some improvement should occur in the first 3–4 weeks, if not, a dose increase is indicated
Comprehensive adverse events check	Weekly for the 1st month of treatment, then biweekly until a stable, well-tolerated dose is found; at least quarterly afterwards
Presence and severity of comorbidities	At least monthly initially, at least quarterly afterwards
Heart rate and blood pressure	At least monthly initially, then every 6 months
Weight	At least monthly initially, then every 6 months
Height	At least yearly

The main differences among SSRIs lie in their pharmacokinetics and in the current level of evidence with which their antidepressant effects have been documented. Thus, fluoxetine has a long elimination life, which allows a once-a-day dosing and minimizes the risk of withdrawal symptoms upon discontinuation. Other SSRIs have a much shorter half-life, require a twice-a-day dosing, and abrupt discontinuation can cause withdrawal symptoms, such as nausea, vomiting, headache, lethargy, and flu-like symptoms. With respect to efficacy in depression, only fluoxetine has been demonstrated to be better than placebo in two or more controlled clinical trials, while for other SSRIs the evidence for efficacy is less conclusive, being supported by only one controlled trial.

As for all the antidepressants, the SSRI antidepressant effects usually take several weeks to become manifest, and full response can take several months. Improvement of depressive symptoms becomes apparent in the first 4–8 weeks, but only a few patients reach remission after 2–3 months of treatment. In many cases, full remission may require continuous treatment for 4–6 months.

The magnitude of the antidepressant effect of the SSRIs can be described in statistical terms as "small to moderate." In fact, the improvement rate is around 50–60% during SSRI treatment and around 35–45% on placebo. The improvement on placebo includes both spontaneous remission of symptoms and expectation of improvement (which is the true "placebo response"). Because of this relatively modest difference between antidepressant and placebo treatment, many clinical trials have not been able to detect statistically significant differences between treatment groups. There is clearly substantial intersubject variability in treatment response, but no clinically useful predictors of treatment effect have been thus far identified. It is to be hoped that future advances in pharmacogenetics will allow a better individualization of the treatment of depression.

Fluoxetine

Fluoxetine is currently the only medication that has regulatory approval for the treatment of depression in children and adolescents, at least in the US. Fluoxetine has been shown to be statistically superior to placebo in decreasing depressive symptoms in more than one controlled trial (Emslie et al, 1997, 2002; TADS Team, 2004).

Consequently, fluoxetine is the first-line medication for the pharmacologic treatment of depression in childhood and adolescence.

Besides the documented evidence of antidepressant efficacy, fluoxetine differs from the other antidepressants in that it has an especially long elimination plasma half-life, which is about 2–3 days for fluoxetine itself and about 7–16 days for its active metabolite norfluoxetine. This slow elimination has several implications. It takes about a month of continuous treatment to reach plasma (and brain tissue) steady-state levels and about the same time for the body to completely eliminate the drug when treatment is discontinued. Dosing can be once a day or even once every few days, and missing a daily dose does not result in a substantial decrease in plasma levels or in withdrawal symptoms.

For both children and adolescents, the recommended starting dose is 10 mg/day, increased to 20 mg/day after 1–2 weeks (Table 4.7). Controlled trials have utilized 20 mg as the target therapeutic dose for both children and adolescents. However, after administration of fluoxetine 20 mg, plasma levels of fluoxetine were about 2-fold higher in children (mean 171 ng/ml) than in adolescents (mean 86 ng/ml), but similar after adjustment for differences in weight (Wilens et al, 2002). The clinical consequence is that for children 10 mg may be an effective dosage. Thus, based on pharmacokinetics data, children could be tried on 10 mg for 3–4 weeks before considering a dose increase if there is no improvement. In adolescents, the average effective dose is around 30–35 mg/day (TADS Team, 2004). Some patients require higher doses, up to 60 mg/day.

Fluoxetine is metabolized by multiple hepatic isoenzymes, including the cytochrome P450 (CYP) 2D6 and CYP 2C9. There is a genetic polymorphism for CYP 2D6 that determines the enzymatic activity. Slow metabolizers account for about 7% of the general population. These subjects have substantially higher levels of fluoxetine (and other drugs metabolized by the CYP 2D6) than the rest of the population. Unusual intolerance to drug side-effects may be due to impaired elimination. Concomitant administration of other drugs that also utilize the CYP 2D6 isoenzymes for their metabolism leads to competition for the same metabolic pathway and can result in increased plasma levels. For instance, based on data in adults, concomitant administration of fluoxetine and a tricyclic medication in adults results in increased plasma levels of the tricyclic.

Table 4.7   Antidepressants used in the treatment of children and adolescents with major depression

Step	Medication	Starting dose (mg/day)	Usual therapeutic dose (mg/day)	Dosing
1	Fluoxetine	10	10–40 (children) 20–60 (adolescents)	Once a day
2[a]	Sertraline	25	50–200	bid
	Citalopram	10	20–40	bid
3–5[b]	Bupropion	75–100	100–300	bid
	Venlafaxine	37.5	112.5–150	bid for immediate release formulation
				Once a day for extended release formulation
	Mirtazapine	30	30–45	Once a day at bedtime

[a]Second step should be another SSRI, such as sertraline or citalopram. If no response to two SSRIs, move to step 3–5 drugs.

[b]These three medications can be tried sequentially, in any order, in case of non-response. Paroxetine is not included, despite some evidence of efficacy, because other SSRIs currently offer a better balance between possible benefits and risk. If a patient does not respond to two SSRIs, a trial of non-SSRI antidepressant is recommended.

Sertraline

Sertraline constitutes with citalopram a second line of antidepressant treatment for children and adolescents after fluoxetine. The efficacy of sertraline in pediatric depression is less well documented than for fluoxetine. Two parallel placebo-controlled trials showed a statistically significant difference from placebo when the data were merged, while each trial in isolation failed to find a difference (Wagner et al, 2003).

The starting dose of sertraline is 25 mg/day, then it is increased within a week to 50 mg/day (Table 4.7). If no improvement emerges after 3–4 weeks on 50 mg/day, the dosage can be further increased by 25 mg/day increments about every 2 weeks up to a maximum of 200 mg/day. A twice a day administration is recommended for daily doses below 200 mg to avoid any possible withdrawal symptoms (Axelson et al, 2002).

Sertraline is extensively metabolized by liver enzymes. Its main metabolite is N-desmethylsertraline, which has only weak pharmacologic activity. Children tend to metabolize the drug with somewhat greater efficiency than adults at doses of 50–100 mg/day, as shown by an elimination half-life after continuous administration of about 15 hours during treatment with 50 mg/day. After continuous treatment with 200 mg/day the mean half-life was 26 hours in children and 28 hours in adolescents (similar to that in adults: 27 hours).

Citalopram

The efficacy of citalopram in pediatric depression is supported by one controlled trial that showed statistically significant superiority over placebo (Wagner et al, 2004). Another trial, currently unpublished, failed to detect a difference. The starting dose of citalopram is 10 mg/day, then it is increased after about 1 week to 20 mg/day (Table 4.7). A further increase to 30 mg/day is warranted if there is no improvement after 3–4 weeks on 20 mg/day. The maximum dose is about 40 mg/day. A twice a day administration is recommended in children to avoid possible withdrawal symptoms.

Citalopram is metabolized by hepatic isoenzymes, in particular CYP 3A4 and CYP 2C19. Citalopram does not inhibit CYP 3A4 and has few clinically significant interactions with other drugs. The plasma elimination half-life of citalopram is similar in adolescents and adults (about 40 hours), but that of the enantiomer S-citalopram (considered responsible for the antidepressant activity) is shorter (17–19 hours) in 9–17-year-old subjects (Perel et al, 2001).

Other SSRIs

Escitalopram is the pure S-enantiomer of citalopram and shares similar pharmacologic activity with the racemic parent compound, but at half the mg dose of citalopram. There is no clear evidence of advantages of escitalopram over the parent compound. Like citalopram, it is metabolized in the liver by CYP 3A4 and CYP 2C19.

Paroxetine has been shown to have antidepressant activity in adolescents on some, though not all the outcome measures (Keller et al, 2001). But two other studies in depression were unable to demonstrate efficacy versus placebo. The half-life after a single 10 mg dose is about 11 hours, with wide intersubject variability (Findling et al, 1999). Concerns about withdrawal symptoms and tolerability profile with respect to the emergence of irritability, nervousness, and possible suicidality have restricted its use in recent years.

Fluvoxamine has been primarily used for the treatment of obsessive-compulsive disorder or other anxiety disorders, such as generalized anxiety disorder, in children and adolescents. There is little documentation of its possible antidepressant activity. It also has a number of potential metabolic interactions with other drugs, due to the fact that it inhibits the CYP 3A4 isoenzyme.

The current role of other SSRIs in the treatment of depression in children and adolescents is questionable and in any case rather limited. In fact, if two separate trials of SSRI medication are not effective to improve an individual patient, treatment with a non-SSRI antidepressant is recommended.

Non-SSRI, non-tricyclic antidepressants

Bupropion

Bupropion is an antidepressant pharmacologically unrelated to the SSRIs. It is a weak inhibitor of the presynaptic re-uptake of norepinephrine, dopamine, and serotonin. It has basically no clinically significant serotonergic activity and can be a logical alternative for patients with SSRI-induced serotonergic side-effects. It is marketed for the treatment of depression in adults, but there are currently no controlled studies demonstrating the efficacy of bupropion in depressed children or adolescents.

The starting dose is 100 mg/day and maintenance doses range from 100 to 300 mg/day (Table 4.7). A bid dosing is recommended. Buproprion is rapidly absorbed with a plasma peak at about 2 hours after dosing and a mean plasma elimination half-life of 12 hours in youths (Daviss et al, 2005). It is metabolized by CYP 3A4 and 2B6. Of its metabolites, hydroxybuproprion and threohydrobuproporion have in elimination half-life of 21 hours and 26 hours, respectively, and mainly nonadrenergic activity, whereas the parent compared buproprion is dopaminergic (Daviss et al, 2005).

Bupropion can cause nausea, insomnia, and palpitations, but these side-effects are not frequent and seldom intolerable. Bupropion can also trigger tics and cause dermatologic reactions, such as rash and urticaria, at times severe enough to lead to discontinuing the drug. Bupropion increases the overall risk for seizures, but this effect is minimal if the dose is maintained within 300 mg/day. It is also important to increase the dose gradually, with increments of no more than 100 mg/day every 7–10 days. If restlessness, agitation, tremor, or insomnia emerge, the dose should be decreased or in any case not further increased. The possible effect of age on the risk for seizures during treatment with bupropion has not been investigated.

Venlafaxine

Venlafaxine belongs to the SNRI class, as it inhibits the presynaptic re-uptake of serotonin and, at higher doses, also that of norepineph-rine. This dual action is hypothesized to result in faster and more powerful antidepressant activity. There are in fact a number of studies that suggest that venlafaxine may be more effective than certain SSRIs, but no conclusive evidence of its superiority has been produced. However, in clinical practice, patients who have not responded to one or more SSRI antidepressants are often treated with venlafaxine.

The efficacy of venlafaxine in depressed children and adolescents remains unproven and currently supported only by open-label, uncontrolled studies, and clinical experience. Two placebo-controlled trials were unable to find a statistically significant difference from placebo. For this reason, venlafaxine can be considered only a drug of third choice (Table 4.4).

The side-effects of venlafaxine are similar to those of the SSRIs. In addition, however, this drug can increase blood pressure in a dose-related manner. In adults, a sustained increase in blood pressure was observed at daily doses above 100 mg and more frequently (13%) at doses above 300 mg/day. Monitoring of blood pressure before and periodically during treatment is part of the clinical management of the patients taking venlafaxine. Based on the two available placebo-controlled trials of venlafaxine in major depression, the relative risk of suicidal behavior or ideation on venlafaxine versus placebo was 8.8 (95% CI: 1.12–69.51), which was the highest among antidepressants. Thus, careful monitoring is needed during treatment with venlafaxine. The rationale for retaining this drug as a step 3 or higher treatment (Table 4.4) is because it offers an alternative pharmacologic profile through the combined serotonergic and norepinephric activity that may be helpful to patients who have not responded to treatment with SSRIs.

Venlafaxine is primarily metabolized by the CYP 2D6 and in small part also by CYP 3A4. Of the metabolites, only O-desmethylvenlafaxine is pharmacologically active. The genetic polymorphism involving CYP

2D6 does not seem to have clinical implications for the use of venlafaxine. As for fluoxetine, concomitant administration of medications that inhibit CYP 2D6, such as the tricyclics, can increase venlafaxine plasma levels. This combination, however, is not likely to be used. The plasma elimination half-life of venlafaxine is about 5 hours and that of its active metabolite about 11 hours, in adults.

The initial dose is 37.5 mg/day, to be increased in a week to 75 mg/day and then by increments of 37.5 mg/day each week to a total dose of about 112.5 mg/day in children and about 150 mg/day in adolescents. A therapeutic effect is expected at these dose levels. For some patients, further increases up to a maximum of 225 mg/day can be considered. The daily dose should be given in two separate doses, morning and evening, in the case of the immediate-release formulation. Less frequent dosing can result in withdrawal symptoms. The extended-release formulation can be given once a day in the morning.

Mirtazapine

Mirtazapine has a pharmacologic profile that is different from that of the drugs thus far discussed. It acts as an antagonist to the presynaptic alpha-2 receptor, thus increasing norepinephrine and, through adrenergic activation of the raphe nuclei, increasing serotonergic transmission. In addition, it blocks the serotonin 5HT2A and 5HT2C receptors. Mirtazapine is marketed for the treatment of depression in adults.

Open-label, uncontrolled data are suggestive of efficacy in adolescents with major depression at doses of 30–45 mg/day, but two, still unpublished, controlled clinical trials have failed to show a difference from placebo. It is metabolized primarily by the CYP 2D6 and CYP 3A4 isoenzymes. The plasma elimination half-life is about 20–40 hours in adults, so that a once-a-day dosing, usually at bedtime to minimize the negative effect of sedation, is sufficient. One of the metabolites, methylmirtazapine, is pharmacologically active.

Mirtazapine is quite safe in overdose, but it can cause sedation, increased appetite, and weight gain. Rare instances of severe neutropenia (about 1.1 per thousand treated patients) have also been reported, so that emergence of sore throat, fever, and infection during treatment should be carefully evaluated as possible signs of agranulocytosis. This is clearly an antidepressant to be considered only in the case of non-response to other antidepressants with better documented efficacy and safety in pediatric populations.

Tricyclic antidepressants

Before the introduction of the SSRIs, tricyclic antidepressants were commonly used to treat children and adolescents with a variety of conditions, such as depression, anxiety, attention deficit hyperactivity disorder (ADHD), and enuresis. There is proven efficacy from controlled studies in ADHD, enuresis, and some forms of anxiety, but, despite a dozen placebo-controlled trials, not in pediatric depression (Hazell et al, 2002). Open studies and anecdotal clinical experience suggest that these drugs can be of help to individual patients, but the available data overall indicate that they are not generally effective for depressed youths as a group. Their considerable toxicity in overdose due to delay in heart conduction is a major safety problem that discourages their use, except in selected cases unresponsive to other treatments. Information about their pharmacology, pharmacokinetics, and dosage is provided in the chapter on the treatment of ADHD. (see Chapter 9)

Other non-SSRI, non-tricyclic antidepressants

Reboxetine is a selective noradrenergic re-uptake inhibitor and as such has a distinctive pharmacologic activity, similar to that of atomoxetine (see Chapter 9). It is marketed in Europe, but not in the US, for the treatment of depression in adults. Little is known about its effects in children. It is metabolized by the CTYP 2D6 and CYP 3A4 isoenzymes and has a half-life of about 12–16 hours in adults.

Nefazodone is an antidepressant related to trazodone. It has a complex pharmacologic activity that includes inhibition of the re-uptake of serotonin and norepinephrine, in addition to acting as an agonist and antagonist at different serotonergic receptors. It has been shown to have effective antidepressant activity in adolescents as well in a currently unpublished controlled trial (while another failed to show a difference from placebo), but it is seldom, if ever, used because of its rare but potentially lethal liver toxicity.

Contraindications to antidepressant treatment

The presence of a bipolar disorder of type I (with history of mania) is a contraindication to the use of antidepressant treatment unless the patient is also receiving a mood stabilizer. Use of antidepressant medication without a mood stabilizer can trigger mania. The contraindication is less absolute in the case of a bipolar disorder of type II (with a history of hypomania), but caution is required if the antidepressant is used without a mood stabilizer.

Certain antidepressants have specific contraindications, such as a history of a seizure disorder in the case of bupropion. Tricyclics are not to be used in subjects with cardiac conduction abnormalities, such as different levels of heart blocks or prolongation on the QTc interval. SSRIs, venlafaxine, and mirtazapine are not to be used concurrently with monoamino oxidase inhibitors (MAOIs) or within 2 weeks of their discontinuation. But MAOIs are, in any case, not recommended for use in pediatric patients.

When antidepressant medication does not seem to work

Antidepressant treatment requires time to start showing efficacy. It is not unusual for an antidepressant to take 3–4 weeks at full therapeutic dosage in order to show clinically significant effects. At times, the response seems to be almost immediate, with relief of symptoms in the first few days of treatment. In these cases, while a true early pharmacologic effect cannot be excluded, a non-specific "placebo effect" due to the expectation of improvement is also likely, especially if the improvement is not sustained over time.

If no response emerges in 3–4 weeks at a therapeutic dose, the dosage should be gradually increased, unless there are tolerability problems, up to the maximum recommended dose. If there is no clinically significant improvement after 4 weeks at maximum dose, the drug should be gradually discontinued and the next line of treatment instituted. The clinician is also invited to review the case to ensure accuracy of diagnosis, the possible presence of medical or psychiatric comorbidities, or problems with treatment adherence (Table 4.8).

In case of partial response to an antidepressant, several alternative courses of actions are possible:

- discontinuation and replacement with another antidepressant
- augmentation with psychotherapy
- augmentation with another medication (such as lithium 300–600 mg/day), or
- continuation with the same antidepressant in the hope that more prolonged treatment will eventually result in full improvement.

Table 4.8 What to consider doing in the case of a non-response to antidepressant treatment

1. Reassess the patient and verify the correctness of the diagnosis of major depression
2. Assess for possible psychiatric comorbid conditions, in particular hypomania, mania, and substance abuse
3. Make sure that the antidepressant trial was of adequate duration (4–6 weeks) at the maximum recommended and tolerated dose
4. Make sure that treatment adherence by the patient was adequate
5. Exclude concomitant medications that might interfere with the antidepressant
6. Exclude underlying medical conditions such as hypothyroidism
7. Assess for possible ongoing environmental stressors and interpersonal conflicts, which may contribute to depression and require targeted psychotherapy

All the four courses of action can be justified based on the individual characteristics of the patient, the experience of the clinician, the preferences of the patient and family, and the available resources. No controlled studies have actually examined the relative advantages of one strategy over the other.

Combination with psychotherapy

In the Treatment for Adolescents with Depression Study (TADS Team, 2004) which studied youths with moderate to severe major depression, fluoxetine had a success rate of 61% when used alone as monotherapy and 71% when used in combination with cognitive-behavioral therapy (CBT), as compared with 43% on CBT alone and 35% on supportive clinical management with pill placebo (Table 4.1). Obviously, combined treatment is more expensive and requires the availability of a therapist trained in CBT in adolescents. No similar studies have been conducted in prepubertal children.

Special populations

Psychotic depression

If depression is accompanied by psychotic symptoms, such as delusions or hallucinations, concomitant administration of antidepressant and antipsychotic medication is usually indicated.

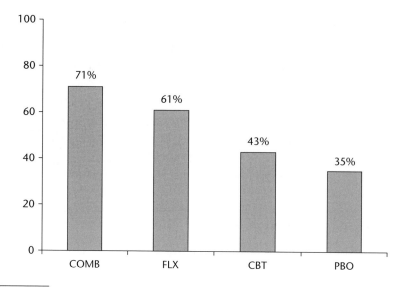

Figure 4.1   *Percent treatment response in the Treatment for Adolescents with Depression Study (TADS Team, 2004). (FLX: fluoxetine; CBT: cognitive behavioral therapy; COMB: combination of FLX and CBT; PBO: placebo.)*

Depression in the context of bipolar disorder

No controlled studies have been conducted to determine treatment efficacy and safety. Based on adult data and clinical experience, it is recommended that treatment with a mood stabilizer be instituted when depression occurs in the context of a bipolar disorder type I (i.e. with a history of mania). An antidepressant can then be added to the mood stabilizer for the depressive component. Use of an antidepressant without a mood stabilizer can trigger mania and further destabilize the clinical picture. Less clear is the course of action in the case of bipolar disorder type II (i.e. with a history of hypomania). The use of a mood stabilizer is probably the safest approach given the reported high rate of switch to mania in adolescent depression (Geller et al, 2001).

Depression in the context of substance abuse

Antidepressants are not drugs of potential abuse and can be safely used in youths with substance abuse. To be successful, however, antidepressant treatment must be accompanied by specific psychosocial treatment for the substance abuse.

Young children

Little research has been conducted on the validation of the diagnosis of depression under age 7. Depression can certainly occur in preschool years, but the diagnostic tools and assessment methods are still in need of adaptation to this age group. No controlled treatment studies have been conducted in depressed children under age 7. Pharmacologic treatment may be considered for selected patients if psychotherapeutic interventions have proven insufficient, but no general guidelines can be formulated at this time.

Comorbidity with ADHD

It is not uncommon for a child with ADHD to suffer also from depression. The most common pharmacologic treatment of ADHD is stimulant medication, which can be administered concurrently with an antidepressant. No specific drug interactions have been reported, but special care should be paid to monitor for the possible emergence of adverse events, in particular agitation, anxiety, nervousness, and insomnia.

Frequently asked questions

1. Q: An adolescent who started treatment with an SSRI antidepressant 4 days ago complains of nausea and headache. What to do?

    A: Nausea and headache can be caused by the SSRI. Unless symptoms are intolerable or cause functional impairment (e.g. unable to attend classes in school), the patient should be encouraged to continue treatment with the expectation that the body will gradually adjust to the SSRI and these side-effects will disappear. If after 7–10 days the patient still has similar complaints, consider switching to another SSRI, which may be better tolerated, or to a non-SSRI antidepressant.

2. Q: An adolescent who started treatment with an SSRI 4 days ago presents with agitation, insomnia, and anxiety attacks. What to do?

A: Given the severity of the negative behavioral activation most likely caused by SSRI-induced serotonergic stimulation, SSRI treatment should probably be discontinued. After a complete resolution of these adverse effects, SSRI could be restarted at a much lower dose and under close monitoring. If similar symptoms emerge even at a reduced dose, a non-SSRI antidepressant should be considered instead.

3.   Q: A child is taking sertraline 50 mg every morning. At the end of the day, he looks very tired and lethargic and complains of feeling sick. This has happened every day now for at least a week. Can these symptoms be side-effects of sertraline?

A: It is more likely that these symptoms are signs of withdrawal from the SSRI. Sertraline has a shorter half-life in children than in adults. A twice a day dosage (25 mg bid in this case) would prevent withdrawal symptoms.

4.   Q: A child has been taking fluoxetine 20 mg/day for 4 weeks and no clinically significant improvement has emerged yet. Should the dose be continued or increased?

A: It may be reasonable to increase the dose to 30 mg/day if there are no important side-effects.

5.   Q: A teenager has been treated with fluoxetine for 2 months and has been doing very well for the last month. She is not depressed any more and is functioning well at home and school. Can the medication be discontinued?

A: This patient has reached remission (absence of depression for at least 2 weeks) but not recovery (absence of depression for at least 2 months). Discontinuing medication now would put this patient at higher risk for relapse. Continuous pharmacotherapy is recommended for at least 6 months after full recovery has been reached.

6.   Q: A teenager has been treated with an SSRI antidepressant and has now recovered from his second episode of major depression. For how long should he continue antidepressant treatment?

A: Given the history of recurrent depression, it may be appropriate to continue treatment for one year after complete remission of depression.

7. Q: A teenager has been in treatment with fluoxetine for 4 months and, although clearly improved, still has clinically significant depression. He has been taking 60 mg/day of fluoxetine for about a month now. What approaches could be considered?

    A: Augmentation with a specific antidepressant psychotherapy, such as cognitive-behavioral therapy, could be added to the current medication. If the response is still insufficient, pharmacologic augmentation with lithium 300–600 mg/day could be considered based on studies in adults (no controlled studies to test augmentation treatment have been conducted in children or adolescents).

8. Q: A teenager has attempted suicide. She had started treatment with an SSRI antidepressant about one week ago. Was the attempt caused by the SSRI?

    A: It cannot be determined if an individual subject's suicidal behavior was due to the underlying depressive disorder, the SSRI treatment, or both. Depression itself is a major risk factor for suicidal behavior. Antidepressant treatment usually decreases depression, but, in some subjects, it can increase the risk for suicidal behavior. At this time, however, it is not possible to separate the possible contribution of these factors at the individual patient level.

References

American Psychiatric Association. *Diagnostic and Statistical Manual of Mental Disorders*, 4th edn. Washington, DC: American Psychiatric Association, 1994.

Axelson DA, Perel JM, Birmaher B, et al. Sertraline pharmacokinetics and dynamics in adolescents. *J Am Acad Child Adolesc Psychiatry* 2002; **41**: 1037–44.

Beck AT, Steer RA, Brown GK. *Manual for the Beck Depression Inventory-II*. San Antonio, TX: The Psychological Corporation, 1996.

Birmaher B, Ryan ND, Williamson DE, Brent DA, Kaufman J. Childhood and adolescent depression: a review of the past 10 Years. Part I. *J Am Acad Child Adolesc Psychiatry* 1996; **35**: 1427–39.

Brent DA, Holder D, Kolko D, et al. A clinical psychotherapy trial for adolescent depression comparing cognitive, family and supportive therapy. *Arch Gen Psychiatry* 1997; **54**: 877–85.

Daviss WB, Perel JM, Rudolph GR, et al. Steady-state pharmacokinetics of bupropion SR in juvenile patients. *J Am Acad Child Adolesc Psychiatry* 2005; **44**: 349–57.

Emslie GJ, Rush AJ, Weinberg WA, et al. A double-blind, randomized, placebo-controlled trial of fluoxetine in children and adolescents with depression. *Arch Gen Psychiatry* 1997; **54**: 1031–7.

Emslie GJ, Rush AJ, Weinberg WA, et al. Fluoxetine in child and adolescent depression: acute and maintenance treatment. *Depress Anxiety* 1998; **7**: 32–9.

Emslie GJ, Heiligenstein JH, Wagner KD, et al. Fluoxetine for acute treatment of depression in children and adolescents: a placebo-controlled, randomized clinical trial. *J Am Acad Child Adolesc Psychiatry* 2002; **41**: 1205–15.

Emslie GJ, Heiligenstein JH, Hoog SL, et al. Fluoxetine treatment for prevention of relapse of depression in children and adolescents: a double-blind, placebo-controlled study. *J Am Acad Child Adolesc Psychiatry* 2004; **43**: 1397–405.

European Medicines Agency. European Medicines Agency finalises review of antidepressants in children and adolescents. Doc. Ref. EMEA/CHMP/128918. London, 25 April 2005 (http://www.emea.eu.int).

Findling RL, Reed MD, Myers C, et al. Paroxetine pharmacokinetics in depressed children and adolescents. *J Am Acad Child Adolesc Psychiatry* 1999; **38**: 952–9.

Fombonne E, Wostear G, Cooper V, Harrington R, Rutter M. The Maudsley long-term follow-up of child and adolescent depression. 2. Suicidality, criminality and social dysfunction in adulthood. *Br J Psychiatry* 2001; **179**: 218–23.

Frank E, Prien RF, Jarrett RB, et al. Conceptualization and rationale for consensus definitions of terms in major depressive disorder. Remission, recovery, relapse, and recurrence. *Arch Gen Psychiatry* 1991; **48**: 851–5.

Geller B, Zimerman B, Williams M, Bolhofner K, Craney JL. Bipolar disorder at prospective follow-up of adults who had prepubertal major depressive disorder. *Am J Psychiatry* 2001; **158**: 125–7.

Gibbons RD, Hur K, Bhaumik DK, Mann JJ. The relationship between antidepressant medication use and rate of suicide. *Arch Gen Psychiatry* 2005; **62**: 165–7.

Hammad TA. Results of the Analysis of Suicidality in Pediatric Trials of Newer Antidepressants. Presentation at the Food and Drug Administration, Psychopharmacologic Drugs Advisory Committee and the Pediatric Advisory Committee, 13 September 2004. Available at http://www.fda.gov/ohrms/dockets/ac/04/slides/2004-4065S1_08_FDA-Hammad_files/frame.htm.

Harrington R, Whittaker J, Shoebridge P, Campbell F. Systematic review of efficacy of cognitive behavior therapies in childhood and adolescent depressive disorder. *BMJ* 1998; **316**: 1559–63.

Hazell P, O'Connell D, Heathcote D, Henry D. Tricyclic drugs for depression in children and adolescents. *Cochrane Database Syst Rev* 2002; **2**: CD002317.

Keller MB, Ryan ND, Strober M, et al. Efficacy of paroxetine in the treatment of adolescent major depression: a randomized, controlled trial. *J Am Acad Child Adolesc Psychiatry* 2001; **40**: 762–72.

Kessler RC, Avenevoli S, Ries Merikangas K. Mood disorders in children and adolescents: an epidemiologic perspective. *Biol Psychiatry* 2001; **49**: 1002–14.

Kovacs M. The Child's Depression Inventory (CDI). *Psychopharmacol Bull* 1985; **21**: 995–8.

Lewinsohn PM, Rohde P, Seeley JR, Fischer SA. Age-cohort changes in the lifetime occurrence of depression and other mental disorders. *J Abnorm Psychol* 1993; **102**: 110–20.

Lewinsohn PM, Hops H, Roberts RE, Seeley JR, Andrews JA. Adolescent psychopathology: I. Prevalence and incidence of depression and other DSM-III-R disorders in high school. *J Abnorm Psychol* 1993; **102**: 133–44.

Mufson L, Dorta KP, Wickramaratne P, et al. A randomized effectiveness trial of interpersonal psychotherapy for depressed adolescents. *Arch Gen Psychiatry* 2004; **61**: 577–84.

National Center for Injury Prevention and Control. *Suicide in the United States*. Atlanta, GA: Centers for Disease Control and Prevention, 2002.

Olfson M, Shaffer D, Marcus SC, Greenberg T. Relationship between antidepressant medication treatment and suicide in adolescents. *Arch Gen Psychiatry* 2003; **60**: 978–82.

Perel J, Axelson D, Rudolph G, Birmaher B. Stereoselective PK/PD of ± citalopram in adolescents: comparison with adult findings. *Clin Pharm Ther* 2001; **60**: 30.

Poznanski EO, Mokros HB. *Manual for the Children's Depression Rating Scale – Revised*. Los Angeles, CA: Western Psychological Services, 1996.

Sallee FR, DeVane CL, Ferrell RE. Fluoxetine-related death in a child with cytochrome P-450 2D6 genetic deficiency. *J Child Adolesc Psychopharmacol* 2000; **10**: 27–34.

TADS Team. The Treatment for Adolescents with Depression Study (TADS): short-term effectiveness and safety outcomes. *JAMA* 2004; **292**: 807–20.

Wagner KD, Ambrosini P, Rynn M, et al. Efficacy of sertraline in the treatment of children and adolescents with major depressive disorder: two randomized controlled trials. *JAMA* 2003; **290**: 1033–41.

Wagner KD, Robb AS, Findling RL, et al. A randomized, placebo-controlled trial of citalopram for the treatment of major depression in children and adolescents. *Am J Psychiatry* 2004; **161**: 1079–83.

Weissman MM, Wolk S, Goldstein RB, et al. Depressed adolescents grown up. *JAMA* 1999; **281**: 1707–13.

Whittington CJ, Kendall T, Fonagy P, et al. Selective serotonin reuptake inhibitors in childhood depression: systematic review of published versus unpublished data. *Lancet* 2004; **363**: 1341–5.

Wilens TE, Cohen L, Biederman J, et al. Fluoxetine pharmacokinetics in pediatric patients. *J Clin Psychopharmacol* 2002; **22**: 568–75.

chapter 5

Pharmacotherapy of bipolar disorder in children and adolescents

Gabriele Masi

Clinical features of bipolar disorder

Introduction

Even if bipolar disorder presents a well-established clinical picture, studies of juvenile bipolar disorder are of more recent vintage. Awareness of bipolar spectrum disorders in children and adolescents is rapidly increasing, as well as a more precise definition of their clinical subtypes and early signs. Epidemiologic studies estimate that the point prevalence of early-onset bipolar disorder may be 0.2–0.4% for the prepubertal population, and about 1% in adolescents (Lewinshon et al, 1995, 2003). Studies examining age at onset of the first episode of bipolar illness show that the median age at onset is lower by 4.5 years in subjects born in the last 50 years, and that subjects with prepubertal onset are significantly higher in the more recent cohorts, usually with a depressive episode as the first episode (Chengappa et al, 2003). Early recognition of early-onset bipolar disorder may improve prognosis of this condition by using appropriate treatments and avoiding potentially worsening medications (i.e. antidepressant monotherapy), preventing the development of chronicity and serious functional impairment. When bipolar children reach adolescence they are at higher risk for substance abuse, which is not accounted for by conduct disorder or other comorbidities (Wilens et al, 2004), as well as for suicide (Lewinshon et al, 2003). The goal of our interventions, pharmacologic as well as psychosocial, is to treat the earlier and acute episodes of both mania and depression, to prevent or to decrease the recurrences, and to improve the psychosocial outcome.

Specificity of early-onset bipolar disorder

Atypical presentation of early-onset mania, compared to adult standards, concerns principally two issues: the mood presentation, with severe irritability and dysphoria, affective storms and temper outbursts, rather than with euphoria, grandiosity, and elated mood; and the lack of distinct cycling, with a subcontinuous or chronic course rather than clearly episodic and/or shorter episodes than adults (Wozniak et al, 1995; Geller et al, 2000; Craney and Geller, 2003). Ultrarapid or ultradian (daily) mood cycling is frequently observed instead of clear episodes of mania (Geller et al, 2004).

Considering these putative discrepancies in clinical characterization of adult and early-onset bipolar disorder, recent studies have addressed the subtyping of juvenile mania according to distinguishing clinical features (Masi et al, 2006, in press). The identification of the features, which may reflect meaningful differences among groups of bipolar children and adolescents, can help to define more homogeneous groups, in terms of family history, clinical presentation, comorbidity, course, and response to treatments. The first clinical differentiation was between a "narrow" and a "broad" phenotype, according to a more or less fit to the full DSM-IV diagnostic criteria for adult bipolar disorder. The "narrow" phenotype is characterized by an episodic course with prominent features of elated mood, euphoria, and grandiosity, as well as other typical manic symptoms, meeting the DSM-IV duration criteria. However, atypical features are frequently reported also in concomitance with this "typical" manic picture, such as shorter episodes and partial remissions, with few euthymic periods, or short and acute worsening superimposed on an impaired baseline.

The "broad" phenotype is characterized by a subcontinuous rather than episodic course, irritability and dysphoria being the most prominent features, along with unstable and/or mixed mood, chronic hyperarousal (hyperactivity, distractibility, increased energy, etc.), hostility and temper outbursts, often reactive to negative stimuli. This subgroup is probably not homogeneous, and it clearly poses the greatest nosographic challenges. Further research is needed for a reliable and valid diagnosis in these patients. More recently, Liebenluft and colleagues (2003) have proposed a refinement of this categorization, including intermediate phenotypes from the "narrow" to the "broad."

Another critical issue in early-onset bipolar disorder is the high rate of comorbidity, namely with attention deficit hyperactivity disorder (ADHD) (Biederman et al, 1996; Masi et al, 2003), conduct disorder (Biederman et al, 2003; Masi et al, 2003), and multiple anxiety disorders (Masi et al, 2001, 2004a; Birmaher et al, 2002; Harpold et al, 2005). Patterns of comorbidity, with externalizing or internalizing disorders, may define specific subtypes of bipolar disorder, in terms of response to treatments, even though available data are still inconsistent.

A more developmentally adapted description of the clinical pictures of bipolar disorder in children and adolescents can be found elsewhere (Craney and Geller, 2003; Kowatch et al, 2005).

Pharmacologic treatment of prepubertal bipolar disorder

In the context of a multi-modal approach, including psychosocial and family interventions, and psychotherapeutic interventions, the core treatment of early-onset bipolar disorder is pharmacologic. An adequate pharmacologic treatment should be undertaken within the context of an optimal clinical care, which includes, in the acute phase, hospitalization and provision of a safe environment, appropriate nursing care, personal and family support, education about the illness and its treatments, and, after the acute phase, a careful intervention on academic, social, and familial functioning (Kutcher, 1997). Patients with early-onset bipolar disorder frequently experience partial remissions, no response during the follow-up, and a higher recurrence of manic episodes, compared to adult-onset bipolar disorder (Carlson et al, 2000). A one-year follow-up in young patients with bipolar disorder (mean age 10 years) showed a recovery rate of 37.1% and a relapse rate of 38.3% (Geller et al, 2001a). Similar recovery rates, but a higher relapse rate (67%, with 50% with two or more episodes) have been reported in an Indian study of similar design (Srinath et al, 1998). The relapse rate is strongly influenced by the presence of a maintenance therapy, not only during the first 2 years after the index episode, but also thereafter (Strober et al, 1995).

The marked differences between pediatric- and adult-onset bipolar disorder raise the issue of the continuity/discontinuities of bipolar illness during development. Recent research suggests that early-onset bipolar disorder can be considered a specific subtype, not only in terms of genetic load, clinical picture, and pattern of comorbidity, but also for treatment response. It may be hypothesized that the age-specific features during the development of the neural substrates involved in mood regulation may explain some specificities in both phenotypical presentations and in response to treatments, in terms of both efficacy and tolerability.

One of the possible reasons for treatment refractoriness in children with bipolar disorder is the mixed or dysphoric nature, with short and acute periods of intense mood lability, rather than typical adult-like euphoria or with rapid cyclicity. Another possible explanation is that, similarly to other illness, early-onset mood disorders are more severe and/or more treatment-resistant than the adult forms. Third, in very early-onset disorder a delayed diagnosis and/or a delayed onset of an effective treatment may be more frequent, with negative implications in terms of clinical response. Finally, different patterns of comorbidity (for example with ADHD) may allow for different presentation, natural history, and response to treatments. However, to date, insufficient evidence supports hypotheses about continuities/discontinuities between childhood bipolar disorder and adulthood bipolar disorder and their implications on the development of neural bases of mood regulation, including the role of pubertal development.

The need to address unresolved issues about strategies in psychopharmacologic treatment in child/adolescent onset bipolar disorder is still valid, given that the empirical evidence is scarce, the use of off-label prescriptions of mood stabilizers and antipsychotics is increasing, parallel to the increasing frequency of diagnosis of prepubertal bipolar disorder, and children are often treated with multiple medications, in partial or excessive doses, or for inadequate trial periods. From a research point of view, randomized, controlled studies are very few, and some of the retrospective chart review studies are characterized by the lack of systematic diagnostic, symptomatologic or side-effect measures, and/or poor reliability and validity of clinical charting.

A recent study explored the use of medications in 111 children and adolescents treated in the community for bipolar disorder (Bhangoo et al, 2003). The result of this study shows that these patients were receiving 3.40 ± 1.48 medications, and had had a mean of 6.32 ± 3.67 trials of medications in the past. Ninety-eight percent received a trial of a mood stabilizer or an anticonvulsant, the most common being valproate (79%), lithium (51%), and gabapentin (29%).

A recent report presented recommendations from a working conference on "Methodological issues and controversies in clinical trials with child and adolescent patients with bipolar disorder" (Carlson et al, 2003), including inclusion and exclusion criteria, investigator training needs and site selections, assessment and outcome measures, protocol designs and ethical issues, and regulatory agencies perspectives. Many of these recommendations for research projects may be helpful in clinical practice as well.

In the following sections a critical review of the empirical evidence on pharmacotherapy of pediatric bipolar disorder will be provided, including mono- and polypharmacy. Practical implications for treatment strategy will be discussed in the final section.

A major methodologic flaw in this review is that in most of the empirical studies bipolar children and adolescents are grouped in the same sample, and it is rather difficult to disentangle the developmental issue of differential effects according to age and pubertal status. The evidence on the question of whether or not there are important differences in the efficacy and safety of medications in younger and older children is still inconclusive.

Another important point is that the sample size in many reported studies may have been too small to detect differences between agents or from the baseline. Finally, efficacy of treatments is usually operationally measured as a reduction of the score of a rating scale. This clinical response is often considerably different from a clinical remission. Many of these patients may remain ill enough to require hospitalization, even though they have resulted in responders. Unfortunately, studies considering clinical remission after treatment are still uncommon in child and adolescent psychopharmacology.

Medications for bipolar disorder

Mood stabilizers

Even though several classes of medications are currently used in the pharmacologic treatment of bipolar disorder, the term "mood stabilizer" usually refers to those medications which are effective not only during the acute phase, but also in the prophylaxis of further episodes. This property is strongly supported by empirical evidence for lithium, while the efficacy of anticonvulsants is less well established. However, these two classes are usually included in the mood stabilizers, although they have different chemical structures, and it is unlikely that they act through identical mechanisms. In the following paragraphs we will describe the prototypal mechanism of lithium, and we will compare it to the mechanism of anticonvulsants where data are available.

Lithium

The principal indication for lithium is in the treatment of acute mania, as well as in the prophylaxis of further manic phases. Other possible indications are the management of depressive phases of the bipolar disorder, the augmentation of treatment-resistant unipolar depression, and the management of aggressive and violent behavior within different mental disorders, including conduct disorder and/or severe personality disorders.

The targets for the action of lithium have shifted from the ability to modulate presynaptic components, including the ion transport and presynaptic transmitter synthesis, release and re-uptake, to post-synaptic events, such as receptor regulation, signal transduction, gene expression, and neuroplastic changes (Manji and Lenox, 2000). To date, lithium appears to influence multiple sites which regulate neurotransmission, and it modulates dopaminergic transmission presynaptically (inhibition) and postsynaptically (preventing receptor upregulation and supersensitivity). It also modulates cholinergic transmission (enhancing receptor-mediated responses). In the long term it enhances the GABA inhibitory transmission and limits the glutamatergic excitatory neurotransmission. The properties of lithium may be mediated by its action on intracellular sites, through its action on the second messenger system (phosphoinositide cycle and cAMP), the protein kinases and their substrates, and, finally, after 2 or 3 weeks (the latency of therapeutic effect), gene regulation and the following long-term neuroplastic and neuroprotective effects, through the synthesis of nuclear transcriptional factors.

Lithium carbonate is a soluble salt, rapidly absorbed after oral administration, and peak serum levels are achieved within 2 hours of administration. It circulates in the blood unbound to proteins, and penetrates the blood–brain barrier within one day of administration. It is excreted prevalently by the kidney, and about 80% is re-absorbed by the proximal renal tubules. This re-absorption of lithium competes with that of sodium. When the re-absorption of sodium decreases, because of inadequate salt intake with food, or other conditions reducing the amount of sodium, including diarrhea, dehydration, or during diuretic treatment, an increased absorption of lithium occurs, with increased serum levels and risk of toxicity. Elimination half-time in adults is about 20–24 hours, but children have a shorter elimination half-time, because of their increased ratio of kidney to whole body size.

However, lithium is less well tolerated in young children, with CNS side-effects and cognitive impairment related to higher doses and higher serum levels (Hagino et al, 1995; Geller et al, 1998a). The most frequent side-effects in lithium treatment are gastrointestinal symptoms, including nausea, vomiting, diarrhea, and abdominal discomfort, which can be decreased with gradual increases of dosage and by administering lithium with meals. Patients can also present with fatigue, usually during a fast dosage increase, which usually improves with time, but, when persisting, sometimes requires a decrease of dose. A fine tremor is common during lithium treatment, while a gross tremor in usually indicative of toxicity. Increased appetite and weight gain are common side-effects. Lithium can determine thyroid side-effects, including a hypothyroidism with increased TSH or, more rarely, decreased circulating T_3 and T_4. In these cases, a thyroid echography and possibly thyroxine replacement therapy can be considered, after an endocrinologic consultation. Polyuria and polydipsia can also occur, and sometimes the patient can present a diabetes-insipidus-like syndrome, which should induce discontinuation of treatment and kidney monitoring, when decreasing the dose is not effective. Dermatologic effects, such as acne vulgaris or maculopapular eruptions, or, more rarely, hair loss, can be of particular concern in adolescent patients.

Lithium is contraindicated in renal disease, as it is primarily excreted by kidney. Thyroid disease is a relative contraindication, and it requires careful thyroid monitoring and sometimes supplemental thyroxine. Cardiovascular diseases significantly increase lithium toxicity (AV block).

Antibiotics, carbamazepine, diuretics and non-steroidal anti-inflammatory agents (ibuprofen) increase serum lithium levels. Caffeine decreases serum lithium leads. Alcohol and antipsychotics increase sedation and confusional states.

A complete personal and familial history, a physical examination, an ECG, a complete blood count (CBC) and differential, an electrolyte check, and, when necessary, a pregnancy test (risk of congenital heart disease) should be performed before treatment. Children and adolescents who are candidates for lithium treatment should also be assessed for kidney function (urinalysis for blood urea nitrogen and creatinine) and thyroid disease (T_3, T_4, TSH). Lithium should be avoided in the presence of renal abnormalities. Renal and thyroid function should be monitored one week after the treatment and, when normal, every 4–6 months thereafter (consult with a specialist if levels are abnormal).

Lithium toxicity is related to blood levels, which should be closely monitored, with therapeutic levels ranging from 0.6 to 1.2 mEq/l. Lithium administration should be twice or three times a day per day. Lithium levels should be checked twice a week during the increase of dosage, then monthly over the next 3 months, and thereafter every 4–6 months, when the patient is euthymic and the dose is stable.

Mild intoxication determines gastrointestinal symptoms and dizziness, which improve after a return of blood levels to within the therapeutic range. Acute intoxication is a severe problem, with neurotoxic symptoms (confusion, drowsiness, slurred speech, ataxia, hyperreflexia, muscular fasciculation), up to delirium, stupor, and seizures. Several conditions may increase lithium levels to toxic concentrations, namely excessive sodium loss (by vomiting and/or diarrhea), or inadequate salt or fluid intake, co-administered medications (e.g. ampicillin) which decrease renal clearance, non-steroid anti-inflammatory agents (ibuprofen), or, most dangerously, poisoning. No specific antidote is available. Reversibility of lithium intoxication is related to the serum level of lithium and to the length of time it remains elevated. Severe symptoms can arise suddenly and without warning, after an initial phase with a milder manifestation which may have induced a false sense of security. Death can occur and, in survivors, severe neurologic sequelae can persist, such as ataxia and neuropsychologic deficits. When serum levels are above 2.5 mEq/l, hospitalization in the emergency room should be considered, and vomiting and gastric lavage should be induced, with saline diuresis and monitoring of electrolytes. When serum levels are at or above 4 mEq/l, a hemodialysis should be undertaken, with monitoring of lithium levels.

Anticonvulsants

Anticonvulsants are the treatment for all the epileptic disorders, but it is well established that they have mood-stabilizing properties.

The mechanisms of action of the anticonvulsant and mood-stabilizing effects are not fully understood, and it is likely that different mechanisms are involved. The anticonvulsant properties have been largely attributed to the ability to inhibit repetitive firing by prolonging the recovery of voltage-gated sodium channels from inactivation. This putative action is thus at the cell membrane, where ion channels (sodium, potassium, calcium) regulate the flow of ions through the membrane. This may enhance the effect of the inhibitory GABA neurotransmission (mainly valproic acid), and/or reduce the effect of the excitatory glutamate neurotransmission (mainly lamotrigine). Whether these mechanisms are involved only in anticonvulsant effects or whether they also affect the mood-stabilizing action is still a matter of debate. It is noteworthy that the anticonvulsant activity is neither necessary nor sufficient for mood stabilization, because lithium has a proconvulsant activity at toxic levels. It is probable that, similarly to lithium, an effect on the second messenger system may be involved in one or both of the pharmacologic effects of these medications. For example, long-term treatment with anticonvulsants, namely valproic acid, can affect the postsynaptic intracellular cascade transmissions, affecting the cAMP generating system, the G protein systems, the protein kinases, and gene expression.

Valproate

The term valproate includes valproic acid, sodium valproate, and divalproex sodium. It is used for the acute management of the disorder, as well as the prophylactic properties to prevent recurrent episodes. Another possible indication is in mental disorders with severe impulsiveness and aggression, including conduct disorders and personality disorders. It is rapidly absorbed when the stomach is empty, whereas the absorption is delayed by 5–6 hours when the medication is taken with meals. The half-life is 8–18 hours, thus a twice daily dosing is recommended. It circulates in a protein-bound form, and has a hepatic metabolism. In clinical practice, optimal serum levels for mood-stabilizing effects are similar to those for seizure control, that is 50–100 mg/ml.

Valproic acid is contraindicated in previous bone marrow depression and pregnancy (development of neural tube defect). Valproate is relatively contraindicated in patients with liver diseases (liver function tests (LFTs) are included in baseline and monitoring procedures), and it should be avoided in patients with renal diseases, given that it is cleared principally by the kidney.

Valproate is usually rather well tolerated, and side-effects are usually mild and transitory (first 2 or 3 weeks of treatment), such as modest sedation, nausea, vomiting, increased appetite, and weight gain. More serious side-effects are hair loss (possibly managed with zinc supplementation), menstrual irregularity, and neurologic effects (ataxia and tremor), usually in patients receiving doses higher than 40–50 mg/kg per day. Two main concerns emerge from epilepsy treatment studies. The first is a potential hepatotoxicity in very young children under 2 or 3 years of age (Bryant and Dreifuss, 1996), the second is an increased risk for polycystic ovaries and hyperandrogenism in adolescence (Isojarvi et al, 1993). Dose-related increases in liver function tests are present in as many as 40% of the patients treated with valproate, but these elevations are usually transient, dose reduction often resulting in the liver enzymes returning to baseline. When this is not the case, further examinations are warranted.

Baseline procedures include count blood cells (CBC), LFTs, and pregnancy test, when needed. CBC, LFTs should be repeated every month in children less 10 years, every 3–4 months in older children and adolescents. Valproic acid levels should be checked every 3–4 months.

Effects of valproate can be increased by many antibiotics, methylphenidate, phenotiazines, and tricyclics, and decreased by birth control pills, cortisol, diazepam and neuroleptics. Valproic acid decreases the effects of hepatically metabolized drugs, and increases effects of carbamazepine. The association of valproate and clonazepam should be carefully monitored, as it can increase the risk of a status epilepticus.

Valproate intoxication is usually not very dangerous in overdose, if other medications are not taken in combination. Toxicity is manifest by incoordination, confusion, and drowsiness.

Carbamazepine

Carbamazepine has a chemical structure similar to that of tricyclic antidepressants. It is relatively easy to dose, as it has a linear kinetics, although it has an active metabolite, usually not measured, which complicates the interpretation of serum levels. It is metabolized by the liver and the elimination half-life ranges from 12 to 60 hours, which decreases to 5–20 hours after chronic administration. For this reason it is recommended that serum levels be monitored during the first 5–6 weeks, as they can decrease, accounting for an apparent reduction in effectiveness.

It is used in bipolar disorder, for the acute management, as well as to prevent recurrent episodes. Another possible indication is in mental disorders with severe impulsiveness and aggression, including conduct disorders and personality disorders.

Baseline procedures include CBC, LFTs, urinanalysis, and a pregnancy test, when needed. CBC, LFTs and urinanalysis should be repeated after one month, then every 3 months. Carbamazepine levels should be monitored every 3–4 months. Carbamazepine is contraindicated in previous bone marrow depression and pregnancy. Liver and kidney diseases are a relative contraindication. The most troublesome side effects are mainly blood dyscrasias (aplastic anemia and agranulocytosis) (Pellock, 1987). Leukopenia is common as well, and a value of less than 4000/ml is found in about 13% of the patients, but it is usually non-progressive and it does not requires drug discontinuation. However, when this low level persists, and it is associated with a neutrophil level below 1700cell/mm^3, discontinuation of carbamazepine and a hematologic consultation is needed. Agranulocytosis (<1000/mm^3) and aplastic anemia are potentially life-threatening, and must be suspected in the presence of bleeding, bruising, fever, and lethargy, with prompt medical attention. As carbamazepine induces cytochrome P450, it interacts with many medications which depend on their hepatic metabolism. The effects of carbamazepine are increased by many antibiotics, methylphenidate, phenotiazine, tricyclics and decreased by birth control pills, cortisol, diazepam and neuroleptics. Carbamazepine decreases serum levels of haloperidol and increases serum levels of lithium. Serum levels should be carefully monitored in the case of a cotherapy with sodium valproate, because carbamazepine induces the metabolism of sodium valproate, and sodium valproate can inhibit the metabolism of carbamazepine, with a risk of neurotoxicity. In this association, carbamazepine levels should be kept at 2–6μg/ml.

Diplopia, incoordination, vertigo, and nystagmus are common but usually transient side-effects. Skin rashes, hyponatremia, and water intoxication (carbamazepine can stimulate antidiuretic hormone) with lethargy, headache, nausea/vomiting, edema, and seizures can rarely occur. When administered to children with atypical absence, carbamazepine can induce a status epilepticus.

Behavioral side-effects may occur, with worsening of the clinical condition, but the exact incidence of this is not well known. The side-effects include irritability, agitation, insomnia, and obsessive-compulsive symptoms, and (hypo)manic or psychotic symptoms. In these cases, discontinuation of the medication and monitoring of the clinical status are recommended.

Given the tricyclic structure of carbamazepine, acute toxicity is a medical emergency, even though lethality is less than with imipramine and other tricyclic antidepressants. It is important to remember that peak levels may occur 2 or 3 days after ingestion. Drowsiness, gait disturbance, nystagmus, confusion, and seizures are the most common manifestations of overdose. Cardiac and respiratory monitoring is needed, whereas hemodialysis is of no help.

Newer anticonvulsants

Among the newer anticonvulsants, topiramate, lamotrigine, oxcarbazepine, and gabapentin have to date limited indications in bipolar children and adolescents. Some information will be provided on these medications.

Topiramate
Topiramate is supposed to act through an action on the sodium channels voltage dependent, a potentiation of GABA transmission and an inhibition of excitatory pathway through AMPA glutamate receptor. It can be used at a starting dose of 25 mg/day, with gradual increments 25 mg every week, up to 100–200 mg/day, two or three times per day. Maintenance treatment should be for 12–18 months, with a gradual tapering. Withdrawal seizures for acute discontinuation are rarely reported.

Most important side-effects are sedation, difficulty concentrating, drowsiness, ataxia, anorexia and weight loss, agitation, impulsiveness, and aggressiveness. More severe behavioral disorders, including psychotic-like symptoms, are reported during a fast increase of dosage. Topiramate does not affect serum levels of other anticonvulsants, but induces the metabolism of birth control pills. Carbamazepine reduces serum levels of topiramate.

The clinical practice baseline procedures should include CBC, LFTs and urinanalysis. These procedure should be repeated after one month of treatment, then every 3 months.

Lamotrigine
Lamotrigine may involve voltage-dependent sodium channels and the inhibition of the (excitatory) glutamate and aspartate release. In clinical use (monotherapy) the starting dose should be 25 mg/day for weeks 1 and 2, then 50 mg/day for weeks 3 and 4, then 100 mg for weeks 5 and 6, and eventual further increments every 2 weeks. Slower titration is needed when lamotrigine is used in poly-pharmacy.

Most frequent side-effects are vertigo, dyplopia, ataxia, blurred vision and somnolence. Skin rash occurs in 2–5% within 2 weeks, with recovery after discontinuation. Severe dermatologic side-effects are more frequent in prepubertal children (up to 1–2%), and include Stevens–Johnson syndrome and Lyell syndrome. The risk is greater with high doses and/or cotherapy with valproic acid, this association should be avoided when possible. Lamotrigine does not induce the metabolism of birth control pills. Baseline procedures include CBC, LFTs, urinalysis, and dermatologic assessment. CBC, LFTs, urinalysis should be repeated after one month, then every 3 months. Dermatologic monitoring is warranted.

Oxcarbazepine
Oxcarbazepine is a 10-keto analogous to carbamazepine, in terms of chemical structure and clinical profile. Similarly to carbamazepine, it blocks voltage-dependent sodium channels. As oxcarbazepine, induces cytochrome P450 less than carbamazepine, it may be more manageable, with fewer pharmachologic interactions than with other medications and lower toxicity. Titration should be slow in order to minimize side-effects. The starting dose is 300 mg, with weekly increases up to 600–1200 mg/day, in two or three doses per day.

Most frequent side-effects are incoordination, vertigo and nystagmus, but they are usually transient. Even though blood dyscrasias, neurotoxicity skin rashes and hyponatremia are reported less frequently than with carbamazepine, the same baseline and monitoring procedures should be applied to oxcarbazepine.

Gabapentin
Gabapentin has a chemical structure derived from the GABA, and it probably modulates the GABAergic system, through an enhance of

synthesis and release of GABA, without a direct interaction with the GABA-A and GABA-B receptors, and without an effect on the GABA reuptake. It is cleared prinicipally by kidney. The starting dose can be 200–300 mg/day, with increase of 200–300 mg every 3–4 days up to a possible maximum dose of 900–1500 mg/day.

Gabapentin is usually well tolerated. Sedation, difficulty concentrating, drowsiness, and ataxia are usually mild and limited to the first 2 weeks of treatment. It does not present significant interactions with other anticonvulsants. Given its efficacy in anxiety disorders (panic disorder, social phobia), gabapentin should be particularly indicated in bipolar patients with co-occurring anxiety symptoms.

Antidepressants

See chapters 3 and 4.

Antipsychotics

See chapter 8.

Treatment of bipolar disorder: available literature

Mood stabilizers

The mood stabilizers, including lithium and anti-epileptic drugs, are the most frequently used medications in early-onset as well as in adult-onset bipolar disorder, even though empirical evidence in pediatric bipolar disorder is still limited.

Kowatch and colleagues (2000) explored the effect size of lithium, divalproex, and carbamazepine in 42 outpatient children with bipolar disorder (mean age 11.4 years) randomly assigned to a 6-week treatment. Even though the effect size was higher for divalproex and lower for carbamazepine according to both Young Mania Rating Scale (YMRS) scores and response rates, differences were not significant among the three groups (ranging from 38% to 53%). According to this study, less than half of the patients were satisfactorily controlled by monotherapy with a mood stabilizer.

Davanzo and colleagues (2003) presented a naturalistic study of 44 hospitalized prepubertal children with bipolar disorder (age range

5 to 12 years, mean age 9.2 years), treated with lithium, divalproex, or carbamazepine (without antipsychotics, antidepressants, or other concomitant medications), and rated with the Clinical Global Impression-Improvement (CGI-I) score. The medication groups did not differ according to severity of illness at admission, comorbidity, or length of hospitalization. However, at week 2, lithium and divalproex were both similarly effective, and controlled symptomatology significantly better than carbamazepine.

In the following sections available studies on mood stabilizers in children with bipolar disorder will be reviewed.

Lithium

Lithium has been proven to be effective in adolescent bipolar disorder, as shown by a 10-week, randomized, placebo-controlled trial on 25 bipolar adolescents (age 16.3 ± 1.2 years) with substance abuse (Geller et al, 1998a). Adolescents randomly assigned to lithium did significantly better both in terms of their bipolar disorder and in terms of their substance abuse than did those randomized to placebo. Kafantaris and coworkers (2003) treated 100 acutely manic adolescents with open lithium (mean 0.99 m Eq/l). Sixty-three subjects met response criteria (decline of Young Mania Rating Scale (YMRS) $\geq 33\%$ and CGI-I 1 or 2), and 26 achieved remission at week 4. However, when responders were randomly assigned to continue or discontinue lithium during a 2-week, double-blind, placebo-controlled phase, the difference in symptom exacerbation between the two groups did not reach statistical significance (52.6% versus 61.9%) (Kafantaris et al, 2004). This finding is not consistent with previous studies (Strober et al, 1990, 1995) according to which, in bipolar adolescents, response rate to lithium (0.9–1.5m Eq/l) was 68% (some subjects received cotherapy with carbamazepine and/or antipsychotics), and patients who discontinued lithium against medical advice had higher relapse rates (92.3% versus 37.5%) and a much shorter interval to the next episode than those who continued the treatment.

Some evidence suggests that lithium may be less effective in manic prepubertal children, with rates of response significantly lower than in adolescent patients. In Strober et al's study (1990), response rate in patients aged less than 12 years was 49%, compared to 80% in adolescent patients. Geller and colleagues (1998b) did not find that lithium (0.99±0.16m Eq/l) was superior to placebo in 30 prepubertal children (mean age 10.7±1.2 years) with depression and high risk for bipolar disorder, on the basis of a positive bipolar family history (Geller et al, 1998b). Comorbid ADHD, which is particularly frequent in prepubertal bipolar children compared to bipolar adolescents, has been found to negatively predict lithium efficacy (Strober et al, 1998; State et al, 2004), but this finding was not replicated in another study (Kafantaris et al, 1998). Strober and coworkers (1998) suggested that some cases of prebipolar ADHD may really be an early expression of bipolar disorder, and the partial resistance to treatment may be secondary to the underdiagnosis and undertreatment of the very early-onset mood disorder, due to a "kindling" phenomenon.

Anecdotal data on open lithium treatment are even available on preschool children aged 4 to 6 years, who were hospitalized for aggression and/or mood disorder (Hagino et al, 1995).

Lithium kinetics has been studied in children (Vitiello et al, 1988). Children have a 20% faster elimination rate resulting in a shorter half-life, and a steady state of 7 days.

In summary, open studies suggest that lithium is effective in about 50–60% of patients, although findings from controlled studies in prepubertal children are still conflicting.

Valproate, sodium valproate and divalproex sodium

Valproate has been extensively used in bipolar adults and, according to some reports, it may be more effective than lithium in rapid cycling or mixed mania (Calabrese et al, 1996). Given that very early-onset bipolar disorder presents mixed features and rapid cycling, valproate may be particularly effective in these patients.

Controlled studies are not available for divalproex in bipolar children and adolescents. Papatheodorou and coworkers (1995) reported on a successful treatment with valproate in a series of 15 adolescents with acute mania. Eight patients showed a marked improvement (decrease of at least 75% on the YMRS), four a moderate improvement, and one a minimal improvement. Deltito and colleagues (1998) described the efficacy of divalproex in 36 inpatient adolescents, prevalently hospitalized for affective disorders. Divalproex proved to be effective in all the psychopathologic variables considered, including mania, mood swings, and aggression, and well tolerated. More recently, DelBello et al (2004) reported their clinical experience with divalproex monotherapy in the treatment of the aggressive dimension in 15 bipolar I (prevalently mixed) inpatient adolescents (14.5 ± 2 years). Fourteen of the 15 patients receiving divalproex completed a 6-week treatment period (one patient withdrew after 2 weeks because of lack of efficacy). Mean valproic serum level was 102 mg/dl. A significant reduction in the YMRS aggression item was observed in 11/15 (73%) of the subjects, 11/15 (73%) significantly improved in the YMRS irritability item, and 12/15 (80%) improved in the irritability item of the Childhood Depression Rating Scale. The hostility cluster of the Positive and Negative Syndrome Scale (PANSS) was reduced in 9/15 subjects (60%).

Fewer data are available from studies including prepubertal children. Wagner and colleagues (2002) openly evaluated efficacy and safety of divalproex sodium (mean dose 813 ± 338 mg/day, or 17.5 mg/kg per day) in 40 bipolar subjects (aged 7 to 19 years, mean age 12.1 ± 3.6 years) with a manic, hypomanic, or mixed episode. Mean YMRS score declined from 26.3 to 12; the improvement started from the first week of treatment and continued throughout the open-label period. Sixty-one percent of the patients showed a reduction of at least 50% on the YMRS. Adverse events were mild and transient (headache, nausea, vomiting, diarrhea, somnolence).

Fifteen children and adolescents (age range 4–18 years, mean age 13.3 ± 4.0 years) with bipolar disorder treated with divalproex (dose 966 ± 501 mg/day, blood level 79.4 ± 23.1 mg/l) were followed for 1.4 ± 1.5 years (Henry et al, 2003). Eight patients (53%) responded according to a CGI-I score of 1 or 2, but six (40%) discontinued, mostly because of side-effects, four for weight gain, and one (a 15-year-old adolescent) for liver enzyme elevation (normalized after divalproex was discontinued).

Divalproex was used in a series of nine very young children with mania, whose symptoms were reported to have worsened during stimulant treatment (Mota-Castillo et al, 2001). These young patients improved their mood after divalproex treatment. More recently, Scheffer and colleagues (2004) reported on the open treatment with mood stabilizers, primarily valproic acid, in 26 manic preschool children, aged 2 to 5. Medication significantly decreased manic symptoms, with continued improvements even in the long-term treatment.

Divalproex has been openly studied in 24 offspring of bipolar parents, aged 6 to 18 years (mean 11.3 years), with mood or behavioral disorders and mild affective symptoms, but without a full-blown bipolar disorder

(Chang et al, 2003a). Of the 23 subjects who completed the study, 18 (78%) were considered responders according to the CGI-I score (very much or much improved). A significant decrease from baseline (at least 50%) of the YMRS mean scores or the Hamilton Depression Rating Scale (from 14 to 6 for both the scales) at week 12 was also found in 19 subjects (83%). The majority of responders improved within the first 4 weeks of treatment. The authors hypothesized that divalproex not only improves bipolar prodromal symptoms, but also may reduce the progression to a fully developed bipolar disorder in a high-risk population with a not yet fully developed bipolar disorder.

In summary, evidence from uncontrolled studies suggests that valproate and divalproex may be effective and relatively well tolerated in about 50–60% of patients with pediatric bipolar disorder. No controlled studies are available to date.

Carbamazepine

Evidence supports the efficacy of carbamazepine in bipolar adults. It has been suggested that carbamazepine, as well as valproic acid, may be more effective than lithium in adult bipolar patients with mixed or rapid cycling bipolar disorder (Calabrese et al, 1996). No specific data are available for carbamazepine in prepubertal children with bipolar disorder, and only sparse data support efficacy in adolescents. Bouvard and colleagues (1993) openly treated with carbamazepine 11 bipolar adolescents (aged 10 to 17 years) and followed them up for at least 1 year. According to a response criterion of at least 1 year of euthymia, seven patients were considered responders, two were moderate responders, and two did not respond. Carbamazepine was well tolerated, and the increase of a single liver enzyme was the most frequently reported side-effect.

Two bipolar adolescents (13- and 14-year-olds) successfully treated with carbamazepine were described by Woolston (1999), at doses of 200–300 mg daily and serum levels of 7–8 µg/ml.

Other anticonvulsants

Sparse data are available for other anticonvulsant agents used as mood stabilizer monotherapy in early-onset bipolar disorder. Few anecdotal data are available for bipolar adolescents treated with gabapentin (Soutullo et al, 1998), lamotrigine (Kusumakar and Yatham, 1997; Caradang et al, 2003), topiramate (Davanzo et al, 2001), and oxcarbazepine (Davanzo et al, 2004; Del Bello et al, 2005). To date, there are no sound data to indicate that monotherapy with these agents has a first-line place in the treatment of child and adolescent bipolar disorder.

Only sparse findings are available on their value as add-on therapy with non-mood stabilizers in prepubertal children. Hamrin and Bailey (2001) reported on an effective treatment of a 12-year-old boy with a history of ADHD and a current bipolar disorder type II with a cotherapy of gabapentin (200 mg/day) and methylphenidate (30 mg/day). Pavuluri and colleagues (2002) associated topiramate (slowly up to 25 mg bid) with a previous treatment with risperidone (0.25 mg bid) in a 4½-year-old girl with a diagnosis of mania, with a stabilization of mood swings and a normalization of overweight (15 kg!) in the subsequent 10 weeks.

Combination pharmacotherapy with mood stabilizers

Bipolar children and adolescents are similar to adults in their resistance to monotherapy with mood stabilizers, with at least 40–50% of the patients in both age ranges not being controlled by a single mood stabilizer (Geller et al, 1998a; Kowatch et al, 2000). For this reason the issue of the combination treatment of mood stabilizers has important implications for clinical practice.

The efficacy of a combined lithium–carbamazepine treatment has been explored in 19 treatment-resistant bipolar adolescents with acute or mixed mania, with a positive response in all patients (Garfinkel et al, 1985).

The efficacy of a combined divalproex–lithium treatment was explored in a prospective open-label study including 90 patients aged 5 to 17 years treated for up to 20 weeks (Findling et al, 2003). Combined treatment was well tolerated and effective in terms of significant improvement in all the outcome measures (YMRS, Children's Depression Rating Scale, Children's Global Assessment Scale (C-GAS)) by week 8 as well as at the end of the study. Interestingly, 47% of the patients met criteria for clinical remission.

Kowatch and colleagues (2003) explored the effectiveness of a combination treatment with mood stabilizers in a 6-month prospective, semi-naturalistic study on 35 prepubertal children with bipolar disorder (mean age 11 years), after a 6–8-week acute treatment with one mood stabilizer. In the extension phase of this period, 58% of these patients required an additional treatment with other mood stabilizers, stimulants, antipsychotics, or antidepressants. The response rate of combination therapies of two mood stabilizers was very good (80%).

Efficacy and tolerability of topiramate (104 ± 77 mg/day) as an adjunctive mood stabilizer for children with bipolar disorder were assessed by DelBello et al (2002a) in 26 pediatric patients (mean age 14 ± 3.5 years), with response rates of 73% for mania, and 62% for overall illness, according to both the CGI-I and C-GAS, and without serious adverse events.

These preliminary findings suggest that a combination of mood stabilizers (first divalproex–lithium) may be an effective strategy in bipolar children non-responders to monotherapy with one mood stabilizer. More research is needed to explore the safety of these combination treatments in younger children.

Atypical antipsychotics

In bipolar patients resistant to mono- or polypharmacotherapy with mood stabilizers, especially when psychotic symptoms, hostility, and psychomotor agitation are associated, antipsychotics are indicated as associated medication. In the above-mentioned study addressing the topic of medication use in 111 early-onset bipolar children and adolescents screened by phone interviews (Bhangoo et al, 2003), a majority of patients (77%) had had a trial of an antipsychotic, the most common being risperidone (58%), olanzapine (35%), and quetiapine (26%). Only 12% of the children received a trial of a typical neuroleptic. Whether this is due to the presence of co-occurring psychotic symptoms, or severe behavioral disorders, or treatment-resistance is not clear.

Kafantaris et al (2001) explored the efficacy of lithium and an antipsychotic in adolescents with acute mania and psychotic features. Antipsychotic medication was gradually discontinued after 4 weeks, with resolution of the psychotic symptoms, and maintenance of lithium to therapeutic levels. A significant improvement was seen in 64% of the patients during 4 weeks of the combined therapy. However, only 43% maintained the good response after discontinuation of the antipsychotic, suggesting that a longer antipsychotic treatment may be needed in this kind of patient.

Conventional antipsychotics, that is neuroleptics (e.g. haloperidol) and dopamine receptor antagonists, have been used during the acute manic phases in adult patients with bipolar disorder. High sensitivity to neuroleptic side-effects, namely extrapyramidal symptoms (acute dystonias, acathisia, Parkinson-like symptoms) and tardive dyskinesia, strongly limit the use of neuroleptics in children (Campbell et al, 1997).

Newer antipsychotics, called atypical antipsychotics, with dopamine and serotonin receptor antagonism (clozapine, risperidone, olanzapine, quetiapine, ziprasidone) present significantly lower risks of acute extrapyramidal effects, tardive dyskinesia, and hyperprolactinemia, and their use is increasing in children and adolescents (Toren et al, 1998). Clozapine, the prototype of an atypical antipsychotic, is particularly effective when other antipsychotics have failed, but it presents potentially severe side-effects (agranulocytosis, seizures) which require careful monitoring. Risperidone is atypical at low doses, but can become "conventional" (with extrapyramidal side-effects and hyperprolactinemia) at higher doses or with rapid titration. Olanzapine has a chemical structure similar to clozapine, without significant risks of agranulocytosis and seizures, but it may cause marked weight gain and hyperglycemia. Quetiapine has a more favorable profile of side-effects, but data on effectiveness are fewer. Only anecdotal evidence is available on ziprasidone.

Antimanic effects of atypical antipsychotics in mono- or poly-pharmacy in children and adolescents have been reported in one controlled study and in several open-label trials and case reports. Few data on pharmacokinetics are available in non-bipolar young patients treated with risperidone (Casaer et al, 1994), olanzapine (Grothe et al, 2000), and quetiapine (McConville et al, 2000).

A reason for concern during treatment with atypical antipsychotics in adults is a metabolic syndrome, with weight gain and/or increased levels of glucose and lipids (Masi, 2004). Weight gain is the most significant side-effect in all the studies on risperidone, olanzapine, and clozapine, while quetiapine and ziprasidone are reported to have a lower incidence of weight gain. This side-effect cannot be disregarded, given the increased morbidity in subjects with obesity. Furthermore, the difficult management of food craving in these patients adds further conflict in the families, reducing the compliance to treatment. Dietary recommendations and psychoeducational counseling are needed at the beginning of the treatment. At present there is no standardized pharmacologic treatment for antipsychotic-induced weight gain, even though trials with amantadine, orlistat, metformin, nizatidine, and topiramate are reported in the literature on adult patients (Baptista et al, 2002).

Atypical antipsychotics are associated with higher levels of glucose and lipid. Specific data on children and adolescents are still scarce. The American Diabetes Association (2004) published a protocol for patients who initiate a treatment with atypical antipsychotics, which includes personal and family history of obesity, diabetes, dyslipidemia, hypertension and cardiovascular diseases, weight and height (with Body Mass Index), blood pressure, fasting plasma glucose and fasting lipid profile. Weight should be reassessed 4, 8, and 12 weeks after initiating treatment, and thereafter at least quarterly during the follow-up. Body weight increases should be carefully monitored, and they should suggest the switch to another medication. Considering that this paper was written with the needs of adults in mind, even closer monitoring is recommended in prepubertal children, including a frequent measuring of body mass index and a regular metabolic follow-up (serum lipids, fasting glucose levels, etc.). Liver function tests should be monitored in children who are taking atypical antipsychotics, particularly in obese children or in those with rapid weight gain.

Risperidone

Frazier and colleagues (1999) investigated the efficacy and safety of risperidone treatment (1.7 ± 1.3 mg/day, for an average period of 6.1 ± 8.5 months) in 28 bipolar children (mean age 10.4 ± 3.8 years). According to the CGI-I score of 1 or 2, 82% of the patients showed improved manic and aggressive symptoms, and 69% improved their psychotic symptoms, but in only 8% were ADHD symptoms ameliorated.

As reported above, the combination of risperidone (0.25 mg bid) plus topiramate has been effectively used in a 4½-year-old girl diagnosed as having mania, according to a structured clinical interview for parents of preschool children (Pavuluri et al, 2002). The adjunctive topiramate (25 mg bid) further stabilized mood, and was associated with a normalization of risperidone-induced overweight.

Olanzapine

Soutullo et al (1999) reported on the efficacy and tolerability of olanzapine in seven adolescents with acute mania. Chang and Ketter

(2000) used olanzapine as an adjunctive drug (2.5–5 mg/day) in three acutely manic prepubertal children treated with mood stabilizers. A marked improvement was evident within the first 3–5 days after the start of olanzapine in all these patients, with sedation and weight gain as the main adverse effects.

An 8-week, open-label study addressed the issue of efficacy and tolerability of olanzapine monotherapy (2.5–20 mg/day) in 23 children and adolescents (age range 5–14 years) with bipolar disorder (Frazier et al, 2001). Olanzapine treatment was associated with a significant improvement in YMRS score; furthermore, 63% of the participants were responders, according to a reduction of at least 30% of the YMRS; body weight gain was 5.0±2.3 kg.

Quetiapine

DelBello and colleagues (2002b) examined the efficacy and tolerability of adjunctive quetiapine, compared with placebo, in 30 adolescent patients with bipolar disorder type I treated with divalproex. Divalproex plus quetiapine were more effective than divalproex plus placebo, according to the improvement of the YMRS response rate (87% versus 53%). Sedation was more frequently reported in the quetiapine group.

Marchand et al (2004) openly assessed efficacy and tolerability of quetiapine (397.4±221.4mg/day) in bipolar children and adolescents (mean age 10.8±3.9 years). After a mean duration of treatment of 6.1±5.9 months, 80% of the patients were responders, according to a CGI-I score of 1 or 2. The CGI-S score also significantly improved during the treatment. Similar rates of response were found in subjects with quetiapine monotherapy and in those with associated medication.

Clozapine

Kowatch et al (1995) reported on the efficacy of clozapine treatment in a small series of ten children and adolescents (mean age 9.9±3.3 years) with treatment-resistant schizophrenia or bipolar disorder. Clozapine (mean dosage 128 mg/day) monotherapy or in association with lithium was effective and well tolerated, with a better clinical response in bipolar than in schizophrenic patients.

Clozapine at a dosage of 142.5±73.6mg/day (range 75–300mg/day) has been effectively used in ten severely impaired manic adolescents (12–17 years old) with treatment-refractory mania, followed up for

12–24 months (Masi et al, 2002). The mean changes in all the outcome measures were significant. Side-effects (increased appetite, sedation, enuresis, drooling) were frequent, but not as severe as to determine a dosage reduction. Mean weight gain after 6 months was 6.96±3.08kg (10.7%).

Kant and colleagues (2004) have recently described their clinical experience with clozapine (mean daily dose 102 mg/day) in 39 adolescents (mean age 14 years) with different diagnoses, including seven subjects with bipolar disorder. Clozapine was effective, with a significant reduction of additional medication, but three patients discontinued the medication for neutropenia/agranulocytosis, and two for marked weight gain.

Ziprasidone

Ziprasidone has been used in four young patients, aged 7, 10, 11, and 13 years, respectively, previously and unsatisfactorily treated with mood stabilizers or other atypical antipsychotics (Barnett, 2004). All the patients had a rapid and positive response after switching to ziprasidone (20 mg bid or tid or 60 mg at bedtime or 20 mg in the morning and 40 mg at bedtime), with good tolerability. Only the 13-year-old boy had tachycardia after increasing the dosage up to 40 mg bid, but this rhythm change was later attributed to anxiety rather than to the medication.

Aripiprazole

Aripiprazole has been naturalistically assessed in 30 bipolar children and adolescents, at a starting dose of 9±4 mg/day and a final dose of 10±3 mg/day (Barzman et al, 2004). Sixty-seven percent of the participants were responders (CGI-I 1 or 2), and CGI-S and CGAS scores improved significantly. The medication was well tolerated.

Biederman et al (2005) assessed chart records of 41 bipolar youths (11.4±3.5 years) who received a mean daily dose of 16.0±7.9 mg over an average of 4.6 months. Seventy-one percent of these patients were responders (CGI-I 1 or 2). Treatment was well tolerated.

ADHD–bipolar comorbidity: therapeutic issues

Symptoms of ADHD and bipolar disorder partly overlap, making the differential diagnosis particularly complex (Craney and Geller, 2003), mainly in preschool children. Furthermore, ADHD is the most frequent comorbidity in pediatric bipolar disorder, even though the rate of this comorbidity is still debated in the literature, ranging from 30% to 90%. However, there is consensus that this comorbidity affects age at onset of the disorder, phenomenology, outcome, psychosocial risk, and response to treatment. For these reasons, differential diagnosis and comorbidity between ADHD and bipolar disorder are closely related.

It is important to consider the diagnosis of bipolar disorder in those children with ADHD-like symptomatology, whose clinical picture is unresponsive or worsened by stimulants, especially when a family member with bipolar disorder is present. Children with an apparent ADHD often have an occult and unrecognized affective disorder, especially an unrecognized bipolar illness. In a consecutive series of 104 children referred for ADHD, 59.6% had a mood disorder (Dilsaver et al, 2003). Compared to those without an affective disorder, children with an affective disorder were 3.3 times more likely to have a positive family history of any affective disorder, and 18.3 times more likely to have a family history of a bipolar disorder. These features were also evident when modified diagnostic criteria for mania (presence of euphoria and/or flight of ideas) were used in order to minimize false positives (9.1 times and 7.3 times, respectively).

Concerns about treatment are related to the fear of exacerbating the patient's mood disorder while treating ADHD with psychostimulants. In 1992 Carlson and coworkers reported a synergistic effect of lithium and methylphenidate in seven prepubertal children with bipolar disorder and disruptive behavior disorder (Carlson et al, 1992). The use of stimulants did not appear to worsen behavior or attentional performances.

Biederman and colleagues (1999) reported on 38 ADHD children with bipolar comorbidity, first treated with mood stabilizers and then with methylphenidate, who responded very well to the addition of the stimulant, without any worsening of the manic features.

Kowatch and colleagues (2003) explored the effect of adjunctive low-dose stimulant treatment in bipolar children treated with mood stabilizers, with positive effect on the child's ADHD symptoms, without exacerbating the mood disorder.

Galanter and colleagues (2003), using data from the multi-modal treatment study of ADHD, showed that subjects with a probable diagnosis of mania responded positively to methylphenidate and did not show more side-effects than controls. Similarly, Carlson and Kelly (2003) showed that the presence and severity of stimulant rebound was not related to the bipolar spectrum. Finally, Scheffer and colleagues (2005) randomized 30 bipolar patients (age range 6–17 years) with comorbid ADHD to placebo or mixed amphetamine salts, after mood stabilization with divalproex sodium. Psychostimulant treatment was shown to be safer and more effective than placebo for ADHD symptoms.

These findings run against the clinical concept that stimulants may favor an earlier onset of bipolar disorder, irrespective of ADHD, possibly through a behavioral sensitization mechanism (DelBello et al, 2001). Although some concerns have recently been raised about a possible exacerbating effect of stimulants on an underlying (hypo)mania (Faedda et al, 2004), clinicians should not a priori avoid stimulants in children with ADHD and manic symptoms.

A different but related issue is whether a comorbid ADHD affects the clinical response to mood stabilizers in early-onset mania. Data are available only on bipolar adolescents with comorbid ADHD, who were found to have a poorer response to lithium (Strober et al, 1998), but this finding was not replicated in another study (Kafantaris et al, 1998). State and colleagues (2004) recently found that a history of ADHD was associated with a lower acute response to lithium or divalproex in manic adolescents. Strober and coworkers (1998) suggested that the possible treatment resistance in bipolar young patients with ADHD may be due to a delayed diagnosis and treatment of the manic symptoms, first masked by ADHD symptomatology. Data on prepubertal children are not available, even though they may further clarify this important issue.

Treatment of bipolar depression

Even though empirical findings have accumulated on the treatment of pediatric mania, fewer data are available on the phenomenology and treatment of bipolar depression, in children even more than in adolescents. It is important to underline that a prepubertal-onset depression can be the first manifestation of a bipolar disorder (Akiskal, 1995; Geller et al, 2001b). A 10-year prospective follow-up of a sample of prepubertal 10-year-olds diagnosed with major depressive disorder and followed until age 20 has found a prevalence of 48.6% bipolar disorder during the follow-up. The bipolar outcome was predicted by parental and grandparental mania. This is confirmed by studies of children with very early-onset of bipolar disorder (Luby and

Mrakotsky, 2003), as well as by studies on offspring of bipolar parents (Chang et al, 2003b; Masi et al, 2004b). These high-risk populations should be carefully evaluated when a potentially switching treatment with antidepressants is considered, given the paucity of data on children. This risk is particularly high in adolescents, given the potential suicidal risk in SSRI-induced manic or mixed states.

Regarding the treatment of bipolar depression, although lithium has some antidepressant properties, as well as divalproex and carbamazepine, they all have limited efficacy in acute bipolar depression, even though they may have some efficacy in preventing depressive symptoms during prophylactic treatment. Consistently with some reports on adult bipolar samples, Kusumakar and Yatham (1997) and Caradang et al (2003) reported on the efficacy of lamotrigine in adolescents with refractory bipolar depression.

The issue of whether to use antidepressants in bipolar depression is still open, given the risk for switching to mania, or rapid cycling or mixed states. In a review of the medical chart of 59 patients with bipolar disorder (Biederman et al, 2000), depressive symptoms were 6.7 times more likely to improve when subjects received an SSRI than when they did not. In contrast, tricyclic antidepressants, stimulants, mood stabilizers, and typical neuroleptics did not improve depressive symptomatology. However, subjects receiving SSRIs were three times as likely to develop manic symptoms at the next follow-up visit than subjects who had not received an SSRI. The efficacy of a concomitant treatment with mood stabilizers was not reduced by the SSRI cotherapy.

Given the frequent misdiagnosis of bipolar disorder as a unipolar depressive disorder, an anxiety disorder, a conduct disorder, or an ADHD, treatment with antidepressants and/or stimulants is not rare. Faedda et al (2004) reviewed clinical records of 82 children with bipolar disorder, in order to ascertain the rate of treatment-emergent mania or increased mood cycling during pharmacologic treatment. Fifty-seven (69.5%) received at least once a mood-elevating agent, and 33 of them (58%) presented an elevation of mood with a median latency of 2 weeks, with a large prevalence of antidepressants. Importantly, some of these patients had prominent suicidal, homicidal, or psychotic behaviors. This is an important issue also in children and adolescents with bipolar disorder comorbid with anxiety and/or obsessive-compulsive disorder (Masi et al, 2001, 2004a).

However, in a prospective follow-up of 93 patients with prepubertal or early-adolescence mania, treated by their own practitioners, Geller and colleagues (2002) did not find that antidepressants increased the rates of recovery or relapse.

Serotonergic agents have a potentially destabilizing effect, but they do not reduce the antimanic effect of mood stabilizers, and they may be used after an adequate mood stabilization. It is best to reduce and gradually discontinue the antidepressant in 6 to 12 weeks after euthymia has been achieved, even though some patients may require a combination of antidepressant and mood stabilizer for a longer period.

Predictors of pharmacologic non-response

Predictors of treatment non-response in early-onset bipolar disorder are not well defined. Many potential variables may be considered. Age, gender, and age at onset of bipolar disorder can affect both clinical presentation and pattern of comorbidity, and both these factors may affect the pharmacologic response. Some features, which in adult patients with bipolar disorder are considered predictors of poor treatment response, such as severity, mixed states, psychotic symptoms, and co-morbid substance abuse, are particularly frequent in youths (Carlson et al, 1999), and they also may influence pharmacologic response in children and adolescents as well. Early-onset bipolar disorder is characterized by high rates of comorbid disorders, which may define specific subtypes of bipolar disorder, in terms of response to treatment, even though available data are still inconsistent.

In the Werry and McClellan study (1992), no clinical predictors of poor outcome were found, whereas the best predictors of future functioning were premorbid functioning, IQ < 80, and bipolar family history, suggesting a lower impact of the illness per se, compared to factors external to the clinical picture. Strober and coworkers (1998) and State and colleagues (2004) found that comorbid ADHD predicted lithium inefficacy. In contrast, in Kafantaris et al's study (1998), the presence of childhood psychiatric diagnoses as a whole, as well as specific types of diagnosis, including ADHD, did not affect response to lithium treatment in adolescents with bipolar disorder, while the presence of psychotic symptoms was associated with poor lithium response. Carlson and colleagues (2002) observed that comorbid psychopathology, mainly behavioral disorders, and, to a lesser degree, earlier age at onset, predicted a poor outcome. Geller and coworkers (2002) found that living in an intact biologic family was the best predictor of recovery, and a low level of maternal–child warmth was the best predictor of relapse after recovery.

Masi et al (2004c) explored pharmacologic treatment non-response in 40 children and adolescents (age range 7–18 years, mean age 14.2 ± 3.3 years) with manic or mixed episodes. Predictors of non-response were the presence of comorbidity with conduct disorder and/or ADHD and the baseline CGI Severity score. Demographic variables (mean age, gender ratio, socio-economic status), age at onset of bipolar disorder; and comorbid anxiety disorders did not influence treatment response.

Duffy and colleagues (1998) have described specific clinical features of adolescent offspring of parents with bipolar disorder, responsive or unresponsive to lithium treatment. According to this study, youngsters of parents who were lithium responders showed psychiatric illnesses in the affective domain, lower rates of comorbidity, and a less episodic course. In contrast, offspring from parents who were lithium non-responders showed a broader range of psychopathology, high rates of comorbid conditions, and high rates of episodes. It is not possible to argue whether these features are markers of a refractory form of early-onset bipolar disorder; however, this study suggests that a good response to lithium may be a marker for a specific subtype of bipolar disorder.

Treatment strategy

Acute phase

Acute treatment is aimed at decreasing agitation or aggression, modulating excitement, and normalizing physiologic functioning (sleeping, eating, etc.). Even though the first option in the bipolar child is a mood stabilizer, lithium or divalproex, in acutely agitated patients or in patients with psychotic symptoms an intervention with an atypical antipsychotic may be necessary. When the patient is acutely agitated and non-collaborative, an intramuscular administration may be necessary, with a high-potency neuroleptic (haloperidol) or with olanzapine. In the case of haloperidol, dystonic or other extrapyramidal side-effects should be carefully monitored, and possibly treated with anticholinergic compounds for at least 2–3 weeks. Akathisia is not a rare side-effect during neuroleptic treatment, and it is often neglected or misinterpreted as a worsening of the psychiatric disorder. Akathisia is poorly sensitive to anticholinergic medications, but it can sometimes improve using beta-blockers or benzodiazepines. Benzodiazepines should be used cautiously, because of their propensity to induce disinhibition. After the acute phase, the opportunity of maintaining the antipsychotic should be considered in the presence of psychotic symptoms and/or severe irritability-hostility. It should be remembered that an early discontinuation of the antipsychotic in severely ill bipolar patients is associated with a marked worsening of the emotional and behavioral symptoms (Kafantaris et al, 2001). When an oral antipsychotic treatment must be continued an atypical antipsychotic should be considered, such as olanzapine, risperidone, or quetiapine. Clozapine should be limited to treatment-refractory cases.

Lithium

When the clinical picture is less acute and severe (patient not excessively agitated and/or without psychotic symptoms), and/or after the acute phase, mood stabilizers in monotherapy are the first-line medications, and lithium and divalproex are the most frequently used and better evaluated treatments in children and adolescents. Even though atypical antipsychotics are currently considered as a first-line treatment for adult bipolar disorder, the data are insufficient to make this statement in pediatric bipolar disorder on the basis of a risk/benefit ratio, unless psychotic symptoms and/or hostility/aggressiveness are prominent. The onset of lithium action is about 2 weeks, and the peak is 6 to 8 weeks, at blood levels higher than 0.5 mEq/l, and more often with an optimal range of 0.8–1mEq/l. As a preliminary to lithium treatment, the screening procedure should include electrolytes, blood urea nitrogen, creatinine, electrocardiogram (ECG), and thyroid function (T3, T4, TSH). A pregnancy test may be recommended, given the increased risk of heart disease in infants born to mothers using lithium during pregnancy, with an increased risk in the first trimester. Lithium can start with an initial dose of 150 mg in children and 300 mg in adolescents, with increments related to the clinical severity, up to 300 mg/day in children and 600–900 mg/day in adolescents. Five or seven days after the last dose adjustment (steady state), and 9–12 hours following the last dose, serum levels should be obtained before another dosage increase, given the narrow therapeutic window. The oral dose necessary to obtain an adequate serum level ranging from 0.5 to 1 mEq/l will be the target dose, in two doses (morning and evening), possibly with the largest dose in the evening to limit side-effects. When lithium is associated with an antipsychotic, the risk of neurotoxic effects is markedly increased and it should be carefully monitored. During lithium treatment an adequate level of blood sodium should be ensured, with an adequate salt intake and monitoring in case of vomiting or diarrhea, in order to prevent a rapid rise in lithium blood levels.

Valproate, sodium valproate, and divalproex sodium

Valproic acid, sodium valproate, and divalproex sodium have been well studied in the treatment of adults with mania, and more data are becoming available for children and adolescents, showing an efficacy similar to lithium, and possibly better efficacy in rapid cycling and mixed states. As a preliminary to valproate treatment, the screening procedure should include a liver function test and complete blood cell count. A pregnancy test may be recommended, given the high risk of development of neural tube defects. Valproate can be started at an initial dose of 125 mg in children and 250 mg in adolescents, with increments related to the clinical severity, up to 20–30 mg/kg per day, to achieve a serum level higher than 50 mg/l (but often a level of 80–100 mg/l is necessary for optimal clinical effect), in two or three doses per day. Serum levels should be obtained 5–7 days after the last adjustment (steady state). The onset of clinical efficacy should appear within 2 or 3 weeks of treatment, with a peak after 6–8 weeks.

A gradual tapering is warranted at the end of this period, during a euthymic phase. Withdrawal seizures can occur in non-epileptic patients, even though they are very rare.

Treatment of refractory cases

When treatment with lithium or valproate is ineffective or only partially effective, a combination of both the medications, or one of them plus carbamazepine, may be considered, at the highest doses and for the adequate time. Carbamazepine can be introduced slowly (100 mg every 5–7 days) up to a maximum dose of 200–600 mg in children and 1200 mg in adolescents, corresponding to a therapeutic serum level of 7–12 µg/ml, depending on clinical response and side-effects. Because of a more rapid elimination in younger patients, carbamazepine should be administered in three doses in children and two doses in adolescents. A specific neurologic assessment is recommended during the first days of treatment and after each dosage increase, with weekly monitoring of CBC and WBC, hepatic enzymes, and carbamazepine serum levels, and an ECG after steady state has been reached. Carbamazepine should be discontinued when WBC are below 4000/mm^3 and/or neutrophils are below 1700/mm^3. Diplopia is usually an early manifestation of neurotoxicity, and it should be considered an alarm signal.

When this procedure is not effective, an augmentation with an atypical antipsychotic is recommended, especially when the clinical symptomatology is severe, with aggression and hostility, and/or in presence of psychotic symptoms. Lithium or valproate can be effectively associated to olanzapine, quetiapine and risperidone. In resistant patients the atypical antipsychotic may be associated with both lithium and valproate.

When the association with an antipsychotic has been considered, olanzapine (up to 10 mg/day in children and 20 mg/day in adolescents), risperidone (up to 2–3 mg/day in children and 4–6 mg/day in adolescents), or quetiapine (up to 200–300 mg/day in children and 400–600 mg/day in adolescents) can be used. Increasing data on aripiprazole are promising in terms of efficacy and tolerability. Even though atypical antipsychotics are currently considered as a first-line treatment for adult bipolar disorder, the data are insufficient to make this statement in pediatric bipolar disorder, unless psychotic symptoms and/or hostility/aggressiveness are prominent. When an augmentation with an atypical antipsychotic is not effective, a switch to another atypical antipsychotic among the three previously mentioned medications is recommended.

When these treatment procedures are non effective in controlling mood and behavior, newer medications can be associated, even though they are still not supported by clear evidence of efficacy. Newer anticonvulsants may be considered in alternative to older anticonvulsants, lamotrigine (in presence of depressive features), topiramate (in presence of overweight), oxcarbazepine (in presence of marked impulsivity). Gabapentin is less supported, but it may be considered when anxiety disorders are comorbid. Alternatively, newer atypical antipsychotics are aripiprazole or ziprasidone which can be associated with an older anticonvulsant. Even though typical antipsychotics gave effective results in adult patients with mania, their use in children and adolescents is strongly limited by their less tolerable side-effect profile.

The use of clozapine should be limited to the more treatment-refractory cases, in monotherapy or in association with other mood stabilizers, with the exception of carbamazepine, for the possible effect on the white blood cells. This treatment necessitates a pretreatment full blood count and regular blood tests thereafter. A pretreatment EEG, with periodic controls, is needed as well, especially when high clozapine doses are used. Detailed information on the use of clozapine in children and adolescents in reported in Chapter 8.

Chronic treatment

When treatment is effective, long-term pharmacologic prophylaxis should be considered to prevent relapses, as part of an ongoing treatment plan. However, long-term studies focusing on the duration of prophylaxis are still lacking. In adults with bipolar disorder, discontinuation of lithium maintenance is associated with high rates of relapse and possible secondary refractoriness to lithium treatment in a following relapse. In an 18-month study addressing the issue of lithium maintenance treatment in bipolar adolescents, continuation of lithium decreased the relapse rate from 92.3% to 37.5% (Strober et al, 1990). In a long-term study addressing the issue of lithium maintenance treatment in bipolar adolescents, 63% remained well during lithium, compared with only 8% in those who discontinued (Strober et al, 1995). Patients and their families are often reluctant to undergo a longer treatment to prevent future episodes. The main reasons for treatment non-adherence are weight gain and cognitive dulling. There are no clear guidelines as to how long mood stabilizers should be prescribed in bipolar children, although the severity of the episode and the strength of the personal and family history may affect the decision. Guidelines for adult bipolar patients recommended that treatment should continue for at least 18 months after mood stabilization. After the first episode, a maintenance of at least 12–18 months should be discussed with the patient and his family. After repeated episodes or when the suicidal risk is higher, a longer and careful maintenance period should be recommended. Adequate serum levels of mood stabilizers are recommended (lithium at

0.8–1 mEq/l, divalproex at 80–100 µg/l). The efficacy of associated psychosocial interventions, including psychoeducation, psychotherapy, and scholastic and social support is very important.

Which medications should be used in the maintenance treatment? Usually the medications effective in the acute phase should be continued in the maintenance treatment. Findling and colleagues (2005) have explored efficacy of maintenance monotherapy of divalproex sodium or lithium in 60 youths who stabilized on combination lithium–divalproex. After randomization in a lithium group or a divalproex group, the two groups did not differ in survival time until emerging symptoms of relapse or until discontinuation for any reason.

When a combined treatment with mood stabilizers and an atypical antipsychotic was necessary an attempt to discontinue the antipsychotic should be considered during the follow-up given the possible risk of weight gain, diabetes mellitus, and changes in lipid levels. Unfortunately, sometimes this discontinuation is associated with a worsening of the clinical picture, in terms of both mood and behavioral control.

Bipolar depression

Event though mood stabilizers may be ineffective in the prevention and treatment of depressive relapses in bipolar patients, the first and safer choice in bipolar depression should be a mood stabilizer, namely lithium or a lithium/valproate association. Another mood stabilizer with mild antidepressant properties is lamotrigine, both in the treatment and prophylaxis of depressive episodes. Careful monitoring of dermatologic complications (Steven–Johnson syndrome) is warranted during lamotrigine treatment, especially when associated with valproate.

When this treatment in ineffective, after increasing the mood stabilizer dosage to the highest level, a low dose of an SSRI may be added, monitoring a switch to mania or mixed mania or rapid cycling and suicide risk. The antidepressant bupropion can also be used as second choice, when SSRIs are non-effective and/or non-tolerated. The antidepressant treatment should be continued for at least 8 weeks after the remission of the depressive symptomatology, then gradually tapered. Antidepressants should not be used when the patient is not depressed, according to an antidepressant-sparing strategy.

A cognitive-behavioral treatment can be effectively used as an alternative or in association with antidepressants, or to prevent depressive recurrence.

Low doses of atypical antipsychotics may be used in the treatment-resistant cases.

Comorbidity between bipolar disorder and attention deficit hyperactivity disorder

The above-mentioned findings about stimulant treatment in bipolar children with ADHD run against the clinical concept that stimulants may favor an earlier onset of bipolar disorder, irrespective of ADHD, possibly through a behavioral sensitization mechanism (Del Bello et al, 2001). Although, even recently, some concerns have been raised about a possible exacerbating effect of stimulants of an underlying (hypo)mania (Faedda et al, 2004), clinicians should not a priori avoid stimulants in children with ADHD and manic symptoms. Data from empirical studies indicate that when a bipolar patient is stabilized with one or more mood stabilizers, the addition of a stimulant may further improve the clinical picture through better control of comorbid ADHD symptoms.

However, when this comorbidity is diagnosed, the mood disorder should be treated first, with mood stabilizers and/or atypical antipsychotics, according to the previously reported strategies. When a significant hyperactive, impulsive, and inattentive symptomatology still persists after this treatment, a specific treatment with stimulant medications can be started. Antidepressants with effective action on ADHD symptoms, such as atomoxetine, tricyclics, and bupropion, should be avoided.

Conclusions

In parallel to the increasing evidence on bipolar disorder in prepubertal children, empirical studies on phenomenology, clinical course, prognostic elements, and response to treatment are going to increase as well. However, to date, differences between childhood-onset and adolescence-onset disorders are still unclear, as well as the meaning of the relationship between ADHD and prepubertal bipolar disorder.

These issues have a primary clinical and theoretic relevance for a deeper understanding of the pathophysiology of bipolar disorder, as well as for an optimal treatment strategy.

In designing future studies, a wide variety of clinical approaches, including both placebo-controlled randomized trials and naturalistic studies, will be helpful. Even though the randomized, placebo-controlled clinical trials can be considered the gold standard when data about safety and efficacy are lacking, an interesting issue is how far the results of controlled studies, on very selected populations, intensively studied for short periods, can apply to everyday care. Long-term naturalistic prospective studies might represent an important source of information regarding the effectiveness of a treatment over extended periods of time on unselected samples of bipolar patients treated under routine clinical conditions, with mono- or polypharmacy, and followed up in a routine clinical setting. When strict exclusion criteria are applied for reason of "purity of the sample," often all those comorbid conditions which represent the rule in clinical settings are excluded.

Finally, further research is warranted on several treatment issues, such as:

- Possible differences in clinical response to treatments from early childhood to late adolescence.
- Alternative treatments in episodes resistant to mood stabilizers, and a possible differential response to mood stabilizers in acute mania, rapid cycling, and mixed state.
- Management of the depressive episodes, with mood stabilizers, and/or with SSRIs, and/or with low-dose atypical antipsychotics.
- Efficacy of mood stabilizers for prophylaxis and the optimal duration of prophylaxis.
- Management of associated disorders, such as ADHD, anxiety disorders, sleep disorders, and severe behavioral disorders.

References

Akiskal HS. Developmental pathways to bipolarity: are juvenile-onset depressions pre-bipolar? *J Am Acad Child Adolesc Psychiatry* 1995; **34**: 754–63.

Baptista T, Kin NM, Beaulieu S, DeBaptista EA. Obesity and related metabolic abnormalities during antipsychotic drug administration: mechanism, management and research perspectives. *Pharmacopsychiatry* 2002; **35**: 205–19.

Barnett MS. Ziprasidone monotherapy in pediatric bipolar disorder. *J Child Adolesc Psychopharmacol* 2004; **14**: 471–7.

Barzman DH, DelBello MP, Kowatch RA, et al. The effectiveness and tolerability of aripiprazole for pediatric bipolar disorders: a retrospective chart review. *J Child Adolesc Psychopharmacol* 2004; **14**: 593–600.

Bhangoo RK, Lowe CH, Myers FS, et al. Medication use in children and adolescents treated in the community for bipolar disorder. *J Child Adolesc Psychopharmacol* 2003; **13**: 515–22.

Biederman J, Faraone S, Mick E, et al. Attention deficit and hyperactivity disorder and juvenile mania: an overlooked comorbidity? *J Am Acad Child Adolesc Psychiatry* 1996; **35**: 997–1008.

Biederman J, Mick E, Prince J, et al. Systematic chart review of the pharmacologic treatment of comorbid attention deficit hyperactivity disorder in youth with bipolar disorder. *J Child Adolesc Psychopharmacol* 1999; **9**: 247–56.

Biederman J, Mick E, Spencer TJ, et al. Therapeutic dilemmas in the pharmacotherapy of bipolar depression in the young. *J Child Adolesc Psychopharmacol* 2000; **10**: 185–92.

Biederman J, Mick E, Wozniak J, et al. Can a subtype of conduct disorder linked to bipolar disorder be identified? Integration of findings from the Massachussetts General Hospital Pediatric Psychopharmacology Research Program. *Biol Psychiatry* 2003; **53**: 938–44.

Biederman J, McDonnel MA, Wozniak J, et al. Aripiprazole in the treatment of pediatric bipolar disorder: a systematic chart review. *CNS Spectrum* 2005; **10**: 141–8.

Birmaher B, Kennah A, Brent D, et al. Is bipolar disorder specifically associated with panic disorder in youths? *J Clin Psychiatry* 2002; **63**: 414–19.

Bouvard MP, Bayle F, Dugas M. Open trial of carbamazepine in the prevention of recurrence of bipolar disorder in adolescents. *Encephale* 1993; **19**: 591–600.

Bryant AE III, Dreyfuss FE. Valproic acid and hepatic fatalities: Part 3. US experience since 1986. *Neurology* 1996; **46**: 465–9.

Calabrese JR, Fatemi SH, Kujawa M, Woyshville MJ. Predictors of response to mood stabilizers. *J Clin Psychopharmacol* 1996; **16**: 24S–31S.

Campbell M, Armenteros JL, Malone RP, et al. Neuroleptic-related dyskinesias in autistic children: a prospective, longitudinal study. *J Am Acad Child Adolesc Psychiatry* 1997; **36**: 835–43.

Caradang CG, Maxwell DJ, Robbins DR, Oestherheld JR. Lamotrigine in adolescent mood disorders. *J Am Acad Child Adolesc Psychiatry* 2003; **42**: 750–1.

Carlson GA, Kelly KL. Stimulant rebound: how common is and what does it mean? *J Child Adolesc Psychopharmacol* 2003; **13**: 137–42.

Carlson GA, Rapport MD, Kelly KL, Patakii CS. The effects of methylphenidate and lithium in attention and activity level. *J Am Acad Child Adolesc Psychiatry* 1992; **31**: 262–70.

Carlson GA, Lavelle J, Bromet EJ. Medication treatment in adolescents vs. adults with psychotic mania. *J Child Adolesc Psychopharmacol* 1999; **9**: 221–31.

Carlson AG, Bromet EJ, Sievers S. Phenomenology and outcome of subjects with early- and adult-onset psychotic mania. *Am J Psychiatry* 2000; **157**: 213–19.

Carlson GA, Bromet EJ, Driessens C, et al. Age at onset, childhood psychopathology and 2-year outcome in psychotic bipolar disorder. *Am J Psychiatry* 2002; **159**: 307–9.

Carlson GA, Jensen PS, Findling RL, et al. Methodological issues and controversies in clinical trials with child and adolescent patients with bipolar disorder: report of a consensus conference. *J Child Adolesc Psychopharmacol* 2003; **13**: 13–27.

Casaer P, Walleghem D, Vandenbuscche I, et al. Pharmacokinetics and safety of risperidone in autistic children. *Pediatr Neurol* 1994; **11**: 89.

Chang KD, Ketter TA. Mood stabilizer augmentation with olanzapine in acutely manic children. *J Child Adolesc Psychopharmacol* 2000; **10**: 45–9.

Chang KD, Dienes K, Blasey C, et al. Divalproex monotherapy in the treatment of bipolar offspring with mood and behavioral disorders and at least mild affective symptoms. *J Clin Psychiatry* 2003a; **64**: 936–42.

Chang K, Steiner H, Ketter T. Studies of offspring of parents with bipolar disorder. *Am J Med Gen* 2003b; **123C**: 23–35.

Chengappa KN, Kupfer DJ, Frank E, et al. Relationship of birth cohort and early age at onset of illness in a bipolar case registry. *Am J Psychiatry* 2003; **160**: 1636–42.

Craney JL, Geller B. A prepubertal and early adolescent bipolar disorder-I phenotype: review of phenomenology and longitudinal course. *Bipol Dis* 2003; **5**: 243–56.

Davanzo P, Cantwell E, Kleiner J, et al. Cognitive changes during topiramate therapy. *J Am Acad Child Adolesc Psychiatry* 2001; **40**: 262–3.

Davanzo P, Gunderson B, Belin T, et al. Mood stabilizers in hospitalized children with bipolar disorder: a retrospective review. *Psychiatry Clin Neurosci* 2003; **57**: 504–10.

Davanzo P, Nikore V, Yehya N, Stevenson L. Oxcarbazepine treatment of juvenile-onset bipolar disorder. *J Child Adolesc Psychopharmacol* 2004; **14**: 344–5.

DelBello M, Soutullo C, Hendricks W, et al. Prior stimulant treatment in adolescent with bipolar disorder: association with age and onset. *Bipol Dis* 2001; **3**: 53–7.

DelBello MP, Kowatch RA, Warner J, et al. Adjunctive topiramate treatment for pediatric bipolar disorder: a retrospective chart review. *J Child Adolesc Psychopharmacol* 2002a; **12**: 323–30.

DelBello MP, Schwiers M, Rosenberg H, Strakowski S. Quetiapine as adjunctive treatment for adolescent mania associated with bipolar disorder. *J Am Acad Child Adolesc Psychiatry* 2002b; **41**: 1216–23.

DelBello MP, Adler C, Strakowski SM. Divalproex for the treatment of aggression associated with adolescent mania. *J Child Adolesc Psychopharmacol* 2004; **14**: 325–8.

DelBello MMP, Findling RL, Kushner S, et al. A pilot controlled trial of topiranate for mania in children and adolescents with bipolar disorder. *J Am Acad Child Adolesc Psychiatry* 2005; **44**: 539–47.

Deltito JA, Levitan J, Damore J, et al. Naturalistic experience with the use of divalproex sodium on a in-patient unit for adolescent psychiatric patients. *Acta Psychiatr Scand* 1998; **97**: 236–40.

Dilsaver SC, Henderson-Fuller S, Akiskal HS. Occult mood disorder in 104 consecutively presenting children referred for the treatment of attention deficit hyperactivity disorder. *J Clin Psychiatry* 2003; **64**: 1170–6.

Duffy A, Alda M, Kutcher S, et al. Psychiatric symptoms and syndromes among adolescents children of parents with lithium-reponsive or lithium.nonresponsive bipolar disorder. *Am J Psychiatry* 1998; **155**: 431–3.

Faedda GL, Baldessarini RJ, Glowinsky IP, Austin NB. Treatment-emergent mania in pediatric bipolar disorder: a retrospective case review. *J Affect Disord* 2004; **82**: 149–58.

Findling RL, McNamara NK, Gracious BL, et al. Combination lithium and divalproex sodium in pediatric bipolarity. *J Am Acad Child Adolesc Psychiatry* 2003; **42**: 895–901.

Findling RL, McNamara NK, Youngstrom EA, et al. Double-blind 18-month trial of lithium versus divalproex maintenance treatment in pediatric bipolar disorder. *J Am Acad Child Adolesc Psychiatry* 2005; **44**: 409–17.

Frazier JA, Meyer MC, Biederman J, et al. Risperidone treatment for juvenile bipolar disorder: a retrospective chart review. *J Am Acad Child Adolesc Psychiatry* 1999; **38**: 960–5.

Frazier JA, Biederman J, Tohen M, et al. A prospective open-label treatment trial of olanzapine monotherapy in children and adolescents with bipolar disorder. *J Child Adolesc Psychopharmacol* 2001; **11**: 239–50.

Galanter CA, Carlson GA, Jensen PS, et al. Response to methylphenidate in children with attention deficit hyperactivity disorder and manic symptoms in the multimodal treatment study of children with attention deficit hyperactivity disorder trial. *J Child Adolesc Psychopharmacol* 2003; **13**: 123–36.

Garfinkel M, Garfinkel L, Himmeloch J, McHugh T. Lithium carbonate and carbamazepine: an effective treatment for adolescent manic or mixed bipolar patients. Proceedings of the Annual Meeting of the Am Acad Child Adolesc Psychiatry, New York 1985; 41–2.

Geller B, Cooper TB, Sun K, et al. Double-blind and placebo controlled study of lithium for adolescent bipolar disorders with secondary substance dependency *J Am Acad Child Adolesc Psychiatry* 1998a; **37**: 171–8.

Geller B, Cooper TB, Zimerman B, et al. Lithium for prepubertal and early adolescent bipolar disorder phenotype. *Am J Psychiatry* 1998b; **158**: 303–5.

Geller B, Zimerman B, Williams M, et al. Diagnostic characteristics of 93 cases of prepubertal and early adolescent bipolar disorder phenotype by gender, puberty and comorbid attention deficit hyperactivity disorder. *J Child Adolesc Psychopharmacol* 2000; **10**: 157–64.

Geller B, Craney JL, Bolhofer K, et al. One-year recovery and relapse rates of children with a pre-pubertal and early adolescent bipolar disorder phenotype. *Am J Psychiatry* 2001a; **158**: 303–5.

Geller B, Zimerman B, Williams M, et al. Bipolar disorder at prospective follow-up of adults who had a prepubertal major depressive disorder. *Am J Psychiatry* 2001b; **158**: 125–7.

Geller B, Craney JL, Bolhofer K, et al. Two year prospective follow-up of a prepubertal and early adolescent bipolar disorder phenotype. *Am J Psychiatry* 2002; **159**: 927–33.

Grothe DR, Calis KA, Jacobsen L, et al. Olanzapine pharmacokinetics in pediatric and adolescent inpatients with childhood-onset schizophrenia. *J Clin Psychopharmacol* 2000; **20**: 220–5.

Hagino OR, Weller EB, Weller RA, et al. Untoward effects of lithium treatment in children aged four through six years. *J Am Acad Child Adolesc Psychiatry* 1995; **34**: 1584–90.

Hamrin V, Bailey K. Gabapentin and methylphenidate treatment of a preadolescent with attention deficit hyperactivity disorder and bipolar disorder. *J Child Adolesc Psychopharmacol* 2001; **11**: 301–9.

Harpold TL, Wozniak J, Kwon A, et al. Examining the association between pediatric bipolar disorder and anxiety disorders in psychiatrically referred children and adolescents. *J Affect Disord* 2005; **88**: 19–26.

Henry CA, Zamvil LS, Lam C, et al. Long-term outcome with divalproex in children and adolescents with bipolar disorder. *J Child Adolesc Psychopharmacol* 2003; **13**: 523–9.

Isojarvi JI, Laatikainen TJ, Pakarinen AJ, et al. Polycystic ovaries and hyperandrogenism in women taking valproate for epilepsy. *N Engl J Med* 1993; **329**: 1383–8.

Kafantaris V, Coletti DJ, Dicker R, et al. Are childhood psychiatric histories of bipolar adolescents associated with family history, psychosis, and response to lithium treatment? *J Affect Disord* 1998; **51**: 153–64.

Kafantaris V, Coletti DJ, Dicker R, et al. Adjunctive antipsychotic treatment of adolescents with bipolar psychosis. *J Am Acad Child Adolesc Psychiatry* 2001; **40**: 1448–56.

Kafantaris V, Coletti DJ, Dicker R, et al. Lithium treatment of acute mania in adolescents: a large open trial. *J Am Acad Child Adolesc Psychiatry* 2003; **42**: 1038–45.

Kafantaris V, Coletti DJ, Dicker R, et al. Lithium treatment of acute mania in adolescents: a placebo-controlled discontinuation study. *J Am Acad Child Adolesc Psychiatry* 2004; **43**: 984–93.

Kant R, Chalansani R, Chengappa KN, Dieringer MF. The off-label use of clozapine in adolescents with bipolar disorder and intermittent explosive disorder, or posttraumatic stress disorder. *J Child Adolesc Psychopharmacol* 2004; **14**: 57–63.

Kowatch RA, Suppes T, Gilfillian SK, et al. Clozapine treatment of children and adolescents treated with bipolar disorder and schizophrenia: a clinical case series. *J Child Adolesc Psychopharmacol* 1995; **5**: 241–53.

Kowatch RA, Suppes T, Carmody TJ, et al. Effect size of lithium, divalproex, and carbamazepine in children and adolescents with bipolar disorder. *J Am Acad Child Adolesc Psychiatry* 2000; **39**: 713–20.

Kowatch RA, Sethuraman G, Hume JH, et al. Combination pharmacotherapy in children and adolescents with bipolar disorder. *Biol Psychiatry* 2003; **53**: 978–84.

Kusumakar V, Yatham LN. An open study of lamotrigine in refractory bipolar depression. *Psychiatry Res* 1997; **72**: 145–8.

Kutcher SP. *Child and adolescent psychopharmacology*. Philadelphia: WB Saunders Company; 1997.

Lean ME, Pajonk FG. Patients on atypical antipsychotic drugs: another high-risk group for type 2 diabetes. *Diabetes Care* 2003; **26**: 1597–605.

Lewinshon P, Klein D, Seeley J. Bipolar disorder in a community sample of older adolescents: prevalence, phenomenology, comorbidity, and course. *J Am Acad Child Adolesc Psychiatry* 1995; **34**: 454–63.

Lewinshon PM, Seeley JR, Klein DN. Bipolar disorders during adolescence. *Acta Psychiatr Scand Suppl* 2003; **418**: 47–50.

Liebenluft E, Charney DS, Towbin KE, et al. Defining clinical phenotypes of juvenile mania. *Am J Psychiatry* 2003; **160**: 430–7.

Luby JL, Mrakotsky C. Depressed preschoolers with bipolar family history: a group at high risk for later switching to mania? *J Child Adolesc Psychopharmacol* 2003; **13**: 187–93.

McConville BJ, Arvanitis LA, Thyrum PT, et al. Pharmacokinetics, tolerability, and clinical effectiveness of quetiapine fumarate: an open-label trial in adolescents with psychotic disorders. *J Clin Psychiatry* 2000; **61**: 252–60.

Manji HK, Lenox RH. The nature of bipolar disorder. *J Clin Psychiatry* 2000; **61**: 42–57.

Marchand WR, Wirth L, Simon C. Quetiapine adjunctive and monotherapy for pediatric bipolar disorder: a retrospective chart review. *J Child Adolesc Psychopharmacol* 2004; **14**: 405–11.

Masi G. Pharmacotherapy of pervasive developmental disorders in children and adolescents. *CNS Drugs* 2004; **18**: 1031–52.

Masi G, Toni C, Perugi G, et al. Anxiety comorbidity in consecutively referred children and adolescents with bipolar disorder: a neglected comorbidity. *Can J Psychiatry* 2001; **46**: 766–71.

Masi G, Mucci M, Millepiedi S. Clozapine in adolescent inpatients with acute mania. *J Child Adolesc Psychopharmacol* 2002; **12**: 93–9.

Masi G, Toni C, Perugi G, et al. Externalizing disorders in consecutively referred children and adolescents with bipolar disorder. *Compr Psychiatry* 2003; **44**: 184–9.

Masi G, Perugi G, Toni C, et al. Obsessive-compulsive-bipolar comorbidity: focus on children and adolescents. *J Affect Disord* 2004a; **78**: 175–83.

Masi G, Akiskal HS, Akiskal K. Detecting the risk for affective spectrum disorders in children of bipolar parents. In: Maj M, Lopez-Ibor JJ, Sartorius N, Sato M, Okasha A, eds. *Early detection and management of mental disorders.* World Psychiatric Association Series; 2004b: 163–84.

Masi G, Perugi G, Toni C, et al. Predictors of treatment non-response on bipolar children and adolescents with manic or mixed episodes. *J Child Adolesc Psychopharmacol* 2004c; **14**: 403–12.

Masi G, Perugi G, Toni C, et al. The clinical phenotypes of juvenile bipolar disorder: toward a validation of the episodic-chronic distinction. *Biol Psychiatry* 2006. In Press.

Mota-Castillo M, Torruella A, Engels P, et al. Valproate in very young children: an open case series with a brief follow-up. *J Affect Disord* 2001; **67**: 193–7.

Papatheodorou G, Kutcher SP, Katic M, Szalai JP. The efficacy and safety of divalproex sodium in the treatment of acute mania in adolescents and young adults: an open clinical trial. *J Clin Psychopharmacol* 1995; **15**: 110–16.

Pavuluri MN, Janicak PG, Carbray J. Topiramate plus risperidone for controlling weight gain and symptoms in preschool mania. *J Child Adolesc Psychopharmacol* 2002; **12**: 271–3.

Pellock JM. Carbamazepine side effects in children and adults. *Epilepsia* 1987; **28**: S64–S70.

Scheffer RE, Niskala Apps JA. The diagnosis of preschool bipolar disorder presenting with mania: open pharmacological treatment. *J Affect Disord* 2004; **82**: S25–34.

Scheffer RE, Kowatch RA, Carmody T, Rush AJ. Randomized, placebo-controlled trial of mixed amphetamine for symptoms of comorbid ADHD in pediatric bipolar disorder after mood stabilization with divalproex sodium. *Am J Psychiatry* 2005; **162**: 58–64.

Soutullo CA, Casuto LS, Keck PE Jr. Gabapentin in the treatment of adolescents mania: a case report. *J Child Adolesc Psychopharmacol* 1998; **8**: 81–5.

Soutullo CA, Sorter MT, Foster KD, McElroy SL, Keck PE. Olanzapine in the treatment of adolescent acute mania: a report of seven cases. *J Affect Disord* 1999; **53**: 279–83.

Srinath S, Reddy YCJ, Girimaji SC, et al. A prospective study of bipolar disorder in children and adolescents from India. *Acta Psychiatr Scand* 1998; **98**: 437–42.

State RC, Frye MA, Altshuler LL, et al. Chart review of the impact of attention-deficit/hyperactivity disorder comorbidity on response to lithium or divalproex sodium in adolescent mania. *J Clin Psychiatry* 2004; **65**: 1057–63.

Strober M, Morrel W, Lampert C, Burroughs J. Relapse following discontinuation of lithium maintenance therapy in adolescents with bipolar I illness: a naturalistic study. *Am J Psychiatry* 1990; **147**: 457–61.

Strober M, Schmidt-Lackner S, Freeman R, et al. Recovery and relapse in adolescents with bipolar affective illness: a five-year naturalistic, prospective follow-up. *J Am Acad Child Adolesc Psychiatry* 1995; **34**: 724–31.

Strober M, De Antonio M, Schmidt-Lackner M, et al. Early childhood attention deficit hyperactivity disorder predicts poorer response to acute lithium therapy in adolescent mania. *J Affect Disord* 1998; **51**: 145–51.

Toren P, Laor N, Weizman A. Use of atypical neuroleptics in child and adolescent psychiatry. *J Clin Psychiatry* 1998; **59**: 644–56.

Vitiello B, Behar D, Malone R, et al. Pharmacokinetics of lithium carbonate in children. *J Clin Psychopharmacol* 1988; **8**: 355–9.

Wagner KD, Weller EB, Carlson GA, et al. An open trial of divalproex in children and adolescents with bipolar disorder. *J Am Acad Child Adolesc Psychiatry* 2002; **41**: 1224–30.

Werry JS, McClellan JM. Predicting outcome in child and adolescent (early onset) schizophrenia and bipolar disorder. *J Am Acad Child Adolesc Psychiatry* 1992; **31**: 147–50.

Wilens TE, Biederman J, Kwon A, et al. Risk for substance use disorder in adolescents with bipolar disorder. *J Am Acad Child Adolesc Psychiatry* 2004; **43**: 1380–6.

Woolston JL. Case study: carbamazepine treatment of juvenile-onset bipolar disorder. *J Am Acad Child Adolesc Psychiatry* 1999; **38**: 335–8.

Wozniak J, Biederman J, Kiely K, et al. Mania-like symptoms suggestive of childhood-onset bipolar disorder in clinically referred children. *J Am Acad Child Adolesc Psychiatry* 1995; **34**: 867–76.

chapter 6

Therapeutic strategies of obsessive-compulsive disorder in children and adolescents

Donatella Marazziti, Chiara Pfanner, Mario Catena, Francesco Mungai, Laura Vivarelli and Silvio Presta

Introduction

Obsessive-compulsive disorder (OCD) is a common psychiatric condition during childhood and adolescence which continues to be underestimated and undertreated; in fact, the original assumption was that OCD was quite rare in childhood and that the occurrence of obsessive or compulsive phenomena should be considered a transient developmental pattern.

In spite of the high prevalence early in life, diagnosis is correctly made 17 years after the onset (Hollander and Weilgus-Kornwasser, 1997) with the result that most of the data available refer to clinical and therapeutic findings in adulthood. The limited amount of data from childhood can also be attributed to other factors, such as the absence of egodystonia, which is quite common, the reluctance of parents or relatives to consult a psychiatrist, the frequent misdiagnosis, and the small size of young samples available for reaching reliable conclusions. Nevertheless, OCD is estimated to be the second most common psychiatric disorder (after depression) in both children and adults and one which requires early recognition and assessment because of its significant potential impact on future global social adjustment, as it represents a primary cause of major disabilities in those ages and, sometimes, of permanent impairments later on.

In recent years, childhood and adolescence OCD has attracted an increasing focus which has promoted a deeper awareness of this illness, a better recognition with earlier interventions, as well as the setting up of more tailored and specific strategies, including psychotropic drugs (Karno et al, 1988). Although several questions still remain open and available data in children are meagre, as is the case for most psychiatric disorders, adult data show that current therapeutic stategies can permit effective management of the disorder and improvement in the quality of life of patients. On this basis, therefore, a similar approach might be beneficial in patients of different ages.

Epidemiology

Initial studies on the prevalence of OCD during childhood reported the presence of typical symptoms in only 0.2–1.3% of young psychiatric populations (Berman, 1942; Judd, 1965; Thomsen and Mikkelsen, 1991). Subsequently, a higher prevalence rate, up to 5%, was observed in Japan (Honjo et al, 1989). However, these data were based on studies carried out on children and adolescents who had been referred to psychiatric wards, thus only a small percentage of OCD children and adolescents were registered. Moreover, the authors did not report the prevalence of OCD in the general population, but in psychiatric samples. As far as surveys undertaken in non-referred groups of patients are concerned, epidemiologic evaluations have described an incidence ranging from 0.35% in the USA to 3.6% in Israel (Flament et al, 1988; Zohar et al, 1992); more recent data from the British nationwide survey of child mental health, carried out on a sample of more than 10 000 subjects, showed a prevalence of 0.25% (Heyman et al, 2001). When subsyndromal forms were included, the prevalence increased significantly up to 12.0% (Maina et al, 1999); another study, based on a screening of Danish school children, reported the presence of obsessive symptoms at a subclinical or clinical level in 4% of the sample and amongst 8-year-old German children, between 4 and 5% reported moderate and up to 3% severe obsessive symptoms (Thomsen and Mikkelsen, 1991).

This evidence suggests that OCD is a relatively common disorder during childhood and adolescence; considering the available public surveys, it may be concluded that the frequency of OCD in children and adolescents ranges between 0.5 and 2%. This is consistent with both the prevalence in the general population and the finding that at least 30–50% of adult patients report an onset of their disorder at an early age. It is not clear whether the prevalence of OCD is influenced by cultural factors and whether it changes at different ages.

In 80% of patients, the onset occurs before 18 years of age, but clear-cut OC manifestations in the form of rituals or stereotypes are often observed during early childhood. From the age of 3 years onwards, patients with a very early onset usually show more compulsive behaviors than obsessions. While with female patients the onset generally occurs during puberty (around the age of 11), male patients are more likely to show a prepubertal onset (around the age of 9); they are also more likely to have a family member affected by OCD or tic disorder and to show more severe symptoms and to present more frequent comorbidity with tic disorder (Flament et al, 1988; Leonard et al, 1992).

Clinical features

OCD is a psychiatric condition characterized by the presence either of obsessions or compulsions, or both. Obsessions are defined as recurrent and persistent thoughts, impulses, or images which are experienced in an intrusive and inappropriate way, at some time during the disorder, which cause marked anxiety and distress and which persist despite all attempts to try to ignore, suppress, or neutralize them. Compulsions are defined as repetitive behaviors or mental acts which a person feels driven to perform in response to an obsession or according to rigid rules; such behaviors are aimed at preventing or reducing distress or a dreaded event and are always unrealistic or excessive (American Psychiatric Association, 1994). Comparisons between children with severe OCD and matched normal controls did not suggest significant differences in the number or type of superstitions, but parents of affected subjects reported more marked patterns of early ritualistic behaviors representing early manifestations of the disorder (Leonard et al, 1990). The diagnosis of OCD in childhood can be rendered more difficult by patients hiding or disguising their symptoms or involving family members in the execution of rituals and, subsequently, a short-term decrease in patients' anxiety levels can reinforce and increase their OCD mechanisms. In addition, OCD children often consult non-psychiatric practitioners, such as pediatricians or dermatologists (because of skin conditions caused by excessive washing), neurologists (when tics are present), dentists (because of excessive cleaning of the teeth), and plastic surgeons (because of somatic obsessions or dysmorphophobic fears). As a result, it has been estimated that on average 8 years pass before psychiatric help is sought and that frequently this does not lead to a correct diagnosis.

The majority of OCD children and adolescents typically have both obsessive and compulsive symptoms; insight with regard to the excessive or unreasonable nature of their worries is rare (Catapano et al, 2001). Specific symptomatology does not exist, but, in most cases, there is a tendency over time towards a change in obsessive content and in illness severity (Rapoport, 1989; Swedo et al, 1989; Yarjura-Tobias et al, 1998). The majority of OCD children and adolescents experience both compulsive thoughts and compulsive actions; however, in individual cases, a child can experience compulsive thoughts without compulsive actions and vice versa. The nature of their obsessions is variable and can range from an unreasonable fear of germs and contamination or of personal harm, or an excessive sense of "right" and "wrong," to unrealistic and bizarre thoughts (Berkowitz and Rothman, 1960), such as fear of AIDS contamination during prepuberty (Fisman and Walsh, 1994). The most frequent compulsions (in decreasing order of frequency) include washing, repetition, checking, counting, ordering and arranging, touching, and hoarding (Judd, 1965; Flament et al, 1988; Fisman and Walsh, 1994) and sometimes the "just right" phenomenon is present.

If a child with compulsive washing rituals is hindered from carrying out rituals, he or she experiences a tremendous discomfort, or even shows violent fear. Compulsive washing can be so pronounced that the skin of the hands and feet becomes extremely dry. This is followed by tenderness and scaling, resulting in disintegration and, ultimately, in serious damage. Checking behavior is the second most common compulsive symptom. A child is compelled to check specific items over and over again. For example, the child will check that the front door is locked; even though the child has just found that it was, the nagging doubt that perhaps it was unlocked will creep back, compelling the child to check the door once again.

Several OCD children and adolescents suffer from compulsive thoughts regarding responsibility for the direct or indirect misfortune of others if they refrain from performing specific rituals or actions. A very common compulsive thought relates to sickness and death. Compulsive thoughts regarding sickness can almost be characterized as hypochondria. The child thinks that he or she is suffering from some kind of illness. In less common cases, some children stare at a specific part of the body, which they find extremely abnormal and which they would like to change. The rituals, which the young patient must complete, can involve extreme exaggeration of daily routines, or they can assume a more bizarre appearance. Other compulsive doubts are related to whether something would happen if they were to do or not to do a specific thing, and whether they have interpreted that which has happened correctly: this is generally labeled as "magic thinking."

A need for perfection is seen in many children, particularly at certain stages of their development. However, when it is seen to be exaggerated, it can also be an expression of OCD. In these patients, the homework is repeatedly corrected, or letters are incessantly rubbed and rewritten. Some OCD children have special demands with regard to symmetry: for example everything in the child's room must be placed in a specific and symmetric way and, at the extreme, in the whole house. Sometimes the child/adolescent must order his thoughts constantly until he or she is unable to concentrate on a simple game, or hold a conversation. Some OCD children are compelled to count, either up to a specific number, or a specific interval, or when he or she moves from one situation to another. This form is often so pervasive that the child has to start from the beginning if he has any doubt about how accurately he has counted. Children with OCD may also experience intrusive and unwelcome mental pictures, which can be of a violent, sexual, or obscene nature.

In adult OCD patients, and in rare cases in children and adolescents, the manifestation can be described as compulsive slowness. This symptom can be associated with difficulty in making even minor, everyday decisions.

The child may have a "place of refuge" at home, where compulsive thoughts can be controlled. In most cases, however, they tend to flare up when the child is in the company of others, or in a particular place; generally speaking, the child's own room becomes the only risk-free area.

When OCD onset occurs before puberty, it is characterized by non-impairing symptoms and by a greater number of obsessions and compulsions unrelated to the total duration of the illness, whereas late-onset OCD, starting during puberty, shows relatively fewer obsessions and compulsions which do correlate to the duration of the illness (Sobin et al, 1999). This would suggest that childhood OCD might represent a distinct genotype, with different gender distribution, familial loading, and clinical patterns (Eichstedt and Arnold, 2001). Adults with an early-onset OCD present higher scores on the Yale-Brown Obsessive Compulsive Scale (Y-BOCS) and higher frequencies of tic-like compulsions, sensory phenomena, and comorbid tic disorder. Poor response to clomipramine and selective serotonin re-uptake inhibitor (SSRI) treatment might identify a specific phenotypic subgroup, whose clinical differences are not restricted to childhood (do Rosário-Campos et al, 2001).

However, future studies are needed in order to validate preliminary observations that early-onset OCD might represent a more severe variant of the disorder. In addition, more information on possible clinical subtypes of childhood and adolescence OCD is warranted.

Course and prognosis

An episodic course with periods of full remission occurs in about 10–15% of adult OCD patients and this percentage tends to increase during childhood (Apter and Tyano, 1988), with rapid improvements occurring independently of any treatment in as many as one third of all cases (Flament et al, 1990), and more frequently in female patients (Thomson and Mikkelsen, 1995). In most cases (85%), patients experience changes in their symptoms, which generally take the form of different obsessions and compulsions existing simultaneously, but with the latest to develop gradually dominating those that had begun earlier (Rettew et al, 1992). In the case of very early-onset OCD (before the age of 6), it usually begins with a unique ritual rather than obsessive thinking. However, although Thomsen (1995) recognized severity of OCD in childhood as a key contributing factor to a poor eventual outcome (defined as the presence of OCD in adulthood), symptom severity as such does not necessarily indicate a poor prognosis, which would instead appear to be associated with a comorbidity with tics or odd cluster personality disorders (Peterson et al, 2001).

Comorbidity

Comorbidity seems to be very common in children and adolescents with OCD and may have a negative impact on treatment response and outcome. Childhood OCD may be preceded and/or followed by mood disorders (bipolar disorder, especially type II, or unipolar depression), other anxiety disorders (such as separation anxiety, panic disorder with agoraphobia, social phobia, or pavor nocturnus), eating disorders (anorexia), psychotic disorders (usually diagnosed as schizophreniform or atypical psychosis), tic disorder, disruptive disorders, or by attention deficit hyperactivity disorder (ADHD) (Bulik et al, 1997; Cassidy et al, 1999; Peterson et al, 2001). Chronologic age and age at onset seem to predict different comorbidity patterns, the first associated with the development of mood and psychotic disorders and the second with an increased risk of anxiety disorders and ADHD (Geller et al, 2001a).

A recent study reported that 57% of patients had at least one psychiatric disorder besides OCD and 30% had multiple other disorders. The response rates to antidepressants in patients with comorbid ADHD, tic disorder, or oppositional defiant disorder were significantly less than in patients with OCD only. Psychiatric comorbidity was associated with a greater rate of relapse (Geller et al, 2003a). In another study, comorbidity was found in 69% of the sample; 22% met criteria for disruptive disorders, 20% were diagnosed with mood disorders, 19% had anxiety disorders, and 17% had tic disorders (Reddy et al, 2000).

It is often difficult to determine which disorder, OCD or depression, appeared first. A primary depression should be considered in the presence of insomnia, suicidal ideation, psychomotor inhibition or agitation, melancholic thoughts, and appetite reduction; moreover, depressed adolescents often experience recurrent self-blaming thoughts regarding disasters, such as earthquakes, eruptions, air/train accidents, and feel that they are responsible for these events. At variance with obsessions, depressive thoughts are not egodystonic and reflect the sense of reality of adolescents. Some depressed children and adolescents may also suffer from auditory, visual, or, less frequently, olfactory hallucinations which are generally absent in OCD.

Schizophrenia usually occurs during adolescence or early adulthood; patients tend to isolate themselves, develop unusual interests, and present delusions and hallucinations (more often voices or visions). In contrast to OCD adolescents, schizophrenic patients do not consider these thoughts to be egodystonic. When obsessive thoughts are very severe and are part of the OCD patient's personality, they may achieve a psychotic level so that it may be difficult to distinguish between this "obsessive psychosis" and schizophrenia. In these cases, although patients are extremely involved in their obsessive thoughts and rituals, they experience them as being bizarre and they do not show delusions or thought disturbances. Studies on the long-term outcome of adolescent OCD did not report a higher risk of developing schizophrenia (Flament et al, 1990; Thomsen and Mikkelsen, 1991). Schizophrenia and OCD may co-occur simultaneously in the same patients and, in these cases, the prognosis is worst.

High rates of bipolar disorder (BD) comorbidity have recently been reported in OCD children and adolescents; in fact, 36.3% of patients were diagnosed as BD, 34.3% were diagnosed as OCD, and 29.4% were diagnosed as BD–OCD. Furthermore, BD of type II was more frequent in the BD–OCD patients than in the BD group and the age of onset was significantly earlier than in the pure OCD patients; the number of obsessions was not different between OCD patients with and without bipolar comorbidity, whereas pure OCD patients showed significantly more compulsions. Existential, philosophical, odd, and superstitious obsessions were significantly more frequent in BD–OCD than in pure OCD patients (Masi et al, 2004).

Several studies have underlined that OCD and anorexia nervosa may be related disorders; in fact, adolescents with anorexia show high scores on the obsessive rating scale and vice versa (Bulik et al, 1997). Moreover, similarities regarding neurotransmitter alterations have been demonstrated in patients with OCD and anorexia, which, in some cases, have been successfully treated with OCD medications. Anorexic adolescents often develop OCD symptoms unrelated to weight or food, such as obsessions and rituals, but little is known about their impact on the course of the illness. Although this evidence led some authors to include anorexia nervosa in the obsessive compulsive spectrum, there are however significant differences between the two conditions; in fact, anorexic adolescents usually present a distorted view of the body which may reach a psychotic level, and the fear of increasing weight may be more similar to a delusion than to an obsession, not being egodystonic and undesirable.

Earlier onset of panic disorder has been found in children and adolescents with OCD or obsessive-compulsive symptoms in separation anxiety disorder, but not simple phobia or social phobia; patients with both childhood separation anxiety disorder and OCD had an even earlier onset of panic disorder than those with isolated childhood separation anxiety disorder or OCD; this evidence would suggest the existence of a specific cluster of associations between separation anxiety, OCD, and early-onset panic disorder (Goodwin et al, 2001). Recently, a growing body of evidence has suggested that ADHD is more frequent in pediatric OCD than in control subjects. An incidence of ADHD in OCD children and adolescents as high as 30% has been reported (Heyman et al, 2001). However, it remains unclear whether the decreased attention, distractibility, and restlessness seen in OCD children are secondary to obsessional ideation or due to ADHD. Children with OCD plus ADHD show significantly more social and attentional problems and aggressive behaviors, compared with children with OCD only. Although the nature of the relationship between the two disorders is not clear, the presence of ADHD in OCD children may be considered a subtype of the disorder with different etiology, clinical features, and, perhaps, prognosis.

In childhood, OCD is often seen in association with tic disorder, especially Tourette syndrome (TS). Some investigators have described OCD or obsessive-compulsive symptoms in TS patients with an incidence of between 40 and 70% (Eichstedt and Arnold, 2001; Leanard et al, 1991). Recently 19% of patients with mild to moderate tic disorder were shown to suffer from OCD, with another 46% suffering from obsessive-compulsive symptoms (Eichstedt and Arnold, 2001). Tic-related OCD appears to have an earlier onset, usually prepubertal, than OCD alone and the intensity of tics seems to be related to the severity of obsessive- compulsive symptomatology. It has also been suggested that there might be a genetic overlapping between TS and OCD, in the sense that OCD may represent an alternative phenotypic manifestation of genetic vulnerability to TS.

It seems possible, as in adulthood (Perugi et al, 1997), to identify different course-based subtypes of the disorder. An episodic course of the illness has been related to multiple comorbidity with bipolar II spectrum disorder, panic disorder, social phobia, and alcohol and marijuana abuse

(Douglass et al, 1995), while the co-occurrence of unipolar depression and generalized anxiety seems to predict a chronic evolution.

Treatment options

The treatment of OCD has changed dramatically since the 1980s, with two approaches systematically assessed and empirically shown to improve the core symptoms of the disorder in children and adolescents. Treatment options include psychodynamic psychotherapy, individual and family therapy, behavioral therapy, and pharmacologic treatment.

The significant interpersonal variations in terms of symptomatology, comorbidity, family issues, and psychosocial impairment in childhood OCD presentation require the design of a comprehensive and tailored treatment plan, as this strategy may have a significant influence on compliance and therapeutic results.

Psychodynamic psychotherapy

This is a controversial approach; according to several authors, traditional psychoanalytic intervention has been considered ineffective (Jenike, 1990). However, this approach may be useful in reducing the impact of illness on the patient's self-esteem, relationships, and on other internal conflicts which may accompany true OCD phenomena, and may improve compliance with more specific anti-OC treatments.

Individual and family therapy

The identification of family problems, inappropriate behavioral boundaries amongst family members, or subsyndromal (or even full) psychiatric disorders in the parents of children with OCD may significantly improve the global diagnostic evaluation. These factors may influence both a family's and a patient's functioning, thus affecting long-term outcome (Hoover and Insel, 1984) and, sometimes, completely blocking treatment evolution. An appropriate understanding of the family involvement in the ritual execution may improve behavioral abnormalities. In fact, the family context represents a possible risk factor in the development and maintenance of OCD. More recently, a cognitive-behavioral family treatment protocol, consisting of a series of self-report measures assessing OC features, depressive symptoms, and family involvement in OCD, proved quite effective (Waters et al, 2001).

Behavioral therapy

Some case reports have suggested the effectiveness of cognitive-behavioral therapy (CBT), especially in the form of exposure and response prevention (ERP), not only in adult OCD (Marks, 1987; Baer, 1992; Greist, 1992) but also in paediatric OCD (Bolton et al, 1983; Wolfe and Wolfe, 1991; March et al, 1994). Exposure-based intervention includes gradual exposure or flooding and response prevention acts on blocking rituals or avoidance patterns (Dar and Greist, 1992). Nevertheless, factors such as repetitive family stressors and even inadequacy on the part of the clinician in applying these techniques, may easily cause a premature discontinuation. It is therefore important to determine the way in which patients and parents consider symptoms or experience distress, resistance, and interference. This procedure helps in obtaining a child's cooperation, minimizing initial anxiety, establishing a hierarchy of interventions, and individualizing treatment. In particular, it has been suggested that very young children may respond well to brief CBT (Tolin, 2001).

In addition to ERP, other behavioral techniques (relaxation techniques, anxiety management training, or cognitive restructuring), with special modifications for their use in childhood, should be considered. ERP may be supplemented by additional cognitive therapies (habit reversal, thought stopping, satiation), especially for severe conditions such as "complex tic-like rituals" (Vitulano et al, 1992). The family needs to be involved in the treatment to a varying extent according to individual situations. This therapy usually involves 13–20 weekly individual or family sessions and homework assignments.

Prognostic indicators of treatment response include the presence of motivation, of overt rituals and compulsions, and the absence of complicating comorbid ilnesses (Foa and Emmelkamp, 1983). Behavior modifications would seem to be less effective in patients with dominant obsessions, or in those who are very young or uncooperative. CBT may be useful for the treatment of anxious patients older than 6 years (Cartwright-Hatton et al, 2004). More recent intervention proposals have suggested the effectiveness of the combination of CBT and pharmacotherapy and its preventive effect on relapse when medication is discontinued (March et al, 1994).

A recent randomized, controlled, 12-week study explored the evaluation of CBT alone, sertraline alone, and combined CBT and setraline in a sample of 112 OCD patients aged 7–17 years (Pediatric OCD Treatment Study Team, 2004). Even though CBT alone, sertra-line alone, and combined treatment were superior to placebo, com-bined treatment was superior to both CBT alone and sertraline alone, which did not differ from each other. The remission rate for combined treatment did not differ from that for CBT, but was higher than that for sertraline alone. According to the authors, these results suggest that children and adolescents with OCD should begin treatment with a combination of CBT plus an SSRI or CBT alone.

Pharmacologic treatments

Although the effectiveness of CBT has been widely reported during its global life-span (Barrett et al, 2004), several OCD patients can be refractory to non-pharmacologic interventions. The first observations highlighting the involvement of serotonin in the pharmacologic treatment of OCD were related to the effectiveness of clomipramine, a tricyclic antidepressant (TCA) with a prevalent inhibitory activity on serotonin re-uptake. Studies in adult samples comparing clomipramine with other TCAs, such as nortriptyline, amitriptyline, imipramine, and desipramine, suggested its selective efficacy on OCD symptoms (Fineberg, 1996). Subsequently, the synthesis of selective SSRIs definitively supported the crucial role of the serotonin system in the pathophysiology and treatment of OCD. In fact, several placebo-controlled studies, in adults, demon-strated the efficacy of fluvoxamine, fluoxetine, sertraline, paroxetine, and citalopram in OCD (Zohar and Westenberg, 2000). Although the efficacy of SSRIs in adult OCD has been widely recognized and confirmed, few controlled (and short-term only) studies are currently available on younger OCD patients.

Clomipramine

Clomipramine was the first agent approved by the US Food and Drug Administration for the treatment of OCD. The effectiveness of clomipramine in children and adolescents has been confirmed in two placebo/controlled trials (Flament et al, 1985; De Veaugh-Geiss et al, 1992), and in one study it was compared with desipramine (Leonard et al, 1989), doses ranging between 75 and 200mg per day. A moderate or marked improvement during clomipramine was apparent by 5 weeks of treatment in 75% of subjects, independent from the presence of depressive symptoms at baseline. Clomipramine may provoke several side-effects; the most common observed in children include (in decreasing order of frequency) dry mouth, somnolence, dizziness, fatigue, tremor, headache, constipation, anorexia, abdominal pain, dyspepsia, insomnia, and hypomania (De Veaugh-Geiss et al, 1992; Leonard et al, 1995). A baseline and periodic ECG or plasma level monitoring are, therefore, generally recommended. Abrupt discontinuation may be followed by withdrawal symptoms of gastrointestinal distress, such as a cholinergic rebound syndrome. Special caution should be paid to epileptic children because of the potential risk of seizures.

SSRIs

All SSRIs are considered effective and well tolerated, as shown in controlled trials or in long-term treatments, and, usually, at lower dosages than in adults (Riddle et al, 1992, 2001; Thomsen, 1997). A recent meta-analysis of published randomized, controlled medication trials in pediatric OCD (12 studies, 1044 participants) showed a highly significant difference between medications and placebo, with clomipramine being superior to each of the SSRIs (fluoxetine, paroxetine, sertraline, fluvoxamine), and with the SSRIs being comparably effective (Geller et al, 2003b). Given their similarities, the choice between one SSRI and another largely depends upon personal preference or the possibility of drug interactions. Sertraline and citalopram are relatively weak inhibitors of the hepatic cytochrome P450 enzymes which metabolize commonly prescribed drugs, and may be preferred if drug interactions are likely to be a problem. Fluoxetine and paroxetine are potent inhibitors of the CYP 2D6 isoenzyme which metabolizes TCAs, antipsychotics, anti-arrythmics, and beta-blockers. Fluvoxamine inhibits both the CYP 1A2 and CYP 3A4 enzymes. For all SSRIs, caution should be paid with concomitant medications, especially terfenadine, astemizole, and ketoconazole, which can prolong the QT interval, and also with regard to combinations of serotonin reuptake inhibitors (SRIs), that should be avoided for the absence of controlled studies and because of the increased risk of ECG abnormalities.

The most commonly described side-effects include psychomotor activation, restlessness, insomnia and nervousness, nausea, gastrointestinal complaints, and hypomania. Systematic dose–response data are not available for children, while side-effects generally appear to be dose-dependent.

Fluoxetine The effectiveness of fluoxetine has been shown in three double-blind, placebo-controlled studies (Geller et al, 2001b; Liebowitz et al, 2002). Fluoxetine, fixed-dose (20 mg/day), was also found to be effective in a short- and long-term open-label trial (Semerci and Unal, 2001).

Sertraline In the largest controlled study completed to date, a multi-center placebo-controlled trial, significant differences between sertraline and placebo emerged at week 3 and persisted for the duration of the study (March et al, 1998). Sertraline is effective in long-term open trials (12 months), with an initial acute response converting to remission and improved functional status in a substantial proportion of patients (Wagner et al, 2003).

Fluvoxamine Fluvoxamine is generally well tolerated and has a proven short-term efficacy compared with placebo (Riddle et al, 2001). Reduction in anxiety symptoms during fluvoxamine treatment has been observed for up to one year (Yaryura-Tobias et al, 2000).

Paroxetine Few data are available for the treatment of children and adolescent OCD with paroxetine. Paroxetine has been found to be effective and well tolerated in a short-term, open-label treatment trial (Rosenberg et al, 1999). Continued paroxetine treatment seemed to reduce the relapse rates, as compared with placebo, even in those patients presenting comorbid disorders (Geller et al, 2003a). Paroxetine treatment was associated with a reduction in amygdala volume in pediatric OCD (Szeszko et al, 2004) and in decreased caudate glutamatergic concentrations (Rosenberg et al, 2000).

Citalopram The clinical effectiveness and tolerability of citalopram during short- (Mukaddes et al, 2003) and long-term treatment (Leonard et al, 1991) was similar to the other SSRIs. Placebo-controlled studies are not currently available.

In conclusion, while considering the higher safety, the tolerability profile, and the lower rates of premature discontinuation, SSRIs should be considered the first-line treatment, with clomipramine as a second-line treatment reserved for patients who do not tolerate SSRIs or who have failed to respond to them.

The optimal duration of maintenance treatment is still unclear, since relapses are frequent when medications are discontinued (Leonard et al, 1991). It is generally agreed that anti-obsessional drugs should be maintained for at least 12–18 months after a satisfactory clinical response has been obtained. Once the decision is made to attempt reduction or discontinuation, the tapering should be gradual.

Augmentation strategies

Despite the effectiveness of SSRIs, nearly 40% of OCD adult patients experience poor or no improvement with these treatments; furthermore, a few patients experience full symptom remission (McDougle et al, 1993). It has been reported that, notwithstanding a significant improvement in functioning, interfering symptoms usually persist (Goodman et al, 1989). Several therapeutic strategies in adults have been proposed, including the use of standard pharmacologic agents in higher dosages or administered via an alternative route, combination drug treatment, and the use of novel compounds.

The neurobiologic basis of these augmentation strategies consists in enhancing the serotonin function, or in adding a dopamine receptor antagonist activity, such as that displayed by some typical or atypical antipsychotics, to ongoing SRI drugs; however, most of these strategies are empirical and have not been confirmed at the bedside or by means of controlled studies.

In juvenile OCD, the overall effect size for medication was modest, while suggesting the need for augmenting strategies or novel medications. In fact, adjunctive medications are frequently used in ordinary clinical settings, as augmenting strategies for unsatisfactory response to SRI monotherapy (McDougle, 1997), and/or to manage comorbid mental disorders, even though empirical evidence supporting effectiveness of augmenting strategies in children and adolescents is still meager. Clinical features of children and adolescents responding to SRI monotherapy, as compared with those of patients refractory to SRI monotherapy, are still under debate. If a response is not obtained at maximal tolerated doses in two or more single medication trials, an augmentation with an additional agent may be necessary.

Clomipramine may be added to an SSRI at a low daily dose of 25–50 mg/day (Figueroa et al, 1998); higher doses of clomipramine could potentially lead to toxicity due to competitive inhibition. The blood levels of tricyclic antidepressants should be measured regularly to ensure patient safety if the two classes of drugs are used together.

Investigations of SRI augmentation with serotonin-enhancing agents have also failed to demonstrate substantial benefits for treatment-refractory childhood cases: the drugs proposed include clonazepam (Leonard et al, 1994) and buspirone (Thomsen and Mikkelsen, 1999), but currently no controlled study has been carried out to confirm or reject these strategies.

Combination treatment with SRIs and dopamine receptor antagonist drugs, such as typical (haloperidol and pimozide mainly) and atypical antipsychotics (risperidone mainly), appears to provide an improved response for the subtype of OCD patients who have comorbid tic-spectrum disorders (Keuneman et al, 2005), although large-scale studies of the efficacy and tolerability of these regimens are not yet available. Haloperidol and particularly pimozide are the two most widely used compounds (Shapiro et al, 1989), but their use is limited by the frequent onset of invalidating side-effects.

Risperidone is at least as effective as pimozide in the treatment of TS, with a comparable efficacy also on comorbid conditions, and with a similar efficacy and safety for both children and adults (Bruggeman et al, 2001; Gilbert et al, 2004; Roessner et al, 2004). An open-label case series described a significant reduction in OC symptoms during risperidone augmentation treatment in juvenile resistant OCD (Fitzgerald et al, 1999).

Olanzapine appears to provide an improved response in the treatment of aggression and tics in children with TS (Stephens et al, 2004).

No data are currently available regarding newer antipsychotics, in particular quetiapine, ziprasidone, and aripiprazole, as well as regarding novel compounds which have shown some effectiveness in resistant adult OCD patients, such as inositol, tryptophan, tramadol, flutamide, etc., in augmentation strategies for pediatric OCD patients.

When high levels of generalized anxiety are present (i.e. when patients are unable to complete behavioral goals), benzodiazepines are useful in treatment regimens. It should also be underlined that, sometimes, the correct identification of comorbidity conditions may have relevant treatment implications: for example, a mood stabilizer should be added to an SRI when bipolar disorder co-exists with OCD (Masi et al, 2004). In fact, anti-obsessive treatment with SSRIs alone may, potentially, induce hypomanic or full manic switches, not infrequent with immature brain structures.

PANDAS

A newly described subgroup of children with tics and/or OCD is thought to develop, or have exacerbation of symptoms, following infection with group A-hemolytic streptococci (Swedo et al, 1998). This subgroup has been identified by the name PANDAS (pediatric autoimmune neuropsychiatric disorders associated with streptococcal infections); OCD pathophysiology in these patients is thought to develop through an autoimmune process. The identification of such a subgroup has facilitated the testing of novel treatment and prevention strategies, including antibiotic prophylaxis, intravenous immunoglobulin, and plasmapheresis, which are currently under investigation.

Conclusions

Although OCD is a relatively common disorder in childhood and adolescence, with profound effects during subsequent years, it is not easily diagnosed. This can be due to several factors, such as the common absence of egodystonia during childhood and adolescence, the reluctance of parents to consult a psychiatrist, and frequent diagnostic mistakes, as well as the limited size of young samples.

Follow-up studies on the course of childhood-onset OCD are still required in order to investigate the stability of OCD diagnosis throughout development, adulthood, and later life; the differences in incidence and prevalence between different "special populations;" lifetime comorbidity patterns; the comparable efficacy of anti-obsessive drugs (and augmentation strategies) for pediatric and adult OCD; and the impact of early treatments on clinical and social outcomes (Presta et al, 2003).

Short- and longer-term follow-up studies have provided definite evidence that two types of treatment intervention can markedly improve the core symptoms of OCD and significantly reduce impairment deriving from this pathologic condition. CBT may be the initial treatment of choice in milder cases without significant comorbidity, whereas severity of OC symptoms, presence of comorbid conditions, or insufficient cognitive skills to cooperate in CBT are strong indicators for pharmacologic treatment with SRIs. At the moment, SSRIs can be considered the first-line treatment, for their specific anti-obsessional effectiveness and the favorable side-effect profile, which is relevant in any age, but particularly in children and adolescents.

In addition, further controlled double-blind or crossover studies are required to establish the role of novel compounds and augmentation strategies in juvenile refractory OCD, as well as to identify possible clinical features or comorbid patterns which may be associated with a positive or a negative response.

However, most important is the evidence that further research is needed in order to elucidate the basic neurobiologic mechanisms in OCD, to improve understanding and long-term outcome of what may prove to be a heterogeneous disorder.

References

American Psychiatric Association, *Diagnostic and Statistical Manual of Mental Disorders (DSM-IV)* 4th edn (revised). Washington, DC: American Psychiatric Press, 1994.

Apter A, Tyano S. Obsessive compulsive disorders in adolescence. *J Adolesc* 1988; **11**: 183–94.

Baer L. Behavior therapy for obsessive-compulsive disorder and trichotillomania: implications for Tourette's syndrome. *Adv Neurol* 1992; **58**: 333–40.

Barrett P, Healy-Farrell L, March JS. Cognitive-behavioral family treatment of childhood obsessive-compulsive disorder: a controlled trial. *J Am Acad Child Adolesc Psychiatry* 2004; **43**: 46–62.

Berkowitz PH, Rothman EP. *The disturbed child; recognition and psychoeducational therapy in the classroom.* New York: New York University Press; 1960: 61–5.

Berman L. Obsessive-compulsive neurosis in children. *J Nerv Ment Dis* 1942; **95**: 26–39.

Bolton D, Collins S, Steinberg D. The treatment of obsessive-compulsive disorder in adolescence: a report of fifteen cases. *Br J Psychiatry* 1983; **142**: 456–64.

Bruggeman R, van der Linden C, Buitelaar JK, et al. Risperidone versus pimozide in Tourette's disorder: a comparative double-blind parallel-group study. *J Clin Psychiatry* 2001; **62**: 50–6.

Bulik CM, Sullivan PF, Fear JL, Joyce PR. Eating disorders and antecedent anxiety disorders: a controlled study. *Acta Psychiatr Scand* 1997; **96**: 101–7.

Cartwright-Hatton S, Roberts C, Chitsabesan P, et al. Systematic review of the efficacy of cognitive behavior therapies for childhood and adolescent anxiety disorders. *Br J Clin Psychol* 2004; **43**: 421–36.

Cassidy E, Allsopp M, Williams T. Obsessive compulsive symptoms at initial presentation of adolescent eating disorders. *Eur Child Adolesc Psychiatry* 1999; **8**: 193–9.

Catapano F, Sperandeo R, Perris F, et al. Insight and resistance in patients with obsessive-compulsive disorder. *Psychopathology* 2001; **34**: 62–8.

Dar R, Greist J. Behavior therapy for obsessive compulsive disorder. *Psychiatr Clin North Am* 1992; **15**: 885–94.

De Veaugh-Geiss J, Moroz G, Biederman J, et al. Clomipramine hydrochloride in childhood and adolescent obsessive-compulsive disorder: a multicenter trial. *J Am Acad Child Adolesc Psychiatry* 1992; **31**: 45–9.

do Rosario-Campos MC, Leckman JF, Mercadante MT, et al. Adults with early-onset obsessive-compulsive disorder. *Am J Psychiatry* 2001; **158**: 1899–903.

Douglass HM, Moffitt TE, Dar R, et al. Obsessive-compulsive disorder in a birth cohort of 18-year-olds: prevalence and predictors. *J Am Acad Child Adolesc Psychiatry* 1995; **34**: 1424–31.

Eichstedt JA, Arnold SL. Childhood-onset obsessive-compulsive disorder: a tic-related subtype of OCD? *Clin Psychol Rev* 2001; **21**: 137–57.

Figueroa Y, Rosenberg DR, Birmaher B, Keshavan MS. Combination treatment with clomipramine and selective serotonin reuptake inhibitors for obsessive-compulsive disorder in children and adolescents. J Child Adolesc Psychopharmacol 1998; **8**: 61–7.

Fineberg N. Refining treatment approaches in obsessive-compulsive disorder. *Int Clin Psychopharmacol* 1996; **11**: 13–22.

Fisman SN, Walsh L. Obsessive-compulsive disorder and fear of AIDS contamination in childhood. *J Am Acad Child Adolesc Psychiatry* 1994; **33**: 349–53.

Fitzgerald KD, Stewart CM, Tawile V, Rosenberg DR. Risperidone augmentation of serotonin reuptake inhibitor treatment of pediatric obsessive compulsive disorder. *J Child Adolesc Psychopharmacol* 1999; **9**: 115–23.

Flament MF, Rapoport JL, Berg C, et al. Clomipramine treatment of childhood obsessive-compulsive disorder. *Arch Gen Psychiatry* 1985; **42**: 977–83.

Flament MF, Whitaker A, Rapoport JL, et al. Obsessive compulsive disorder in adolescence: an epidemiological study. *J Am Acad Child Adolesc Psychiatry* 1988; **27**: 764–71.

Flament MF, Koby E, Rapoport JL, et al. Childhood obsessive compulsive disorder: a prospective follow-up study. *J Child Psychol Psychiatry* 1990; **31**: 363–80.

Foa E, Emmelkamp P. *Failures in behavior therapy*. New York: Wiley & Sons; 1983.

Geller DA, Biederman J, Faraone SV, et al. Disentangling chronological age from age of onset in children and adolescents with obsessive-compulsive disorder. *Int J Neuropsychopharmacol* 2001a; **4**: 169–78.

Geller DA, Hoog SL, Heiligenstein JH, et al. Fluoxetine Pediatric OCD Study Team. Fluoxetine treatment for obsessive-compulsive disorder in children and adolescents: a placebo-controlled clinical trial. *J Am Acad Child Adolesc Psychiatry* 2001b; **40**: 773–9.

Geller DA, Biederman J, Stewart SE, et al. Impact of comorbidity on response to paroxetine in pediatric obsessive-compulsive disorder: is the use of exclusion criteria empirically supported in randomized clinical trials? *J Child Adolesc Psychopharmacol* 2003a; **13**: S19–S29.

Geller DA, Biederman J, Stewart SE, et al. Which SSRI? A meta-analysis of pharmacotherapy trials in pediatric obsessive-compulsive disorder. *Am J Psychiatry* 2003b; **160**: 1919–28.

Gilbert DL, Batterson JR, Sethuraman G, Sallee FR. Tic reduction with risperidone versus pimozide in a randomized, double-blind, crossover trial. *J Am Acad Child Adolesc Psychiatry* 2004; **43**: 206–14.

Goodman WK, Price LH, Rasmussen SA, et al. Efficacy of fluvoxamine in obsessive-compulsive disorder. A double-blind comparison with placebo. *Arch Gen Psychiatry* 1989; **46**: 36–44.

Goodwin R, Lipsitz JD, Chapman TF, et al. Obsessive-compulsive disorder and separation anxiety co-morbidity in early onset panic disorder. *Psychol Med* 2001; **31**: 1307–10.

Greist JH. An integrated approach to treatment of obsessive-compulsive disorder. *J Clin Psychiatry* 1992; **53**: 38–41.

Heyman I, Fombonne E, Simmons H, et al. Prevalence of obsessive-compulsive disorder in the British nationwide survey of child mental health. *Br J Psychiatry* 2001; **179**: 324–9.

Hollander E, Weilgus-Kornwasser J. Counting the cost – the psychosocial and economic burden of OCD. *Focus on OCD* 1997; **5**: 3–5.

Honjo S, Hirano C, Murase S, et al. Obsessive-compulsive symptoms in childhood and adolescence. *Acta Psychiatr Scand* 1989; **80**: 83–91.

Hoover CF, Insel TR. Families of origin in obsessive compulsive disorder. *J Nerv Ment Dis* 1984; **172**: 207–15.

Jenike MA. *Psychotherapy of obsessive-compulsive personality disorder.* Chicago, IL: Year Book Medical; 1990.

Judd LL. Obsessive compulsive neurosis in children. *Arch Gen Psychiatry* 1965; **12**: 136–43.

Karno M, Golding JM, Sorenson SB, Burnam MA. The epidemiology of obsessive compulsive disorder in five U.S. communities. *Arch Gen Psychiatry* 1988; **45**: 1094–9.

Keuneman RJ, Pokos V, Weerasundera R, Castle DJ. Antipsychotic treatment in obsessive-compulsive disorder: a literature review. *Aust NZ J Psychiatry* 2005; **39**: 336–43.

Leonard HL, Swedo SE, Rapoport JL, et al. Treatment of obsessive compulsive disorder with clomipramine and desipramine in children and adolescents: a double-blind crossover comparison. *Arch Gen Psychiatry* 1989; **46**: 1088–92.

Leonard HL, Goldberger EL, Rapoport JL, et al. Childhood rituals: normal development or obsessive-compulsive syptoms? *J Am Acad Child Adolesc Psychiatry* 1990; **29**: 17–23.

Leonard HL, Swedo SE, Lenane MC, et al. A double-blind desipramine substitution during long-term clomipramine treatment in children and adolescents with obsessive-compulsive disorder. *Arch Gen Psychiatry* 1991; **48**: 922–7.

Leonard HL, Lenane MC, Swedo SE, et al. Tics and Tourette's syndrome: a 2 to 7–year follow-up study of 54 obsessive-compulsive children. *Am J Psychiatry* 1992; **149**: 1244–51.

Leonard HL, Topol D, Bukstein O, et al. Clonazepam as an augmenting agent in the treatment of childhood-onset obsessive-compulsive disorder. *J Am Acad Child Adolesc Psychiatry* 1994; **33**: 792–4.

Leonard HL, Swedo SE, March J, et al. Obsessive compulsive disorder. In: Gabbard G, ed. *Treatment of psychiatric disorders.* Washington DC: American Psychiatric Press; 1995: 301–13.

Liebowitz MR, Turner SM, Piacentini J, et al. Fluoxetine in children and adolescents with OCD:a placebo-controlled trial. *J Am Acad Child Adolesc Psychiatry* 2002; **41**: 1431–8.

McDougle CJ. Update on pharmacologic management of OCD: agents and augmentation. *J Clin Psychiatry* 1997; **58**: 11–17.

McDougle CJ, Goodman WK, Leckman JF, Price LH. The psychopharmacology of obsessive compulsive disorder. Implications for treatment and pathogenesis. *Psychiatr Clin North Am* 1993; **16**: 749–66.

Maina G, Albert U, Bogetto L, Ravizza L. Obsessive compulsive syndromes in older adolescents. *Acta Psychiatr Scand* 1999; **100**: 447–50.

March JS, Mulle K, Herbel B. Behavioral psychotherapy for children and adolescents with obsessive-compulsive disorder: an open trial of a new protocol-driven treatment package. *J Am Acad Child Adolesc Psychiatry* 1994; **33**: 333–41.

March JS, Biederman J, Wolchow R, et al. Sertraline in children and adolescents with obsessive-compulsive disorder. A multicenter randomized controlled trial. *JAMA* 1998; **280**: 1752–6.

Marks IM. *Fears, phobias and rituals, panic anxiety and their disorders.* Oxford: Oxford University Press; 1987.

Masi G, Perugi G, Toni C, et al. Obsessive-compulsive bipolar comorbidity: focus on children and adolescents. *J Affect Disord* 2004; **78**: 175–83.

Mukaddes NM, Abali O, Kaynak N. Citalopram treatment of children and adolescents with obsessive-compulsive disorder: a preliminary report. *Psychiatry Clin Neurosci* 2003; **57**: 405–8.

Pediatric OCD Treatment Study (POTS) Team. Cognitive-behavior therapy, sertraline, and their combination in children and adolescents with obsessive-compulsive disorder: Pediatric OCD Treatment Study (POTS) randomized controlled trial. *JAMA* 2004; **292**: 1969–76.

Perugi G, Akiskal HS, Pfanner C, et al. The clinical impact of bipolar and unipolar affective comorbidity on obsessive-compulsive disorder. *J Affective Dis* 1997; **46**: 15–23.

Peterson BS, Pine DS, Cohen P, Brook JS. Prospective, longitudinal study of tic, obsessive-compulsive, and attention-deficit/hyperactivity disorders in an epidemiological sample. *J Am Acad Child Adolesc Psychiatry* 2001; **40**: 685–95.

Presta S, Marazziti D, Dell'Osso L, et al. Obsessive-compulsive disorder in childhood and adolescence. *Psychopathology* 2003; **36**: 55–64.

Rapoport JL. *Obsessive compulsive disorder in children and adolescents.* Washington DC: American Psychiatric Press; 1989.

Reddy YC, Reddy PS, Srinath S, et al. Comorbidity in juvenile obsessive-compulsive disorder: a report from India. *Can J Psychiatry* 2000; **45**: 274–8.

Rettew DC, Swedo SE, Leonard HL, et al. Obsessions and compulsions across time in 79 children and adolescents with obsessive-compulsive disorder. *J Am Acad Child Adolesc Psychiatry* 1992; **31**: 1050–6.

Riddle MA, Scahill L, King RA, et al. Double-blind, crossover trial of fluoxetine and placebo in children and adolescents with obsessive-compulsive disorder. *J Am Acad Child Adolesc Psychiatry* 1992; **31**: 1062–9.

Riddle MA, Reeve EA, Yaryura-Tobias JA, et al. Fluvoxamine for children and adolescents with obsessive-compulsive disorder: a randomized, controlled, multicenter trial. *J Am Acad Child Adolesc Psychiatry* 2001; **40**: 222–9.

Roessner V, Banaschewski T, Rothenberger A. Therapy of tic-disorders. *Z Kinder Jugendpsychiatr Psychother* 2004; **32**: 245–63.

Rosenberg DR, Stewart CM, Fitzgerald KD, et al. Paroxetine open-label treatment of pediatric outpatients with obsessive-compulsive disorder. *J Am Acad Child Adolesc Psychiatry* 1999; **38**: 1180–5.

Rosenberg DR, MacMaster FP, Keshavan MS, et al. Decrease in caudate glutamatergic concentrations in pediatric obsessive-compulsive disorder patients taking paroxetine. *J Am Acad Child Adolesc Psychiatry* 2000; **39**: 1096–103.

Semerci ZB, Unal F. An open trial and discontinuation study of fluoxetine in children and adolescents with obsessive-compulsive disorder. *Turk J Pediatr* 2001; **43**: 323–8.

Shapiro E, Shapiro AK, Fulop G. Controlled study of haloperidol, pimozide and placebo for the treatment of Gilles de la Tourette's syndrome. *Arch Gen Psychiatry* 1989; **46**: 722–30.

Sobin C, Blundell M, Weiller F, et al. Phenotypic characteristics of obsessive-compulsive disorder ascertained in adulthood. *J Psychiatr Res* 1999; **33**: 265–73.

Stephens RJ, Bassel C, Sandor P. Olanzapine in the treatment of aggression and tics in children with Tourette's syndrome – a pilot study. *J Child Adolesc Psychopharmacol* 2004; **14**: 255–66.

Swedo SE, Rapoport JL, Leonard H, et al. Obsessive-compulsive disorder in children and adolescents: clinical phenomenology of 70 consecutive cases. *Arch Gen Psychiatry* 1989; **46**: 335–44.

Swedo SE, Leonard HL, Garvey M, et al. Pediatric autoimmune neuropsychiatric disorders associated with streptococcal infections: clinical description of the first 50 cases. *Am J Psychiatry* 1998; **155**: 264–71.

Szeszko PR, MacMillan S, McMeniman M, et al. Amygdala volume reductions in pediatric patients with obsessive-compulsive disorder treated with paroxetine: preliminary findings. *Neuropsychopharmacology* 2004; **29**: 826–32.

Thomsen PH. Obsessive compulsive disorder in children and adolescents: predictors in childhood for long-term phenomenological course. *Acta Psychiatr Scand* 1995; **92**: 255–9.

Thomsen PH. Child and adolescent obsessive-compulsive disorder treated with citalopram: findings from an open trial of 23 cases. *J Child Adolesc Psychopharmacol* 1997; **7**: 157–66.

Thomsen PH, Mikkelsen HU. Children and adolescents with obsessive-compulsive disorder. The demographic and diagnostic characteristics of 61 Danish patients. *Acta Psychiatr Scand* 1991; **83**: 262–6.

Thomsen PH, Mikkelsen HU. Course of obsessive-compulsive disorder in children and adolescents: a prospective follow-up study of 23 Danish cases. *J Am Acad Child Adolesc Psychiatry* 1995; **34**: 1432–40.

Thomsen PH, Mikkelsen HU. The addition of buspirone to SSRI in the treatment of adolescent obsessive-compulsive disorder. A study of six cases. *Eur Child Adolesc Psychiatry* 1999; **8**: 143–8.

Tolin DF. Case study: bibliotherapy and extinction treatment of obsessive-compulsive disorder in a 5-year-old boy. *J Am Acad Child Adolesc Psychiatry* 2001; **40**: 1111–14.

Vitulano LA, King RA, Scahill L, Cohen DJ. Behavioral treatment of children and adolescents with trichotillomania. *J Am Acad Child Adolesc Psychiatry* 1992; **31**: 139–46.

Wagner KD, Cook EH, Chung H, Messig M. Remission status after long-term sertraline treatment of pediatric obsessive-compulsive disorder. *J Child Adolesc Psychopharmacol* 2003; **13**: S53–60.

Waters TL, Barrett PM, March JS. Cognitive-behavioral family treatment of childhood obsessive-compulsive disorder: preliminary findings. *Am J Psychother* 2001; **55**: 372–87.

Wolfe RP, Wolfe LS. Assessment and treatment of obsessive-compulsive disorder in children. *Behav Modif* 1991; **15**: 372–93.

Yarjura-Tobias JA, Stevens KP, Neziroglu F. A review of childhood and adolescent obsessive-compulsive disorder. Associaçao Brasileira de Psiquiatria Biologica. *Psiquiatria Biologica* 1998; **6**: 19–27.

Yaryura-Tobias JA, Grunes MS, Walz J, Neziroglu F. Parental obsessive-compulsive disorder as a prognostic factor in a year long fluvoxamine treatment in childhood and adolescent obsessive-compulsive disorder. *Int Clin Psychopharmacol* 2000; **15**: 163–8.

Zohar J, Westenberg HG. Anxiety disorders: a review of tricyclic antidepressants and selective serotonin reuptake inhibitors. *Acta Psychiatr Scand* 2000; **403**: 39–49.

Zohar AH, Ratzoni G, Pauls DL, et al. An epidemiological study of obsessive-compulsive disorder and related disorders in Israeli adolescents. *J Am Acad Child Adolesc Psychiatry* 1992; **31**: 1057–61.

chapter 7

Tourette syndrome: treatment

Ana G Hounie, Maria C Rosário-Campos, Lucas Quarantini,
Aline S Sampaio, Pedro G Alvarenga, Juliana B Diniz,
Antonio C Lopes, André A Seixas, Adriana Pinto,
Priscilla Chacon, Helena S Prado, Cristina Belotto, Márcia Motta,
Mária A De Mathis, Maria E De Mathis, Sonia Borcato,
Maura Carvalho, and Eurípedes C Miguel

Brief historical review

Howard Kushner, one of the greatest historians on Tourette syndrome (TS) did an important review on the history of TS which served as the basis for this introduction (see Kushner, 1999, for review). He performed detailed research in which he personally translated several French documents, including the first article by Gilles de la Tourette, published in 1885 and which reports a case series of patients who presented a combination of multiple motor tics and "involuntary" vocalizations with the eventual appearance of eruptive cursing that he designated "coprolalia" (Tourette, 1885). Gilles de la Tourette labeled this disorder *maladie des tics convulsifs avec coprolalie*, insisting that it was distinct from choreas and hysterias. Based on nine patients' case histories, Gilles de la Tourette concluded that, although its signs and symptoms might wax and wane, the disease ultimately resisted all interventions (Kushner, 1999). Many theories were postulated to explain the origin of this strange disease, such as psychologic (a type of hysteria), degenerative, infectious (a type of chorea, or rheumatic fever, or secondary to encephalitis), and hereditary. As a result, patients with similar medical histories and symptoms received different treatments depending on the philosophy and training of their particular physicians (Kushner and Howard, 2000).

Until the 1960s the prevailing etiologic theory was psychoanalytic. However, from 1963 to 1967, some authors reported success with haloperidol on a group of patients with tics and coprolalia, for whom all previous interventions had failed (Chapet et al, 1964). In 1968 Shapiro and Shapiro reported their successful treatment of a 24-year-old woman with several motor tics and vocalizations using haloperidol. Although they emphasized Gilles de la Tourette's 1885 description of symptoms, the Shapiros rejected his view that tics had a degenerative etiology. This case story relieved parents unwilling to accept blame for their children's symptoms. By the early 1970s, similar stories began to appear in newspapers and magazines throughout North America about children with motor movements and eruptive vocalizations. After years of failed psychotherapeutic and behavioral modification treatments, each family learned that these odd behaviors were caused by a chemical imbalance or neurotransmission malfunction, which was most likely amenable to treatment with haloperidol (Shapiro et al, 1978).

Several families of the Shapiros' patients organized a group to form the Tourette Syndrome Association (TSA). The TSA pursued a variety of strategies: they referred ticing patients to the Shapiros and later to like-minded colleagues, publicized the disease in a variety of venues, and recruited influential psychiatrists and celebrities to their cause. They also persuaded researchers to investigate the biologic factor of tics by providing generous sources of funding for research. These activists established a national network and support group (Shapiro et al, 1975; Wertheim, 1982; Shapiro, 1982). Similar associations have been created in different parts of the world, such as France, England, Australia, Canada, Czech Republic, Germany, Finland, Ireland, Iceland, Israel, Japan, the Netherlands, Peru, Poland, Scotland, Sweden, Switzerland, Argentina, and Brazil.

Increasing energy has focused on the search for a genetic component, but disputes over the TS phenotype continue to hinder attempts to locate a genetic substrate. Pauls and Leckman (1986) and their colleagues at Yale have led the search for a genetic etiology of TS. However, after more than a decade of intensive investigations, initial hope for a simple Mendelian (dominant) genetic etiology has been dashed and replaced by the more difficult task of exploring the genome for polygenic factors (Barr et al, 1999). The most recent findings on genetics will be described later in this chapter.

Simultaneously, although not necessarily in contradiction to genetic research, there has been a rediscovery and renewed interest in an infectious substrate, particularly the role of antibodies to group A beta hemolytic streptococcus (GABHS) based on Sydenham's model (Taranta and Stollerman, 1956; Husby et al, 1976; Swedo, 1994). This research has implicated GABHS as possibly providing the environmental trigger in genetically susceptible families for a variety of movement disorders including TS (Swedo et al, 1997). If the neuronal antibody theory is sustained, there may be a variety of routes to the development of TS symptoms; and rather than looking at one disease, there may be several different routes to similar sign/symptom clusters (Kurlan et al, 1991; Allen et al, 1995; Leckman et al, 1997; Hounie et al, in press).

Epidemiology

Until the 1970s, TS was considered to be a very rare condition with few research studies published, most of all consisting of case studies (Abuzzahab and Anderson, 1973; Robertson, 1989, 1994). In the 1980s, large-sample epidemiologic studies changed this view, reporting that tics and TS are a lot more frequent than the once imagined rate of 5/10000. For instance, Robertson (2003) suggested that 1% of school age children would fulfill criteria for TS. When considering all kinds of tics, the studies suggest rates ranging from 2.9% to 18%, with a mean prevalence rate for tics of 10% among children (Carroll and Robertson, 2000; Lanzi et al, 2004).

Differences in the prevalence of tics are observed according to gender, being more frequent in males than in females. Lanzi et al (2004) reported rates of 4.4% and 1.1% in school-age boys and girls, respectively. The male/female ratio for TS has ranged from 4:1 to 6:1, according to the sample characteristics (Kadesjo and Gillberg, 2000).

It has also been reported that the frequency of tics is significantly higher in children with special education needs than in children in regular programs. Eapen et al (1997) compared the rates of tics in four different groups, with ages ranging from 5 to 16 years old. The first group was composed of 20 children with behavioral/emotional problems, and tics were present in 13 of them (65%). In the second group, composed of 25 children with reading disabilities, tics were present in 24% ($P<0.05$). The third group was composed of 17 "difficult" children, with 6% of them presenting tics ($P<0.003$). In the randomly selected normal control group none of the children had tics ($P<0.0006$).

Kurlan et al (2001) also found significantly higher rates of tics in 341 children in special needs school programs, compared to 1255 children in regular school programs (27% and 19.7%, $P=0.008$). These authors hypothesized that the higher rates of tics in these children might be a consequence of the same developmental brain problem causing the learning disabilities.

Eapen et al (2001) investigated the frequency of tics among 200 psychiatric hospitalized patients and did not find any higher rates of tics among them compared to community studies, refuting the theory that psychiatric disorders in general are associated with tics.

It is important to mention that TS has not been associated with lower IQ rates (Apter et al, 1993). Similarly, no racial and/or socio-economic status differences have been reported for TS patients.

Clinical features

A tic is a sudden, repetitive movement, gesture, or utterance that typically mimics some fragment of normal behavior. Tics have brief duration and often tend to occur in bouts or brief inter-tic intervals so that they have a character. They vary in intensity or forcefulness (Lekman et al, 1997).

Tics typically diminish during sleep or activities that need concentration. On the other hand, anxiety, stress, fatigue, and excitement are often associated with an increase in tic severity. Tics can be suppressed by voluntary effort, but this leads to high emotional tension. The warning given by premonitory urges (sensory phenomena) may contribute to this ability (Hounie and Petribú, 1999).

Motor tics vary from simple tics such as eye blinking, head jerks, or shoulder shrugs to complex tics with apparently purposeful behaviors such as facial expressions or gestures. Complex tics are usually slower than simple tics and involve non-related muscular groups. Complex tics may also involve ritualized behaviors, resembling compulsions. The difference between complex tics and compulsions can be subtle.

Phonic or vocal tics are sounds, noises, or utterances made by the air flow through the nose or mouth. They can range from simple throat clearing sounds to more complex vocalizations, which may include echolalia, palilalia, or coprolalia (obscene speech) in about 30% of the cases (Hounie and Petribú, 1999).

The presence of tics along the lifespan is the main characteristic of all tic disorders. Several diagnostic classification systems describe tic disorders, including DSM-IV (American Psychiatric Association, 1994), the ICD-10 (World Health Organization, 1992), and the classification of tic disorders by the Tourette Syndrome Association (The Tourette Syndrome Classification Study Group, 1993). Although some differences exist among these classification manuals, they are broadly congruent, with each containing three major categories: Tourette syndrome, chronic motor or vocal tic disorder, and transient tic disorder (Lekman et al, 1997).

According to the DSM-IV, TS is characterized by the presence of both multiple motor tics and one or more vocal tic, which have been present at some time during the illness, although not necessarily concurrently (American Psychiatric Association, 1994). The diagnosis is made on the basis of clinical observation and judgment since there are no diagnostic tests for TS or other tic disorders at the present time.

The average age of onset of symptoms is 7 years, but typically ranges from 2 to 15 years, and no more than 18 years according to the DSM-IV or 21 years according to the TSA. Tics initially may come and go, but eventually become persistent for at least a year, with tic-free intervals of no longer than 3 months.

TS typically begins with transient bouts of simple motor tics of the eyes, face, or head, often progressing to shoulders, trunk, and extremities. Although some patients have a "rostra-caudal" progression of motor tics (head, neck, shoulders, arms, torso), the course is not predictable. As the syndrome develops, complex motor tics may appear and might involve dystonic movements. In a small fraction of cases (<5%), complex motor tics have the potential to be self-injurious and to further complicate management since the symptoms may be relatively mild, for example, slapping or tapping, or quite dangerous, for example punching one side of the face, biting a wrist, or gouging eyes to the point of blindness (Lekman et al, 1997).

On average, phonic tics begin 1 to 2 years after the onset of motor tics and are usually simple in character, for example, throat clearing, grunting, and squeaks. Coprolalia presents as the initial symptom in only a small minority of patients. Similarly, echolalia is present in approximately 10 to 40% of patients. Other complex vocal symptoms include dramatic and abrupt changes in rhythm, rate, and volume of speech. Studies in China, Korea, and Japan show that vocalizations are present in two thirds of the subjects, but vary from 47% to 89% across samples. These values are higher than those reported in Western studies, which identified vocalizations as the initial symptoms in approximately 13 to 39% of subjects. This difference could be explained by the fact that in some cultures there is still the myth that coprolalia is needed for the diagnosis of TS (Staley et al, 1997).

The frequency of tics varies from rare events occurring a few times a week to uncountable bursts occurring more than 100 times per minute. Motor and phonic tics tend to occur in bouts (Lekman et al, 1997).

The forcefulness of motor tics and the volume of phonic tics can also vary tremendously from behaviors that are not noticeable (a slight shrug or hushed guttural noise) to strenuous displays (arm thrusts or loud barking) that are frightening and exhausting (Lekman et al, 1997).

Tic severity is frequently influenced by environmental factors. Some precipitating stress factors include arguments with parents, school exams, and public situations. Other factors such as infectious diseases and febrile episodes may also worsen tics or trigger their onset (Staley et al, 1997).

The factors that determine the degree of disability versus resiliency are largely unknown, but are likely to include the presence of additional disorders, the level of support and understanding from parents, peers, and educators, and the presence of special abilities (as in sports) or personal attributes (intelligence, social abilities, and personal traits).

Although most children with TS are loving and affectionate, many patients have difficulties with their social skills. Whether this is due to the stigmatizing effects of the tics, the patients' own uneasiness, or some more fundamental difficulty linked to basic neurobiologic mechanisms is still unknown. In the interpersonal area, social isolation, difficulty in making friends, and family conflicts are examples of frequent problems. Staley and colleagues (1997) reported that aggressive (e.g. throwing objects and hitting others) and self-injurious behavior (including suicide attempts) was present in 18% and 10% of the cases, respectively. Sleep disturbances, such as insomnia, and employment difficulties in maintaining a job were both identified in 8% of the sample.

Consistent with available epidemiologic data, tic disorders tend to improve in late adolescence and early adulthood. In many instances, the phonic symptoms become increasingly rare or may disappear, and motor tics may be reduced in frequency and intensity. Complete remission of both motor and phonic symptoms has also been reported (Lekman et al, 1997).

Neuroimaging

The goal of neuroimaging studies in TS is to identify the neural bases for symptoms of the disorder and to define the neural systems that modulate or compensate for the presence of those core symptoms. Identifying these systems will ultimately help in the design and monitoring of new therapeutic interventions. The previous decade has seen the birth and rapid maturation of neuroimaging investigations in TS.

Studies using computed tomography (CT) scanning of the brain have found no specific anatomic abnormalities in children with TS (Robertson et al, 1988; Robertson, 1989). On the other hand, magnetic resonance imaging (MRI) studies have pointed out specific volumetric changes in TS patients, when compared to normal controls, especially smaller volumes of the left putamen and globus pallidus (Peterson et al, 1993; Singer et al, 1993). Aberrant laterality in TS was suggested by the reduced or reversed basal ganglia asymmetry, mainly in male TS subjects. TS subjects have also shown significantly smaller caudate nucleus volumes and, in the case of comorbid obsessive-compulsive disorder (OCD), reduced lenticular nucleus volumes were observed. Reduced caudate and lenticular nucleus volumes might constitute candidates for trait markers of TS (Peterson et al, 2003).

Morphometric changes in other brain regions have also been described, such as larger dorsal prefrontal volumes in TS patients, especially in children, as well as larger parieto-occipital areas in TS males and smaller inferior occipital volumes. TS boys tend to show smaller orbitofrontal, subgenual, and premotor volumes. Tic severity is associated with smaller orbitofrontal and parieto-occipital volumes (Peterson et al, 2001).

Regarding white matter changes, a TS group showed a reduced cross-sectional corpus callosum (CC) area when compared to normal controls (Peterson et al, 2003). On the other hand, TS children showed larger volumes in four subregions of the CC (mainly in the rostral body) (Baumgardner et al, 1996). This latter subregion of the CC is formed by axons connecting premotor and supplementary motor areas of both hemispheres (Witelson, 1989).

Positron emission tomography (PET) and single photon emission tomography (SPECT) studies have thus far resulted in similar findings. It was initially suggested that TS patients presented reduced glucose utilization in brain areas such as the frontal, cingulum, and insula cortices, and ventral striatum, when compared to normal controls in a fluorodeoxyglucose (FDG) PET study (Chase et al, 1986). Others have pointed out an increased right frontal regional blood flow (rBF) in TS subjects, as well as reduced left putamen and globus pallidus rBF, using hexamethyl-propylene amine oxide (HMPAO) SPECT, or lower rBF in the left caudate, cingulum, right cerebellum, left dorsolateral prefrontal, and left orbital region (George et al, 1992; Riddle et al, 1992; Diler et al, 2002).

In a comparison 16 TS patients with 16 normal controls under FDG PET, TS subjects showed a higher metabolism in the superior sensorimotor cortices, and reduced metabolism in the paralimbic, ventral prefrontal, ventral striatal, and brainstem areas, especially in the left hemisphere (Braun et al, 1993). A similar HMPAO SPECT study found the left caudate nucleus, anterior cingulum, and left dorsolateral prefrontal cortex to have reduced perfusion. Tic suppression under a functional MRI study was correlated to higher signal intensity in the ventral right caudate and right midfrontal, right middle temporal, bilateral superior temporal, right anterior cingulate, and bilateral occipital cortices. Lower signal intensity was observed in the ventral globus pallidus, ventral putamen, midbody of each hemithalamus, right posterior cingulate, left hippocampus and parahippocampus, bilateral cuneate, left sensorimotor, and left inferior parietal cortices (Peterson et al, 1998). The smaller the difference between right caudate activation and deactivation of other subcortical areas, the greater the symptom severity.

Radioligand studies initially indicated no changes in dopamine (DA) precursor metabolism or DA receptor binding (Brooks et al, 1992; Singer et al, 1992; Turjanski et al, 1994). On the other hand, higher striatal DA transporter levels and higher caudate D2-receptor densities have been found (Madison et al, 1995; Wolf et al, 1996).

Genetics

The familial nature of Gilles de la Tourette syndrome was first observed in 1885 by Gilles de la Tourette himself. However, it was not until the late 1970s that studies (Eldridge et al, 1997; Shapiro et al, 1978) demonstrated an increased frequency of a positive family history of tics, both TS and chronic tics (CT), in the families of TS patients.

In the early 1980s, five separate studies (Baron et al, 1981; Kidd and Pauls, 1982; Comings et al, 1984; Devor, 1984; Price et al, 1988) used family-history data to test specific genetic hypotheses regarding the inheritance of TS and CT. All studies reported that the pattern of inheritance within families was consistent with a genetic hypothesis that postulated the existence of a single gene of major effect that conferred susceptibility to TS and/or CT.

As indicated, all these studies relied on family-history data. It has been demonstrated that family-history data underestimate the "true" rates of TS and CT obtained with direct interviews (Pauls et al, 1984). To address the potential problem of reporting biases in family-history studies, the Yale Family Study of TS was undertaken in 1981. In this study, all available first-degree relatives were personally assessed using a structured psychiatric interview. The results from this study reinforce the idea that TS is familial and that CT and some forms of OCD are variant expressions of the syndrome (Pauls et al, 1991).

The hypothesis that OCD is a variant manifestation of the syndrome grew out of a number of studies with TS patients (Kelman, 1965; Fernando, 1967; Morphew and Sim, 1969; Nee et al, 1980, 1982; Yaryura-Tobias et al, 1981; Jagger et al, 1982; Montgomery et al, 1982; Stefi, 1984; Cummings and Frankel, 1985; Robertson et al, 1988; Robertson, 1989) that documented the increased frequency of obsessive-compulsive symptomatology in TS patients and was reinforced by the Yale Family Study data suggesting that OCD could represent a variant expression of TS (Pauls and Leckman, 1986; Pauls et al, 1986). Several subsequent studies (Frankel et al, 1986; Pitman et al, 1987; Walkup et al, 1988; Robertson et al, 1988; Pauls et al, 1991) have supported these findings. These studies report that the rate of OCD is significantly higher in the families of TS probands regardless of whether the proband has a concomitant diagnosis of OCD.

Additional evidence that at least some TS and OCD patients share the same genetic vulnerability has come from OCD genetic family studies (Pauls et al, 1995; Grados et al, 2001; do Rosário-Campos et al, in press). These studies present higher rates of tics and/or TS in first-degree relatives of OCD patients, when compared to control relatives. A clearer understanding of the familial relationship between OCD and

TS came from studies with relatives of OCD probands, suggesting that there are several different forms of OCD, some familial and others not familial. Among the familial forms of OCD, some are tic-related (Pauls et al, 1995).

A recent family study conducted in Japan reported lower rates of TS (2%), CT (14.6%), OCD (1.6%), and sub-clinical OCD (7%) in the 165 first-degree relatives of 52 TS probands, when compared with the rates reported in Western family studies (Kano et al, 2001).

To examine whether these family-study data would result in different genetic hypotheses being supported, segregation analyses were undertaken. Pauls and Leckman (1986) demonstrated that the pattern within families was consistent with autosomal dominant transmission. Segregation analyses were also undertaken with data collected for a linkage study of TS (Pauls et al, 1990). In both sets of analyses, an autosomal dominant hypothesis was supported when:

- only relatives with TS were included as affected
- relatives with TS or CT were included as affected, and
- relatives with TS, CT, or OCD were included as affected.

While more recent segregation analyses generally continue to support the presence of a major locus, the reported characteristics of this predisposition gene have varied (Kurlan et al, 1994; Hasstedt et al, 1995; Walkup et al, 1996; McMahon et al, 1996; Seuchter et al, 2000). Despite the differences in findings, methodologies, and proposed models of inheritance, the bulk of family and segregation analysis studies supports the idea that genes play a major role in the etiology of TS and related disorders (State et al, 2000).

Additional support for a genetic component in the etiology of TS has come from twin studies (Price et al, 1985; Hyde et al, 1992), which show concordance rates for TS in monozygotic (MZ) twins to range between 60 and 80%, compared to less than 20% for dizygotic (DZ) twins (Price et al, 1985; Hyde et al, 1992). When the phenotype assessed is the presence of all kinds of chronic tics, the concordance rate increases to almost 100% in MZ twins (Walkup et al, 1988).

The search for the genes

The overt nature of tics, the belief that TS was a homogeneous disorder, the hypothesis of an autosomal dominant pattern of inheritance, and the advances in molecular biology techniques caused researchers to be very enthusiastic about using linkage and association methods to find the susceptibility gene(s) causing TS. Unfortunately, to date, no genetic loci have been identified.

The initial studies assuming autosomal dominant transmission and genetic homogeneity have excluded almost 90% of the genome (Barr et al, 1999; State et al, 2000). Nevertheless, even performing a model-based linkage analysis, a recent study of a large French Canadian family identified evidence for linkage with a LOD score of 3.24 on chromosome 11 (11q23) (Mérrette et al, 2000). It is important to mention that this study used markers previously identified in linkage studies of population isolates in South Africa (Simonic et al, 1998). The initial scan of chromosome 17 performed on two large pedigrees provided a non-parametric LOD score of 2.41 near D17S928. Fine mapping with 17 additional microsatellite markers increased the peak to 2.61 ($P=0.002$) (Paschou et al, 2004).

Given current uncertainties regarding the inheritance parameters, non-parametric methods, such as the sib-pair approach, were undertaken by the Tourette Syndrome International Consortium for Genetics (TSICG) (Walkup et al, 1988; TSICG, 1999). This study reported two regions of the genome (on chromosomes 4q and 8p) with LOD scores higher than 2 (TSICG, 1999).

A genome scan using the affected pedigree method (APM) was completed on a series of multi-generational families and revealed eight markers with possible linkage in at least one of the families (Barr et al, 1999). Interestingly, one of the regions presented in this study (19p), also reached a LOD score higher than 1 in the sib-pair study (TSICG, 1999; Singer, 2000).

Several association studies have examined a variety of candidate genes in TS patients and controls. Some of the evaluated genes include dopamine receptors (DRD1, DRD2, DRD4, and DRD5), the dopamine transporter, various noradrenergic genes (ADRA2a, ADRA2C, and DBH) and some serotoninergic genes (5-HTT) (Comings et al, 1991, 1993, 1996; Nöthen et al, 1994a, 1994b; Grice et al, 1996; Simonic et al, 1998; Thomson et al, 1998). Nevertheless, their results must be interpreted with caution given the known potential pitfalls of this approach.

An additional approach is the search for cytogenetic abnormalities in TS patients. Some of the findings include breakpoints in chromosome 7 (Petek et al, 2001) and fragile sites on chromosome 16q22–23 (Kerbeshian et al, 2000; Seuchter et al, 2000). Unfortunately, none of the chromosomal regions in which cytogenetic abnormalities have been found to cosegregate with TS have shown any convincing evidence for linkage in the high-density families, the sib-pair study, or the population isolates studies. State et al (2003) described an (18q21.1–q22.2) inversion in a patient with CT and OCD. Another case report of a 14-year-old girl associated severe OCD with a t(2;18) (p12;q22) translocation (Cuker et al, 2004).

Another explanation for the limited success in the search for genes is that TS is in fact a heterogeneous disorder. Amongst the frequent comorbid diagnoses, OCD has been constantly identified as representing an alternative expression of the TS phenotype. With the aim of further clarifying the phenotype of these TS plus OCD patients, two recent studies have shown interesting results (Zhang et al, 2002; Leckman et al, 2003). One did a genome scan of the hoarding phenotype and reported significant allele sharing for markers at 4q34–35, 5q35, and 17q25. The other study completed univariate and complex segregation analyses using obsessive-compulsive (OC) dimensions scores, and showed interesting results. For instance, segregation analyses were consistent with dominant major gene effects for both factor 1 (aggression obsessions and related compulsions) and factor 2 (symmetry obsessions and related compulsions), whereas for factor 3 (contamination/cleaning) and 4 (hoarding symptoms), the most parsimonious solution was consistent with recessive inheritance (Leckman et al, 2003). These dimensions had been previously identified by Leckman et al (1997c) and have proven to be valuable in genetic studies (Mataix-Cols et al, 2005).

Future work

The localization of a gene or genes responsible for the expression of TS will be a major step forward in our understanding of the genetic/biologic risk factors important for the expression of this syndrome. In addition, this work will allow the potential identification of non-genetic factors associated with the manifestation or the amelioration of the symptoms of the disorders (Leckman et al, 1990; Pauls et al, 1990). Once the location of a gene or genes has been verified, it will be possible to type the unaffected children in high-risk families to determine with a high probability who is carrying a susceptibility gene. It will then be possible to examine in more detail the interaction between genotype and the environment (Kidd, 1984).

Until this day comes, all efforts will be directed towards improving existing genetic techniques such as the identification of more specific markers, as well as developing more advanced and accurate ones. At the same time, the search for more homogeneous phenotypes and more comprehensive assessment tools needs to be emphasized.

Psychopharmacologic treatment

Not all TS patients will require medication. In mild cases psycho-education will suffice. Tics should be treated only when they interfere with children's routines. Several medications have been studied in TS, but only a few have been evaluated in placebo-controlled studies. Several other medications have at least open-label data supporting their use for reducing tics. Medications that have been reported in isolated cases or have not been replicated will be described as "experimental drugs." Alpha-adrenergic drugs are considered the first-line treatment for TS. Typical neuroleptics, once the treatment of choice, are now second-line agents.

Alpha-adrenergic drugs

Possible explanations for the involvement of noradrenergic systems in TS symptomatology are based on findings in animal models, neurophysiologic studies, and treatment response. For example, the stimulation of locus ceruleus noradrenergic activity in animals elicits behaviors that present similarities with the TS clinical picture (Redmond, 1977) and some TS patients may present elevated levels of the major metabolite of norepinephrine in the cerebral spinal fluid (Cohen et al, 1980). On the other hand, sites of the ventral striopallidal complex which regulate the motor behavioral response to emotional stimuli seem to be regulated by noradrenergic afferents (Chappell et al, 1990).

The alpha-2 agonists clonidine and guanfacine may benefit TS patients by ameliorating tics, ADHD symptoms, and OC symptoms. Clonidine is an imidazoline derivative used for the treatment of arterial hypertension. In low doses, clonidine seems to reduce central noradrenergic functioning by its pre- and postsynaptic effects (Cohen et al, 1980). In patients who did not tolerate previous treatment with haloperidol, clonidine has been shown to be an effective alternative treatment, for reducing not only tic severity but also compulsive behavior, irritability, and attentional deficit in some studies of a single research group (Cohen et al, 1979, 1980; Young et al, 1981). However, these results were based on the judgment of the senior author (Cohen DJ) and attentional difficulties and behavioral problems seemed to respond better to medication than did tics. Some posterior, double-blind, clinical trials support clonidine efficacy (McKeith et al, 1981; Borison et al, 1983; Leckman et al, 1991) although some reported negative results (Dysken et al, 1981; Goetz et al, 1987). Leckman et al (1991) reported that oral clonidine at a dose of 3 to 5 µg/kg seems to be more effective than placebo in the treatment of tics, especially motor tics, and other compulsive and disruptive behaviors. Main side-effects of clonidine include "sedation" or "fatigue," reported by up to 90% of the patients, "dry mouth," and "faintness" or "dizziness," reported by approximately half of the patients, and irritability, reported by one third of the patients. An initial dose of 0.025 mg once or twice daily with a gradual increase to 0.1–0.3 mg per day in three divided doses might help to develop tolerance to its sedative effects (Peterson and Cohen, 1998a).

Compared to typical neuroleptics such as haloperidol and pimozide, clonidine was not more effective in one uncontrolled clinical trial, although a small number of patients who did not tolerate haloperidol showed some benefit from this medication (Shapiro et al, 1983). In a clinical trial with 24 TS patients comparing risperidone versus clonidine (Gaffney et al, 2002) both drugs were effective for the treatment of tics, OC symptoms, and ADHD symptoms. Risperidone tended to show better results regarding reduction in severity scale measures, although this difference was not statistically significant. Both drugs were well tolerated, although adverse effects such as dizziness and sedation were reported less frequently by patients taking risperidone.

In conclusion, clonidine is a potentially effective alternative for TS patients who do not tolerate or do not respond to neuroleptics. Due to its safer profile it is considered the first-line treatment. It can be used in combination with neuroleptics, although special attention might be directed to worsening of side-effects and hypotension. There might be a group of TS patients that responds better to this medication, however future studies are still needed to define which characteristics of this group of patients should guide clinicians in their treatment decisions.

Guanfacine is an alpha-2 agonist similar to clonidine that was first studied in patients with ADHD because of its longer excretion half-life, lower sedative side-effects, and more selective binding profile. Preliminary data on the treatment response of ADHD patients showed a beneficial response of behavioral alterations (Horrigan and Barnhill, 1995; Hunt et al, 1995). In patients with comorbid TS and ADHD, Chappell et al (1995) and Walkup et al (1995) also reported an improvement in phonic and motor tics as well as a behavioral response to guanfacine treatment. In these studies few side-effects, such as transient sedation and headaches, were reported. However, Horrigan and Barnhill (1999) drew attention to five cases of possible guanfacine-induced mania in children with risk factors for bipolar disorder. In one randomized clinical trial with TS patients, guanfacine was not superior to placebo regarding improvement on tic severity and neuropsychologic measures (Cummings et al, 2002).

Thus, guanfacine might be a good treatment option for TS patients, especially those with comorbid ADHD. However, data on guanfacine treatment are still preliminary and future studies are needed to confirm these findings.

Typical neuroleptics

Typical antipsychotics are the most effective treatment for tics. Rates of improvement reach 80% in several reports. However, due to the severe potential adverse reactions, such as tardive dyskinesia, they are now considered second-line agents (Robertson, 2000). We will report on double-blind trials and examine the drugs separately in detail. Trade names have been obtained from British National Formulary (1998) and Martindale Pharmacopoeia (1996).

Neuroleptics are most often used as antipsychotic agents and are also misleadingly referred to as major tranquilizers. They act primarily by interfering with dopaminergic transmission in the brain by blocking dopamine receptors. Neuroleptics decrease the dopaminergic input to the basal ganglia. They also affect cholinergic, alpha-adrenergic, histaminergic, and serotonergic receptors (British National Formulary, 1998).

Haloperidol

Haloperidol, a butyrophenone derivative, is primarily a dopamine D2-receptor blocker (Messiha, 1988). It was one of the most widely used agents used in treating TS. Many case reports of its successful use exist (Caprini and Melotti, 1961; Challas and Brauer, 1963; Chapel et al, 1964; Stevens and Blachly, 1966; Fernando, 1967; Lucas et al, 1967;

Boris, 1968; Shapiro and Shapiro, 1968; Shapiro et al, 1973; Stanciu et al, 1972; Perera, 1975; Feinberg and Carroll, 1979; Singer et al, 1986; Wright and Peet, 1989). Shapiro and colleagues reviewed 41 reports of its use over a 14-year period and found its efficacy to be between 78 and 91% (Shapiro et al, 1988).

Although it is unequivocally effective, haloperidol produces important side-effects in approximately 84% of patients and therefore only a minority of 20–30% of TS patients continue treatment for extended periods (Sallee et al, 1997). In addition, in many studies, haloperidol has been shown to produce more side-effects when compared with other neuroleptics (Ross and Moldofsky, 1977, 1978; Singer et al, 1982; Shapiro and Shapiro, 1982b; Goetz et al, 1984; Sallee et al, 1997).

Borison and colleagues conducted placebo-controlled, double-blind studies using fluphenazine and trifluoperazine which were as efficacious as haloperidol, but with fewer side-effects. In other studies, clonidine was shown to be equally as efficacious as haloperidol, but with no adverse side-effects (Borison et al, 1983). The same group also compared amantadine and benztropine in a cross-over study and found amantadine to be superior in treating the side-effects of haloperidol treatment in TS (Borison et al, 1983).

Given its potency as a postsynaptic D2-receptor blocker, haloperidol is often effective at low doses. In current clinical practice haloperidol is usually started at 0.25 mg or 0.5 mg in the evening, with the addition of 0.25 mg or 0.5 mg in the morning 4 to 7 days later. The total daily dose can be raised every 4 to 7 days, alternating between the morning and evening dose as tolerated to a total daily dose of 0.75 mg to 2.0 mg. The therapeutic effects and adverse responses should be monitored closely in the dose-adjustment phase (Scahill et al, 2000). The use of a low starting dose and a slow upward adjustment protects against acute dystonic reactions, although parents should be educated about this possibility. If dystonic reactions occur, anti-parkinsonian agents such as benztropine should be used. Other adverse effects can often be managed by reducing the dose. Beta-blockers such as propranolol or pindolol may be useful to treat akathisia (Chandler, 1990).

Pimozide

Pimozide is a diphenylbutylpiperidine derivative with postsynaptic dopamine blocking activity (Messiha, 1988). Ross and Moldofsky

(1978) conducted a placebo-controlled, double-blind study, in which both pimozide and haloperidol significantly decreased tic frequency in nine TS patients. Follow-up at 4–20 months later showed that six of seven patients receiving pimozide and one of two receiving haloperidol had over 75% improvement in symptoms (Ross and Moldofsky 1978).

Regeur and colleagues (1986) reviewed the medical charts of 65 TS patients. Fifteen patients (23%) received no medication. Pimozide was their most popular medication (given in 46 out of the 65 cases, or 71%) due to its low side-effect profile. Thirty-seven were treated with pimozide alone, five with pimozide and tetrabenazine, and four with pimozide and clonidine. The dose ranges of pimozide were 0.5–9 mg per day. Eighty-one percent experienced a good clinical response without side-effects.

Shapiro and colleagues treated 57 TS patients in a double-blind study comparing haloperidol, pimozide, and placebo. Haloperidol and pimozide were more effective than placebo, but haloperidol was slightly more effective than pimozide. Adverse effects occurred more frequently with haloperidol than with pimozide, but this frequency was not significantly different. Clinically significant cardiac effects did not occur at a maximum dosage of 20mg/day for pimozide and 10mg/day for haloperidol (Shapiro et al, 1989). Sallee and colleagues, in a 24-week, placebo-controlled, double-blind study, with double cross-over comparison of pimozide and haloperidol, measured prolactin levels, tic severity, and extrapyramidal side-effects (EPS) in 22 TS children and adolescents. Pimozide produced a 40% improvement in tics from baseline compared to 27% for haloperidol. Haloperidol produced a higher frequency of side-effects and significantly more EPS than pimozide. Patients experienced clinical response rates of 69% on 3.4mg/day of pimozide and 65% on 3.5mg/day of haloperidol. Pimozide responders demonstrated significantly raised prolactin compared with pimozide non-responders and haloperidol-treated patients, suggesting that prolactin may be a marker for tic response to pimozide and, conversely, a potential marker for haloperidol-related incidence of EPS (Sallee et al, 1997). Sallee and colleagues had previously reported results of cognitive testing in 66 TS patients (of whom one third had comorbid ADHD). The authors concluded that pimozide was found to be significantly superior to haloperidol in improving cognitive functioning in these patients (Sallee et al, 1994).

Sandor and colleagues described a long-term follow-up study of 33 TS patients treated with pimozide (2–18 mg), haloperidol (2–15 mg), or no drugs. Both drugs produced comparable relief of symptoms at follow-up. Significantly more patients receiving haloperidol (47%), compared with pimozide (8%), discontinued treatment. Haloperidol resulted in significantly more acute dyskinesias and dystonias than did pimozide. Otherwise, the adverse side-effect profile was similar for the two agents. This study did not demonstrate increased incidence of ECG abnormalities with pimozide (Sandor et al, 1990).

The typical starting dose is 0.5 mg in young children or 1 mg per day in older children. The dosage may be increased every 4 to 7 days in 0.5 mg to 1 mg increments over a 2–4-week period. The total dose in children typically ranges from 2 mg to 4 mg per day given in divided doses (Scahill et al, 2000) although it can be administered once a day due to its long half-life. Use of pimozide requires caution regarding the possibility of QT prolongation. Electrocardiograms at baseline, during dose adjustment, and annually during maintenance therapy are recommended. Concomitant treatment with drugs that inhibit the cytochrome P450 3A4 isoenzyme (e.g. erythromycin, ketoconazole, cisapride, fluvoxamine, sertraline, citalopram) should be avoided because of the predictable and potentially dangerous rise in pimozide serum levels at the same oral dose (Desta et al, 1999).

Substituted benzamides

The substituted benzamides, selective D2 antagonists, have also become popular worldwide, excluding the USA and Canada, for the treatment of motor and vocal tics. This group is popular as the drugs produce fewer EPS and less tardive dyskinesia (Robertson, 2000). Sulpiride and amisulpride, previously classified as typical antipsychotics, are better classified as atypical.

Sulpiride

The most widely documented benzamide in the treatment of TS is sulpiride, which was first used in 1970 (Yvonneau and Bezard, 1970) and has been extensively used and documented thereafter (Robertson et al, 1990a; George et al, 1993). Robertson and colleagues treated 63 out of 114 (55%) TS patients with a mean age of 29.3 years (range 10–68 years) with sulpiride and worthwhile beneficial effects occurred in 59%. Positive effects were decreased motor and vocal tics, decreased obsessive-compulsive symptoms, decreased aggressiveness, decreased echophenomena and tension, and, finally, an improved mood. The dose of sulpiride started at 200 mg daily and increased to a maximum of 1 g daily (Robertson et al, 1990a). Although those authors started with 200 mg/day, in our practice we usually start with 50 mg/day. George and colleagues undertook a double-blind study with a placebo-controlled cross-over of fluvoxamine versus sulpiride, followed by single-blind combined therapy in 11 subjects with comorbid TS and OCD. Sulpiride monotherapy significantly reduced tics and non-significantly improved OCD. Fluvoxamine, either alone or combined with sulpiride, non-significantly ameliorated tics and reduced obsessive-compulsive symptoms (George et al, 1993).

Tiapride

Tiapride, not licensed in the USA, Canada, or UK, is widely used in Europe for the treatment of TS. A case report of a 17-year-old TS female (Lipcsey, 1983) and a study including extrapyramidal hyperkinetic syndromes (Klepel et al, 1988) have shown the efficacy of tiapride. Eggers and colleagues conducted a placebo-controlled study on 10 children followed by a double-blind crossover study on 17 children using tiapride; it was shown to have a positive therapeutic effect on tics and no adverse effects on neuropsychologic cognitive performance in children. Neurophysiologic parameters such as the EEG frequency analysis and sensory evoked potentials were not affected by tiapride, nor was the neurosecretory, hypothalamic–hypophyseal regulation of the sex hormones, thyroid stimulating hormone, growth hormone, or thyroid hormone impaired. The hyperprolactinemia induced by tiapride was moderate and restricted to the duration of therapy (Eggers et al, 1988).

A double-blind, placebo-controlled study showed significant benefit of tiapride in dyskinesia management. Maximal dosage was 900 mg/day. The forms of dyskinesia which responded best to tiapride included those of TS patients. Tiapride-induced parkinsonism occurred in a few patients (Chouza et al, 1982).

Other benzamides

Amisulpride has been demonstrated to be beneficial in tic management (Trillet et al, 1990; Fountoulakis et al, 2004). Other benzamide trials in smaller numbers of TS patients include metoclopramide

(Desai et al, 1983) and remoxipride (Sandor et al, 1996). In the UK, remoxipride can only be prescribed on a named patient basis because of blood dyscrasias (aplastic anemia, cytopenia). To the best of the author's knowledge, there have been no reports of the use of the other benzamides such as raclopride and nemonapride for TS treatment (Robertson, 2000).

Other typical neuroleptics

The traditional neuroleptic fluphenazine was evaluated in an open-label trial in 21 refractory patients (age 7 to 47 years). Eleven of the 21 subjects reported a better response to fluphenazine compared to previous treatment with haloperidol, six patients showed a similar response to fluphenazine, and two patients preferred haloperidol. The mean dose of fluphenazine was 7 mg per day (range 2 to 15 mg per day). Of the six patients who reported akathisia on haloperidol, only one reported akathisia on fluphenazine (Goetz et al, 1984). Fluphenazine therapy may begin with 0.5 mg to 1 mg per day, increasing to bid dosing in 5 to 7 days. In children, the likely dose range is 2 mg to 5 mg per day in divided doses (Scahill et al, 2000). Other neuroleptics such as the diphenylbutylpiperidine penfluridol (Stanciu et al, 1972), and the phenothiazines, trifluoperazine (Polites et al, 1965; Fernando, 1967; Prabhakaran, 1970), and thioproperazine (Lechin et al, 1982) have also been used successfully. In a few patients, depot neuroleptics such as haloperidol (Paolucci et al, 1984; Clarke and Ford, 1988) or flupenthixol (Robertson, 2000) have been used successfully.

Atypical neuroleptics

The risk of tardive dyskinesia in treating TS with typical neuroleptics has increased interest in the atypical neuroleptics, although they are still scarcely studied in TS. Atypical neuroleptics are effective in blocking D2-receptors and also act as 5HT2 antagonists. A recently published systematic review on the use of off-label indications for atypical antipsychotics found 10 papers on Tourette treatment (and included risperidone, olanzapine, and quetiapine) (Fountoulakis et al, 2004).

Risperidone

The best-studied atypical antipsychotic for the treatment of TS is still risperidone. Van der Linden et al (1994), in an open trial with 11 patients, showed a 36 to 56% reduction in tics. Similarly, a case series by Lombroso et al (1995) found similar results. Brunn and Budmann (1996) replicated those findings in a larger sample. One double-blind, randomized trial compared risperidone to pimozide (Bruggeman et al, 2001). Risperidone was found to be equally effective for TS with a mean dose of 3.8mg/day. Dion et al (2000) in a double-blind, placebo-controlled trial with 48 TS patients, found that risperidone, in doses ranging from 1 to 6mg/day, was more effective than placebo. Scahill et al (2003), in a double-blind placebo-controlled trial, found risperidone to be a safe and effective option for TS treatment. Gaffney et al (2002) found risperidone as effective as clonidine in a short single-blind study. Risperidone is used in a dose range from 1.0 to 6.0 mg/day in divided doses. Adverse effects include sedation, acute dystonic reactions, weight gain, dysphoria, and galactorrhea (Kossoff and Singer, 2001).

Olanzapine

Olanzapine has a greater affinity for 5HT2 receptors than for D2 receptors. There are some case reports (Bhadrinath, 1998; Bengi Semerci, 2000; Karam-Hage and Ghaziuddin, 2000; Lucas Taracena and Montanes Rada, 2002) of the effectiveness of olanzapine in Tourette patients. There are two open-label studies (Stamenkovic et al, 2000; Budman et al, 2001) and one double-blind cross-over study with pimozide (Onofrj et al, 2000), all of them favoring olanzapine in doses ranging from 2.5 to 20 mg/day. Stephens et al (2004) found olanzapine superior to placebo both for tics and aggressive behavior. Adverse effects include weight gain, sedation, akathisia, hypoglycemia (Budman and Gayer, 2001), and hyperlipidemia.

Quetiapine

Quetiapine is an atypical antipsychotic with peculiar properties such as a low D2 and 5HT2A affinity and it has been cited in three case reports (Chan-ob et al, 2001; Parraga and Woodward, 2001; Schaller and Behar, 2002; Matur and Ucok, 2003) and one open-label study (Bruggeman et al, 2001) on quetiapine in TS, all with favorable results. The doses used in the case reports were 400 mg/day, 150 mg/day, 100 mg/day, 50 mg/day, and 75 mg/day. Hyperglycemia and hypertriglyceridemia were associated with quetiapine in a case report (Domon and Cargile, 2002).

Ziprasidone

Ziprasidone has a unique effect on 5HT1A receptors in addition to the D2 and 5HT2 antagonistic properties, suggesting a safer use in comorbid depression and anxiety (Kossoff and Singer, 2001). Ziprasidone was reported as effective in one TS case (Meisel et al, 2004) and in one pilot double-blind and placebo-controlled study (Sallee et al, 2000) with TS patients (doses ranging from 5 to 40 mg/day). Ziprasidone has the advantage of lesser propensity to weight gain, but has a greater propensity to prolong QT interval, as does pimozide. Other side-effects are sedation, insomnia, and akathisia.

Aripiprazole

Aripiprazole has been described as a stabilizer of the dopamine/serotonin system. Its suggested mechanism of action is the partial agonism on D2 receptors, as it binds more to D2 G-protein-bound receptors than to those which are not (Burris et al, 2002). The affinity of the drug for D2 is 4 to 20 times lower than that of haloperidol, chlorpromazine, or other typical antipsychotics (Lawer et al, 1999). In addition, it shows a partial agonist activity on 5HT1A receptors and antagonism on 5HT2A receptors. Most neocortex 5HT1A receptors are situated in glutamatergic pyramidal neurons. These receptors have an inhibitory action, which would reduce the excitatory glutamatergic output. It is believed that part of the control of tics would stem from this control in the glutamatergic projection pathways.

There are two published studies on the treatment of TS with aripiprazole. One study reports one case (Hounie et al, 2004a) and the other (Kastrup et al, 2005) two cases, both with good results, which suggest it may be a promising alternative. Double-blind, placebo-controlled studies with aripiprazol are warranted.

Experimental drugs

In this section we will cover some of the drugs or procedures that have been reported in isolated cases, or case series, or even in well-designed studies which have not been replicated or are not as extensively studied as alpha-adrenergic drugs and antipsychotics were. As well as neuroleptics, other antidopaminergic drugs have been studied, such as tetrabenazine, which acts by depleting dopamine stores, and has been found efficacious in a small open-label trial (Jankovic and

Table 7.1   Experimental trials in the treatment of Tourette syndrome

Drug	Reference	Type of study	Results on tics
Topiramate	Abuzzahab and Brown, 2001	Case report	Positive
Marihuana	Muller-Vahl et al, 2002, 2003	DBPC SDT; DBPC	Positive (trend)
Baclofen	Awaad, 1999; Singer et al, 2001	Open trial; DBPC	Inconclusive
Selegiline	Feigin et al, 1996	DBPC	Positive
Nicotine + antipsychotics	Silver et al, 2001; Howson et al, 2004	DBPC; DBPC	Inconclusive
Ondansetron	Toren et al, 1999	Open-label	Positive
Metoclopramide	Acosta and Castellanos, 2004	Open-label	Positive
Naloxone	van Wattum et al, 2000	Case report	Positive
Tramadol	Shapira et al, 1997	Case report	Positive
Ketanserin	Bonnier et al, 1999	Case series	Positive
Mecamylamine	Silver et al, 2001	DBPC	Negative
Talipexole	Goetz et al, 1994	DBPC	Negative
Buspirone	Dursun et al, 1995	Case report	Positive
Flutamide	Peterson et al, 1998b	DBPC	Positive
Vigabatrin	Stahl et al, 1985	Case report	Negative
Cyproterone	Izmir and Dursun, 1999	Case report	Positive
Lithium	Hamra et al, 1983; Kerbeshian and Burd, 1988	Case report; case series	Positive
Methadone	Meuldijk and Colon, 1992	Case report	Positive
Levodopa	Black and Mink, 2000	Single high-dose challenge	Positive
Clonazepam	Kaim, 1983; Merikangas et al, 1985	Case report, single-blind study	Positive
Donepezil	Hoopes, 1999	Case report	Positive
Nifedipine	Micheli et al, 1990	Case series	Negative
Flunarizine	Micheli et al, 1990	Case series	Positive
Clozapine	Caine et al, 1979	DBPC	Negative
Aripiprazole	Hounie et al, 2004a; Kastrup et al, 2005	Case report; Case report	Positive; Positive

DBPC: double-blind, placebo-controlled trial; SDT: single-dose trial; case report (one or two cases); case series (three or more cases).

Orman, 1988). Pergolide, used primarily for Parkinson's disease, is a dopamine agonist and has been found effective and safe, both in an open-trial (Lipinski et al, 1997) and in a randomized clinical trial (Gilbert et al, 2003). Other drugs used in the treatment of tics are shown in Table 7.1.

Non-pharmacologic experimental procedures

This section covers postinfectious, autoimmune-mediated, neuropsychiatric disorders: treatment and prophylaxis perspectives.

The PANDAS hypothesis

TS and OCD have been associated with rheumatic fever (RF) with (Swedo et al, 1993, 1997; Swedo, 1994; Asbahr et al, 1998; Mercadante et al, 2000; Hounie et al, 2004b) and without Sydenham's chorea (Mercadante et al, 2000; Hounie et al, 2004b). A subgroup of childhood-onset OCD and tic disorders has been found to have a postinfectious, autoimmune-mediated etiology. Clinical observations and systematic investigations have shown that a subgroup of OCD and/or tic disorder patients has the onset and subsequent exacerbations of their symptoms following infections with group A beta-hemolytic streptococci (rheumatic fever implicated agent). Swedo and colleagues designated this subgroup by the acronym PANDAS: pediatric autoimmune neuropsychiatric disorders associated with streptococcal infections (Swedo et al, 1998). PANDAS may arise when antibodies directed against invading bacteria cross-react with basal ganglia structures, resulting in exacerbations of OCD or tic disorders (Swedo et al, 1993). The existence of PANDAS, however, is not free from controversy. No prospective epidemiologic study has confirmed that an antecedent streptococcal infection is specifically associated with either the onset or exacerbation of tic disorders or OCD, although such a study is in progress (Singer, 1999).

Immunologic aspects

Recent studies support the hypothesis that there is an immune-related pathogenesis for a subgroup of patients with tic disorders triggered by streptococcal infections. Giedd and colleagues (1996) reported severe worsening of obsessive-compulsive symptoms and tics in an adolescent boy following infection with group A beta-hemolytic streptococci, with basal ganglia enlargement in magnetic resonance imaging scans. Significant elevated expression of a β-lymphocyte monoclonal protein called D8/17 (that is a known susceptibility marker of rheumatic fever) has been reported in patients with tic disorders (Hoekstra et al, 2004a). Moreover, Muller and collaborators reported higher titers of antibodies against M proteins (the major virulence factor of group A streptococci) in 25 TS adult patients but not in 25 healthy controls (Muller et al, 2001).

Antibiotic prophylaxis

Because penicillin prophylaxis has proven to be effective in preventing recurrences of rheumatic fever, it was postulated that it might also prevent streptococcal-triggered neuropsychiatric symptom exacerbations. Garvey and colleagues conducted a cross-over study and found no significant change in neuropsychiatry symptom severity, which they related to the failure in penicillin to achieve streptococcal prophylaxis (Garvey et al, 1999).

Immunomodulatory therapies

Pearlmutter and colleagues (1999) assessed 30 children with severe, infection-triggered exacerbations of OCD or tic disorders, including TS, which were randomly assigned treatment with plasma exchange, intravenous immunoglobulin, or placebo. Twenty-nine completed the trial. Ten subjects received plasma exchange, nine intravenous immunoglobulin, and ten placebo. At one month, the intravenous immunoglobulin and plasma exchange groups showed striking improvements in obsessive-compulsive symptoms and anxiety. Tic symptoms were also significantly improved by plasma exchange. Curiously, there was no relation between therapeutic response and the rate of antibody removal titers.

Despite the apparent success of Perlmutter's trial, in a recent double-blind, placebo-controlled trial assessing 30 children with tic disorder, Hoekstra and collaborators (2004b) observed no significant differences between intravenous immunoglobulin and placebo in tic severity. Intravenous immunoglobulin was associated with significantly more side-effects.

Allen and colleagues reported on four boys (aged 10 to 14) undergoing clinical assessment. One had TS, and two had TS plus OCD. Two were treated with plasmapheresis, one with intravenous immunoglobulin, and one with immunosuppressive doses of prednisone. The authors reported clinically significant responses immediately after treatment (Allen et al, 1985). However, this study presents major limitations such as the lack of control group and blinding to the treatment assignments.

Although potentially promising for the highly selected patient, active immunomodulatory therapy is not ready for routine use. Thus, this treatment should be given only as part of controlled double-blind protocols (Singer, 1999).

Neurosurgery

Neurosurgical interventions for TS were first conducted by Baker, in 1962, using a bimedial leucotomy technique (Baker, 1962). In spite of tic improvement, a serious complication was described (frontal lobe abscess). Since then, different techniques have been employed (e.g. chemothalamectomy of the ventrolateral nucleus (Cooper, 1962), prefrontal lobotomy (Stevens, 1964), dentatotomy (Nadvornik et al, 1972), and bilateral campotomy (Beckers, 1973)), with no adequate assessment of improvement measures. Other surgical techniques (such as stereotactic limbic leucotomy or cingulotomy) have also been conducted, without good evidence of symptom improvement (Kurlan et al, 1988, 1990; Robertson et al, 1990b; Rauch et al, 1995). Severe side-effects were also described in combined infrathalamic and cingulotomy lesions (Leckman et al, 1993; Rauch et al, 1995).

In 1970, three patients were operated on in the intralaminar and medial thalamic nuclei, and in the ventro-oralis internus (Voi), with tic improvement ranging from 70 to 100% (Temel and Visser-Vandewalle, 2004). Similar thalamic lesions in the zona incerta and thalamus (ventrolateral nuclei – VL/lamella medialis thalamus – LM) resulted in a 50% reduction of tics in 6 of 11 patients (56%). However, some important side-effects were present (cerebellar signs, dystonia, dysarthria, and hemiballism) (Babel et al, 2001).

In 1999, deep-brain stimulation was first employed in three TS patients, in similar regions as those described by Hassler and Dieckmann (Vandewalle et al, 1999). A greater than 80% reduction in tics was observed, with a few minor side-effects.

Neurosurgery for TS possibly acts by interrupting cortico–striatal–thalamic–cortical loops, including projections to both the premotor/prefrontal cortex and the striatum. In spite of recent positive results, neurosurgery for the treatment of TS is still an extreme therapeutic option. Its use should be restricted to very severe TS patients, refractory to all major drug and psychotherapeatic alternatives.

Psychotherapeutic treatment

The usual behavioral intervention for TS is a package of multi-component treatment known as habit reversal (HR). This procedure was first developed by Azrin and Nunn in 1973, and had successful results in the treatment of nervous habits, tics and stuttering (Miltenberger et al, 1998).

The original procedure consisted of nine major techniques. The first four techniques were focused on increasing the awareness of the tics. They included response description, response detection, early warning, and situation awareness. A fifth technique consisted of developing a competing response to replace the target tic when the patients first became aware that the tics were about to occur. To increase and sustain compliance motivation three additional techniques were used (habit inconvenience review, social support procedure, and public display) and another one was designed for generalization training (Azrin and Nunn, 1973).

During the early research on HR in the 1970s, all procedure components were implemented at the same time to produce immediate and lasting decreases in the occurrence of habit behaviors. As a consequence, it was difficult to differentiate which behavioral mechanism(s) was (were) responsible for the results of the procedure (Miltenberger et al, 1998).

During the last 25 years of research, HR has been shown to be effective and replicable (Miltenberger et al, 1998), restricting the use of other procedures only to those cases which have not responded to an HR trial. In a case study, Wagaman et al (1995) used differential reinforcement (giving praise or something that the child liked after a period without tics) after an unsuccessful HR, and reported a significant decrease in the frequency of tics.

More recently, research studies investigating variations, simplified versions, and the role of each component of HR have been undertaken.

In 1996, Woods et al used a mixed multiple baseline design across participants and behaviors to investigate how each component of HR acts for results. They concluded that, in some cases, awareness of the tic makes its occurrence an aversive event that some individuals would escape or avoid by suppressing the tic, probably by engaging in a competing response to avoid the tic. These authors reported that there may be success in some cases by just using awareness training (Woods et al, 1996). Another finding was that by training competing responses, one can enhance the response to treatment. With respect to self-monitoring and social support, they found limited results, probably as a consequence of the study design (Woods et al, 1996).

Case studies have observed that some tics may be partially maintained by social reinforcement contingencies (positive or negative – such as attention), or by multiple control of social and automatic reinforcement contingencies (Carr et al, 1996). Positive automatic reinforcement happens when, after the tic, the person feels a sensorial stimulation that may enhance the probability of responding in the same way (tic) in the future. Negative automatic reinforcement occurs by the reduction of the tension after the tic, also maintaining the occurrence of tics in further similar occasions.

Additional research on HR is needed, with bigger sample sizes, in order to better explore its limitations, to program and enhance the generalization of results across places and time, and to identify maintainers of the problem (Miltenberger et al, 1998). For instance, Wilhelm et al (2003) suggested that relapse prevention and booster sessions could help patients maintain their benefits.

Self-help groups and coaching

Participation in self-help groups is an important part of tic treatment. Coaching is also fundamental for learning and maintaining the techniques used to deal with tics. We will didactically separate this item into awareness, strategies to deal with tics, and family group coaching.

Awareness

The first goal is to help patients develop awareness of their tics. Patients are taught to increase their awareness through self-monitoring training, in order to better understand the pattern of the behavior. Then, it will be possible to develop some strategies to deal with tics, sometimes taking into account some subjective experiences named sensory phenomena – a procedure that will be explained in the section on strategies. The self-monitoring training helps patients to become aware of these subjective experiences.

To introduce the self-monitoring training, it is helpful to explain clearly why it is a necessary step:

> *"It is important for us to know what exactly the movements you make are, as well as their frequency and intensity. Sometimes you may tic and do not realize it! And you cannot control something that you do not even know. The rule is: keep tracking your tics and write down your feelings/perceptions that may occur before or during your performance. When you register time/intensity/frequency you can evaluate how you are doing."*

There are many environmental stressors that may influence the waxing and waning of tics. Professional help (therapist/coaching group) is extremely important to aid in tracking those stressor factors, i.e. identifying the specific situations that may trigger an increase/decrease in tics. For instance, it is quite common to find an exacerbation of tics in a period of anxiety before an important test in school, or when the family is distressed, or at the end of an important relationship. In contrast, the patient may perform fewer tics when doing homework or playing football.

Whenever the patient is aware of the environmental triggers of tics, it is easier to lower expectations regarding their occurrence. The family and therapist are also important in helping with the identification of the stressors and giving support to the patient.

Although habit reversal is a recommended training for chronic tic disorders, it is extremely important to be very clear that the purpose of this technique is to deal with tics in such a way as to diminish their complexity and make them less noticeable, and not to get rid of them at all. Moreover, this is a kind of training that requires time and persistence, especially if tics are too complex, and it can be stressful and tiring as it demands a constant observation and self-monitoring of body and mind. For this reason, family members should reward any improvement or efforts in this direction, even if small ones, and motivate patients to keep doing all the exercises.

Strategies to deal with tics: coaching

The Professional and Personal Coaches Association defines coaching as an ongoing relationship which focuses on clients taking action toward the realization of their visions, goals, or desires. Put simply, coaches help people to meet the challenges and opportunities life presents (http://www.americoach.org/).

Our goal is to help patients to control their tics, and we will describe how the sensory phenomena may be a tool to improve their quality of life.

Many patients with TS and/or OCD refer subjective experiences that may trigger or accompany their repetitive behaviors and those experiences cause uncomfortable and disturbing sensations, feelings, or urges that can be experienced physically or mentally. Those experiences are called sensory phenomena (see Table 7.2). Described in the literature first in TS patients, sensory phenomena have also been reported as part of OCD (Leckman and Cohen, 1994; Miguel et al, 1995, 1997, 2000).

A research group from Yale University introduced the concept of "just right" perceptions, which corresponds to the sensation that some patients refer to of not feeling well, balanced, or "just right," which makes them perform the repetitive behaviors until they feel "just right". This sensation would be, in most cases, related to visual, tactile, and auditory sensory stimuli, i.e. patients would perform the compulsions until objects are "just right" visually, until they hear a specific sound, or feel a tactile sensation that makes them feel "just right." Such perceptions have been reported by up to 81% of OCD associated with TS patients (Leckman et al, 1992, 1997a; Miguel et al, 1995).

Other examples of sensory phenomena described in the literature correspond to a mental sensation of inner tension or energy that builds up and needs to be released through the performance of the repetitive behaviors; and to feelings of incompleteness, imperfection, and insufficiency (Miguel et al, 1995).

The following examples illustrate patients' statements, behaviors, and their own perceptions concerning their tics and some of our suggestions that might help them. However, it is very important to emphasize, again, that we are not trying to eliminate tics but to show that patients can have a better control over them by being aware of those subjective experiences. Patients are able to model some tics with the technique of habit reversal and make them more socially adequate.

Table 7.2   Examples of sensory phenomena

Physical sensation	*Mental sensation*
1. Tactile physical sensation	1. Internal "just right"
Example:	Example:
My hands or other parts of my body feel oily, sticky, or greasy and I need to wash them to relieve or get rid of this sensation	I have feelings/perceptions of not being "just right" and these feelings/perceptions make me re-read or repeat movements or arrange objects until I feel "just right" inside myself
2. Muscle-skeletal or visceral physical sensation	2. "Just right" feeling/perception triggered by visual stimuli
Example:	Example:
I have a sensation in my muscles that makes me tense my muscles in a certain pattern, like from right to left and then on the other direction. I feel the need to do a repetitive behavior until achieving a specific sensation in my mouth	Objects in my room need to be placed and organized in a certain way, or symmetrically, so that they "look just right"
	3. "Just right" feeling/perception triggered by tactile stimuli
	Example:
	I need to touch or rub objects until I get this "just right" feeling in my hands
	4. Feelings or perceptions of incompleteness
	Example:
	I have feelings or perceptions of incompleteness, of imperfection, or insufficiency, as if something was missing in myself, and these feelings/ perceptions make me perform the repetitive behavior until I feel relieved, although I may never feel complete
	5. "Just an urge" – no sensations or feelings, just an urge to do the repetitive behaviors
	Example:
	I have the urge to stare at certain places, people, or certain parts of people's bodies, without any kind of sensory phenomena or any obsession preceding or accompanying this behavior

Habit reversal consists of awareness training, self-monitoring, relaxation training, competing response training, and contingency management (Wilhelm et al, 2003). The first example is shown here. For more examples please see the Appendix.

Example

Behavior: a 17-year-old adolescent taps everything around him: floor, walls, tables and puts his fingers in his mouth to lick them afterwards.

Statement: I feel the need to touch smooth surfaces (like velvet, rocks, plastic), until I get a specific physical sensation in my fingers and then I lick two of them, of each hand, to release the warm sensation on it and I do this until I have a balanced feeling, the same refreshing sensation in my fingers of both hands. This really bothers me because people stare at me and make a sick face when I lick my fingers. Since this tic began I just can't go dating anymore!

Sensory phenomena: tactile physical sensation and a mental sensation of tactile stimuli, a need to even up, a need to feel things "just right."

Therapist/Coach: in this statement we can see social blame and significant emotional impairment. However, we may suppose that he might not have a need to touch different surfaces, he probably has a need to relieve a distressing sensation and, then, he touches! Furthermore, he licks to release a consequent sensation, a "side-effect" sensation, i.e. the heat in his fingertips after so many touches.

Considering this behavior, we could suggest to him that he keeps objects that provide him with relief, such as keeping in his pocket some marbles with different surfaces in order to touch them and so relieve those sensations. However, there are some steps we should go through before reaching this final suggestion. These steps are a technique called habit reversal, which should be done at home first until his self-confidence allows him to generalize the practice outdoors. A family member trained in the group of family coaching may act as a cotherapist.

Steps suggested:

1. Choose *with him* three or four different kinds of marbles with sizes that he may handle comfortably, and let him "try" them, "taste with the fingers."
2. Teach him how to discriminate his sensations and realize that he is going to tic.
3. As soon as he begins the tic, let him continue and gently give him the marbles so he can *finish* the relief of his sensations by playing

with the marbles. Try to do this as much as possible, but do it in an easy-going way, otherwise he will get anxious and his tics may worsen as well as his mood. Don't be lax, just gentle.

4. After he gets used to his marbles, he has to pick up those marbles *before* starting to tap surfaces, that is, he *begins to relieve* his sensations with the marbles and he may tap one or two surfaces.

5. He must relieve his sensations only with his marbles.

This may take a few days and thus it is important to carry his marbles with him every time he goes out, as he *may want to try* using them while he's outside, that is, he *must have the option* of preserving himself from the exposure. By the time he is ready to be trained outdoors, he will probably have been training alone with some success! Our three main goals were reached: relieving the sensation, not being people's curiosity, and making tics socially adequate.

In conclusion, patients may or may not have sensory phenomena that trigger tics. If we understand the stressing factors plus the pattern of tics, including the subjective experiences associated with them, sensory phenomena may become a useful tool.

Family group coaching

What is going on with my child? What can I do to help? I am so tired. Is there any help?

Those are the most common questions that parents and the family, as a whole, ask when they search for counseling for TS. Sometimes parents are afraid that their children will get "labeled" if they let the school know that they have TS. However, if symptoms are significant enough to receive a diagnosis, those symptoms may be so severe as to cause impairment and interference in school/social life. Sometimes there are also comorbid disorders such as dysthymia, low self-esteem, disruptive behaviors, and learning disabilities. Some patients with mild forms of chronic tics do not recognize or notice their presence or their intensity. Parents and family can be very important in helping them to recognize tics and by providing support. On the other hand, some children with chronic tic disorder become aware at an early age that they are different. They become aware that they have something that other children do not have and they need to understand these bizarre behaviors. The first step is to teach them how to deal with themselves by explaining the disorder, why it happens, that it's not a rare disorder, and that they still have many things that they can do to improve themselves. Parents also need psychoeducation (Miguel et al, 2000). For instance, if a child/adolescent has disruptive behaviors as soon as they get home, this may be influenced by the suppression of symptoms while they were at school (or away from home). Parents must be aware of this possibility and be supportive and, with professional help, learn how to help their children without being too severe or too lax.

The first step to help is to recognize people with tics as persons who have natural abilities and who may be frustrated with the difficulties and disabilities that interfere in their lives, preventing them from being successful. When parents are educated about the disorder, and become part of the team that supports their children in attaining an education and social life, the goals are much more easily reached. As far as TS symptoms appear to be within the control of the children, it is easy to believe that negative consequences will be an incentive for them to change the behavior. However, punishment generally does not work because tics are due to a chemical imbalance in the brain and, as such, are not deliberate misbehaving, even though they may appear that way. Research has proven that punishment, humiliation, and negative consequences are counterproductive in teaching children with TS strategies to replace difficult behavior. The best approach begins with knowledge.

School problems are quite common in as far as school is a setting where children will spend much of their daily life, experiencing social life in micro environment. Thus parents and teachers must be aware of bizarre behaviors, and avoid punishing them but try and help, as the "side-effects" can be lifelong. The aim is eventually that the children may become socially adequate adults. Parents of children with TS have to walk a fine line between understanding and overprotection. They are constantly faced with deciding whether or not certain actions are the expression of TS, poor behavior, or blackmail behavior. It is not easy for parents to make the "right choice" and this is extremely distressing. This is the reason why they really need to have support from a family coaching group. For socially unacceptable behavior, children should be encouraged to control what they are able to, whenever possible, and try to make their behaviors more socially acceptable, as explained in the section on strategies. Parents are urged to give their

TS children the opportunity for as much independence as possible, while gently but firmly limiting attempts by some children to use their symptoms to control those around them.

Whether in school or in their social life, TS children will require support in dealing with difficult situations. However, if every obstacle were eliminated (by parents or school) they would lose the opportunity of learning how to deal with similar situations as an adult. It is important that children be allowed to experience many hurdles, so school and parents may provide them with strategies that overcome these hurdles, to help them be successful later in life.

Patients' associations

As with other chronic diseases, TS and OCD have a great impact on patients' lives and aspirations, as well as on their family members. The limitations imposed by the disease can result in an impoverished way of life, which often leads to compromised social relationships, difficulties at the work place or school, and many hurdles in daily routines.

Patient associations such as the Tourette Syndrome Association (TSA) have been fundamental in divulging information about TS. The search for the correct diagnoses and successful treatment strategies was the main fuel for the mothers who founded the Brazilian Association of TS, tics and OCD (ASTOC). ASTOC followed the structure of and advice from the TSA and the Obsessive Compulsive disorder Foundation (OCF). ASTOC is a non-profit association created for the support of carers and related families. ASTOC's main goal is to provide and spread knowledge of these disorders and improve the quality of life of people suffering from them. ASTOC was created with a partnership with the OCD Spectrum Disorder Project (PROTOC), a group of mental health professionals specializing in OCD and TS, which provides the scientific and technical support to ASTOC, enabling a team of volunteers to assist the population.

Thus, ASTOC has been promoting symposiums for professionals from different fields and also for the patients and their families. Other activities involving ASTOC members include assistance to families about school acceptance issues and legal rights, the creation of self-help support groups, and the organization and editing of books.

The support groups for patients and families follow the model of the OCF. These groups were created with the objective of bringing people closer together, to provide the certainty that they are not alone since there are other people with similar problems, to facilitate discussion of their problems, and offer mutual support. On the basis of suggestions from members of the support groups, ASTOC has been organizing art workshops and group physical exercises.

ASTOC believes that barriers can and must be overcome. Therefore, it seeks to act as a motivational force to its associates, to enable them to be able to control, more and more effectively, the limitations that TS and OCD attempt to impose in their lives. It is our hope that the actions we have taken can, in fact, remove these barriers.

References

Abuzzahab FS, Brown VL. Control of Tourette's syndrome with topiramate. *Am J Psychiatry* 2001; **158**: 968.

Abuzzahab FE, Anderson FO. Gilles de la Tourette's syndrome. *Minn Med* 1973; **56**: 492–6.

Acosta MT, Castellanos FX. Use of the "inverse neuroleptic" metoclopramide in Tourette syndrome: an open case series. *J Child Adolesc Psychopharmacol* 2004; **14**: 123–8.

Allen AJ, Leonard HL, Swedo SE. Case study: a new infection-triggered, autoimmune subtype of pediatric OCD and Tourette's syndrome. *J Am Acad Child Adolesc Psychiatry* 1995; **34**: 307–11.

American Psychiatric Association. *Diagnostic and statistical manual of mental disorders* – 4th edn *(DSM-IV)*. Washington DC; American Psychiatric Press, 1994.

Apter A, Pauls DL, Bleich A, et al. An epidemiologic study of Gilles de la Tourette's Syndrome in Israel. *Arch Gen Psychiatry* 1993; **50**: 734–8.

Asbahr F, Negrão AB, Gentil V, et al. Obsessive-compulsive and related symptoms in children and adolescents with rheumatic fever with and without chorea: a prospective 6-month study. *Am J Psychiatry* 1998; **155**: 1122–24.

Awaad Y. Tics in Tourette syndrome: new treatment options. *J Child Neurol* 1999; **14**: 316–19.

Azrin NH, Nunn RG. Habit reversal: a method of eliminating nervous habits and tics. *Behav Res Therapy* 1973; **11**: 619–28.

Babel TB, Warnke PC, Ostertag CB. Immediate and long term outcome after infrathalamic and thalamic lesioning for intractable Tourette's syndrome. *J Neurol Neurosurg Psychiatry* 2001; **70**: 666–71.

Baker EFW. Gilles de la Tourette syndrome treated by bimedial leucotomy. *Can Med Assoc J* 1962; **86**: 746–7.

Baron M, Shapiro E, Shapiro A, Ranier JD. Genetic analysis of Tourette Syndrome suggesting a major gene. *Am J Hum Genet* 1981; **33**: 767–75.

Barr CL, Wigg KG, Pakstis AJ, et al. Genome scan for linkage to Gilles de la Tourette syndrome. *Am J Med Genet* 1999; **88**: 437–45.

Baumgardner TL, Singer HS, Denckla MB. Corpus callosum morphology in children with Tourette syndrome and attention deficit hyperactivity disorder. *Neurology* 1996; **47**: 477–82.

Beckers W. [Gilles de la Tourette's disease based on five own observations]. *Arch Psychiatr Nervenkr* 1973; **217**: 169–86.

Bengi Semerci Z. Olanzapine in Tourette's disorder. *J Am Acad Child Adolesc Psychiatry* 2000; **39**: 140.

Bhadrinath BR. Olanzapine in Tourette syndrome. *Br J Psychiatry* 1998; **172**: 366.

Black KJ, Mink JW. Response to levodopa challenge in Tourette syndrome. *Mov Disord* 2000; **15**: 1194–8.

Bonnier C, Nassogne MC, Evrard P. Ketanserin treatment of Tourette's syndrome in children. *Am J Psychiatry* 1999; **156**: 1122–3.

Boris M. Gilles de la Tourette's syndrome: remission with haloperidol (letter). *JAMA* 1968; **205**: 648–9.

Borison RL, Arg L, Hamilton WJ, et al. Treatment approaches in Gilles de la Tourette syndrome. *Brain Res Bull* 1983; **11**: 205–8.

Braun AR, Stoetter B, Randolph C, et al. The functional neuroanatomy of Tourette's syndrome: an FDG-PET study. I. Regional changes in cerebral glucose metabolism differentiating patients and controls. *Neuropsychopharmacology* 1993; **9**: 277–91.

British National Formulary. BNF 35, March 1998. London: British Medical Association and Royal Pharmaceutical Society of Great Britain.

Brooks DJ, Turjanski N, Sawle GV, et al. PET studies on the integrity of the pre- and post-synaptic dopaminergic system in Tourette syndrome. *Adv Neurol* 1992; **58**: 227–31.

Bruggeman R, van der Linden C, Buitelaar JK, et al. Risperidone versus pimozide in Tourette's disorder: a comparative double-blind parallel-group study. *J Clin Psychiatry* 2001; **62**: 50–6.

Bruun RD, Budman CL. Risperidone as a treatment for Tourette's Syndrome. *J Clin Psychiatry* 1996; **57**: 29–31.

Budman CL, Gayer AI. Low blood glucose and olanzapine. *Am J Psychiatry* 2001; **158**: 500–1.

Budman CL, Gayer A, Lesser M, et al. An open-label study of the treatment efficacy of olanzapine for Tourette's disorder. *J Clin Psychiatry* 2001; **62**: 290–4.

Burris KD, Molski TF, Xu C, et al. Aripiprazole, a novel antipsychotic, is a high-affinity partial agonist at human dopamine D2 receptors. *J Pharmacol Exp Ther* 2002; **302**:381–9.

Caine ED, Polinsky RJ, Kartzinel R, Ebert MH. The trial use of clozapine for abnormal involuntary movement disorders. *Am J Psychiatry* 1979 Mar; **136**: 317–20.

Caprini G, Melotti V. Un grave sindrome ticcosa guarita con haloperidol. *Riv Sper Freniatr Med Leg Alienazioni Ment* 1961; **85**: 191–6.

Carr JE, Taylor CC, Wallander RJ, Reiss ML. A functional-analytic approach to the diagnosis of a transient tic disorder. *J Behav Ther Exp* 1996; **27**: 291–7.

Carroll A, Robertson M. *Tourette syndrome. A practical guide for teachers, parents and carers.* London; David Fulton Publishers, 2000.

Challas G, Brauer W. Tourette's disease: relief of symptoms with R 1625. *Am J Psychiatry* 1963; **120**: 283–4.

Chan-Ob T, Kuntawongse N, Boonyanaruthee V. Quetiapine for tic disorder: a case report. *J Med Assoc Thai* 2001; **84**: 1624–8.

Chandler JD. Propranolol treatment of akathisia in Tourette's syndrome. *J Am Acad Child Adolesc Psychiatry* 1990; **29**: 475–7.

Chapel JL, Brown N, Jenkins RL. Tourette's disease: symptomatic relief with haloperidol. *Am J Psychiatry* 1964; **121**: 608–10.

Chappell PB, Leckman JF, Pauls DL, et al. Biochemical and genetic studies of Tourette syndrome: implications for treatment and future research. In: Deutsh S, Weizmar A, Weizmar R, eds. *Application of basic neuroscience to child psychiatry.* New York: Plenun Publishing Corp; 1990: 241–60.

Chappell PB, Riddle MA, Scahill L, et al. Guanfacine treatment of comorbid attention-deficit hyperactivity disorder and Tourette's syndrome: preliminary clinical experience. *J Am Acad Child Adolesc Psychiatry* 1995; **34**: 1140–6.

Chase TN, Geoffrey V, Gillespie M, et al. Structural and functional studies of Gilles de la Tourette syndrome. *Rev Neurol* 1986; **142**: 851–5.

Chouza C, Romero S, Lorenzo J, et al. [Clinical trial of tiapride in patients with dyskinesia (author's transl)]: *Sem Hop* 1982; **58**: 725–33.

Clarke DJ, Ford R. Treatment of refractory Tourette syndrome with haloperidol decanoate. *Acta Psychiatr Scand* 1988; **77**: 495–6.

Cohen DJ, Young JG, Nathanson JA, et al. Clonidine in Tourette's syndrome. *Lancet* 1979; **2**: 551–3.

Cohen DJ, Detlor J, Young G, et al. Clonidine ameliorates Gilles de la Tourette Syndrome. *Arch Gen Psychiatry* 1980; **37**: 1350–7.

Comings DE, Comings BG, Devor EJ, Cloninger CR. Detection of a major gene for Gilles de la Tourette syndrome. *Am J Hum Genet* 1984; **36**: 586–600.

Comings DE, Comings BG, Muhleman D, et al. The dopamine D2 receptor locus as a modifying gene in neuropsychiatric disorders. *JAMA* 1991; **266**: 1793–800.

Comings DE, Muhleman D, Dietz G, et al. Association between Tourette's syndrome and homozygosity at the dopamine D3 receptor gene. *Lancet* 1993; **341**: 906.

Comings DE, Wu S, Chiu C, et al. Polygenic inheritance of Tourette syndrome, stuttering, attention deficit hyperactivity, conduct, and oppositional defiant disorder. *Am J Med Genet (Neuropsych Genet)* 1996; **67**: 264–88.

Cooper IS. Dystonia reversal by operation in the basal ganglia. *Arch Neurol* 1962; **7**: 64–74.

Cuker A, State MW, King RA, Davis N, Ward DC. Candidate locus for Gilles de la Tourette syndrome/obsessive compulsive disorder/chronic tic disorder at 18q22. *Am J Med Genet A* 2004; **130**: 37–9.

Cummings JL, Frankel M. Gilles de la Tourette syndrome and neurological basis of obsessions and compulsions. *Biol Psychiatry* 1985; **20**: 1117–26.

Cummings DD, Singer HS, Krieger M, et al. Neuropsychiatric effects of guanfacine in children with mild Tourette syndrome: a pilot study. *Clin Neuropharmacol* 2002; **25**: 325–32.

Desai AB, Doongaji DR, Satoskar RS. Metoclopramide in Gilles de la Tourette's syndrome (a case report). *J Postgrad Med* 1983; **29**: 181–3.

Desta Z, Kerbusch T, Flockhart DA. Effect of clarithromycin on the pharmacokinetics and pharmacodynamics of pimozide in healthy and extensive metabolizers of cytochrome P450 2D6 (CYP2D6). *Clin Pharm Therapeut* 1999; **65**: 10–20.

Devor EJ. Complex segregation analysis of Gilles de la Tourette syndrome: further evidence for a major locus mode of transmission. *Am J Hum Genet* 1984; **36**: 704–9.

Diler RS, Reyhanli M, Toros F, Kibar M, Avci A. Tc-99m-ECD SPECT brain imaging in children with Tourette's syndrome. *Yonsei Med J* 2002; **43**: 403–10.

Dion Y, Annable L, Sandor P, et al. Risperidone in the treatment of Tourette's syndrome: a double-blind, placebo-controlled trial. Annual Meeting of the American Psychiatric Association, 13–17 May 2000; Chicago, Illinois.

Domon SE, Cargile CS. Quetiapine associated hyperglycemia and hypertriglyceridemia. *J Am Acad Child Adolesc Psychiatry* 2002; **41**: 495–6.

do Rosário-Campos MC, Leckman JF, Curi M, et al. A family study of early-onset obsessive-compulsive disorder. *Am J Med Genet* 2005; **136**: 92–7.

Dursun SM, Burke JG, Reveley MA. Buspirone treatment of Tourette's syndrome. *Lancet* 1995; **345**: 1366–7.

Dysken MW, Berecy JM, Samarza A, et al. Clonidine in Tourette syndrome. *Lancet* 1981; **2**: 26–7.

Eapen V, Robertson MM, Zeitlin H, Kurlan R. Gilles de la Tourette's syndrome in special education schools: a United Kingdom study. *J Neurol* 1997; **244**: 378–82.

Eapen V, Laker M, Anfield A, Dobbs J, Robertson MM. Prevalence of tics and Tourette syndrome in an inpatient adult psychiatry setting. *J Psychiatry Neurosci* 2001; **26**:417–20.

Eggers C, Rothenberger A, Berghaus U. Clinical and neurobiological findings in children suffering from tic disease following treatment with tiapride. *Eur Arch Psychiatry Neurol Sci* 1988; **237**: 223–9.

Eldridge R, Sweet R, Lake CR, Ziegler M, Shapiro AK. Gilles de la Tourette's syndrome: clinical, genetic, psychological and biochemical aspects in 21 selected families. *Neurology* 1977; **27**: 115–24.

Feigin A, Kurlan R, McDermott MP, et al. A controlled trial of deprenyl in children with Tourette's syndrome and attention deficit hyperactivity disorder. *Neurology* 1996; **46**: 965–8.

Feinberg M, Carroll BJ. Effects of dopamine agonists and antagonists in Tourette's disease. *Arch Gen Psychiatry* 1979; **36**: 979–85.

Fernando SJ. Gilles de la Tourette's syndrome. A report on four cases and a review of published case reports. *Br J Psychiatry* 1967; **113**: 607–17.

Fountoulakis KN, Iacovides A, St Kaprinis G. Successful treatment of Tourette's disorder with amisulpride. *Ann Pharmacother* 2004; **38**: 901.

Fountoulakis KN, Nimatoudis I, Iacovides A, Kaprinis G. Off-label indications for atypical antipsychotics: a systematic review. *Ann Gen Hosp Psychiatry* 2004; **3**: 4.

Frankel M, Cummings JL, Robertson MM, et al. Obsessions and compulsions in the Gilles de la Tourette syndrome. *Neurology* 1986; **36**: 379–82.

Gaffney GR, Perry PJ, Lund BC, et al. Risperidone versus clonidine in the treatment of children and adolescents with Tourette's syndrome. *J Am Acad Child Adolesc Psychiatry* 2002; **41**: 330–6.

Garvey MA, Perlmutter SJ, Allen AJ, et al. A pilot study of penicillin prophylaxis for neuropsychiatric exacerbations triggered by streptococcal infections. *Biol Psychiatry* 1999; **45**: 1564–71.

George MS, Trimble MR, Costa DC, et al. Elevated frontal cerebral blood flow in Gilles de la Tourette syndrome: A 99Tcm-HMPAO SPECT study. *Psychiatry Res* 1992; **45**:143–51.

George MS, Trimble MR, Robertson MM. Fluvoxamine and sulpiride in comorbid obsessive-compulsive disorder and Gilles de la Tourette syndrome. *Hum Psychopharmacol* 1993; **8**: 327–34.

Giedd JN, Rapoport JL, Leonard HL, et al. Case study: acute basal ganglia enlargement and obsessive-compulsive symptoms in an adolescent boy. *J Am Acad Child Adolesc* 1996; **35**: 913–15.

Gilbert DL, Dure L, Sethuraman G, et al. Tic reduction with pergolide in a randomized controlled trial in children. *Neurology* 2003; **60**: 606–11.

Goetz CG, Tanner CM, Klawans HL. Fluphenazine and multifocal tic disorders. *Arch Neurol* 1984; **41**: 271–2.

Goetz CG, Tanner CM, Wilson RS, et al. Clonidine and Gilles de la Tourette syndrome: double-blind study using objective rating methods. *Ann Neurol* 1987; **21**: 307–10.

Goetz CG, Stebbins GT, Thelen JA. Talipexole and adult Gilles de la Tourette's syndrome: double-blind, placebo-controlled clinical trial. *Mov Disord* 1994; **9**: 315–17.

Grados MA, Riddle MA, Samuels JF, et al. The familial phenotype of obsessive-compulsive disorder in relation to tic disorders: the Hopkins OCD family study. *Biol Psychiatry* 2001; **50**: 559–65.

Grice DE, Leckman JF, Pauls DL, et al. Linkage disequilibrium between an allele at the dopamine D4 receptor locus and Tourette syndrome, by the transmission–disequilibrium test. *Am J Hum Genet* 1996; **59**: 644–52.

Hamra BJ, Dunner FH, Larson C. Remission of tics with lithium therapy: case report. *J Clin Psychiatry* 1983; **44**: 73–4.

Hasstedt SJ, Leppert M, Filloux F, van de Wetering BJM, McMahon WM. Intermediate inheritance of Tourette syndrome, assuming assortive mating. *Am J Hum Genet* 1995; **57**: 682–9.

Hoekstra PJ, Bijzet J, Limburg PC, et al. Elevated binding of D8/17-specific monoclonal antibody to B lymphocytes in tic disorder patients. *Am J Psychiatry* 2004a; **161**: 1501–2.

Hoekstra PJ, Minderaa RB, Kallemberg CG. Lack of effect of intravenous immunoglobulins on tics: a double-blind placebo-controlled study. *J Clin Psychiatry* 2004b; **65**: 537–42.

Hoopes SP. Donepezil for Tourette's disorder and ADHD. *J Clin Psychopharmacol* 1999; **19**: 381–2.

Horrigan JP, Barnhill LJ. Guanfacine for treatment of attention-deficit hyperactivity disorder in boys. *J Child Adolesc Psychopharmacol* 1995; **5**: 215–23.

Horrigan JP, Barnhill LJ. Guanfacine and secondary mania in children. *J Affect Disord* 1999; **54**: 309–14.

Hounie A, Petribú K. Síndrome de Tourette – revisão bibliográfica e relato de casos. *Rev Bras Psiquiatr* 1999; **21**: 50–63.

Hounie A, De Mathis A, Sampaio AS, et al. Aripiprazole and Tourette syndrome. *Rev Bras Psiquiatr* 2004a; **26**: 213.

Hounie AG, Pauls DL, Mercadante MT, et al. Obsessive-compulsive spectrum disorders in rheumatic fever with and without Sydenham's chorea. *J Clin Psychiatry* 2004b; **65**: 994–9.

Hounie AG, do Rosário-Campos MC, Dinix J, et al. Obsessive-compulsive disorder in Tourette syndrome. *Adv Neurol* (in press).

Howson AL, Batth S, Ilivitsky V, et al. Clinical and attentional effects of acute nicotine treatment in Tourette's syndrome. *Eur Psychiatry* 2004; **19**: 102–12.

Hunt RD, Arnsten AF, Asbell MD. An open trial of guanfacine in the treatment of attention-deficit hyperactivity disorder. *J Am Acad Child Adolesc Psychiatry* 1995; **34**: 50–4.

Husby G, Van de Rijn I, Zabriskie JB, et al. Antibodies reacting with cytoplasm of subthalamic and caudate nuclei neurons in chorea and rheumatic fever. *J Exp Med* 1976; **144**: 1094–110.

Hyde TM, Aaronson BA, Randolph C, Rickler KC, Weinberger DR. Relationship of birth weight to the phenotypic expression of Gilles de la Tourette's syndrome in monozygotic twins. *Neurology* 1992; **42**: 652–8.

Izmir M, Dursun SM. Cyproterone acetate treatment of Tourette's syndrome. *Can J Psychiatry* 1999; **44**: 710–11.

Jagger J, Prusoff BA, Cohen DJ, et al. The epidemiology of Tourette's syndrome: a pilot study. *Schizophrenia Bull* 1982; **8**: 267–78.

Jankovic J, Orman J. Tetrabenazine therapy of dystonia, chorea, tics, and other dyskinesias. *Neurology* 1988; **38**: 391–4.

Kadesjo B, Gillberg C. Tourette's disorder: epidemiology and comorbidity in primary school children. *J Am Acad Child Adolesc Psychiatry* 2000; **39**: 548–55.

Kaim B. A case of Gilles de la Tourette's syndrome treated with clonazepam. *Brain Res Bull* 1983; **11**: 213–14.

Kano Y, Ohta M, Nagai Y, Pauls DL, Leckman JF. A family study of Tourette Syndrome in Japan. *Am J Med Genetics* 2001; **105**: 414–21.

Karam-Hage M, Ghaziuddin N. Olanzapine in Tourette's disorder. *J Am Acad Child Adolesc Psychiatry* 2000; **39**: 139.

Kastrup A, Schlotter W, Plewnia C, et al. Treatment of tics in Tourette syndrome with aripiprazole. *J Clin Psychopharmacol* 2005; **25**: 94–6.

Kelman DH. Gilles de la Tourette's disease in children: a review of the literature. *J Child Psychol Psychiatry* 1965; **6**: 219–26.

Kerbeshian J, Burd L. Differential responsiveness to lithium in patients with Tourette disorder. *Neurosci Biobehav Rev* 1988; **12**: 247–50.

Kerbeshian J, Severud R, Burd L, Larson L. Peek-a-boo fragile site at 16d associated with Tourette syndrome, bipolar disorder, autistic disorder, and mental retardation. *Am J Med Genet* 2000; **96**: 69–73.

Kidd KK. New genetic strategies for studying psychiatric disorders. In: Sakai T, Tsuboi T, eds. *Genetic aspects of human behavior.* Tokyo: Igaku-Shoin; 1984: 325–46.

Kidd KK, Pauls DL. Genetic hypotheses from Tourette syndrome. In: Friedhoff AJ, Chase TN, eds. *Gilles de la Tourette syndrome.* New York: Raven Press; 1982: 243–9.

Klepel H, Gebelt H, Koch RD, et al. Treatment of extrapyramidal hyperkineses in childhood with tiapride. *Psychiatr Neurol Med Psychol (Leipz)* 1988; **40**: 516–22.

Kossoff EH, Singer HS. Tourette syndrome: clinical characteristics and current management strategies. *Paediatr Drugs* 2001; **3**: 355–63.

Kurlan R, Caine ED, Lichter D, Ballantine HT Jr. Surgical treatment of severe obsessive-compulsive disorder associated with Tourette syndrome. *Neurology* 1988; **38**: 203.

Kurlan R, Kersun J, Ballantine HT Jr, Caine ED. Neurosurgical treatment of severe obsessive-compulsive disorder associated with Tourette's syndrome. *Mov Disord* 1990; **5**: 152–5.

Kurlan R, Majumdar L, Deeley C, et al. A controlled trial of propoxiphene and naltrexone in patients with Tourette's syndrome. *Ann Neurol* 1991; **30**: 19–23.

Kurlan R, Eapen V, Stern J, McDermott MP, Robertson MM. Bilineal transmission in Tourette's syndrome families. *Neurology* 1994; **44**: 2336–42.

Kurlan R, McDermott MP, Deeley C, et al. Prevalence of tics in schoolchildren and association with placement in special education. *Neurology* 2001; **57**: 1383–8.

Kushner HI. *A Cursing Brain? The Histories of Tourette Syndrome.* Cambridge, Mass: Harvard University Press; 1999.

Kushner, HI. A brief history of Tourette syndrome. *Rev Bras Psiquiatr* 2000; **22**: 76–9.

Lanzi G, Zambrino CA, Termine C, et al. Prevalence of tic disorders among primary school students in the city of Pavia, Italy. *Arch Dis Child* 2004; **89**: 45–7.

Lawer CP, Prioleau C, Lewis MM, et al. Interactions of the novel antipsychotic aripiprazole (OPC-14597) with dopamine and serotonin receptor subtypes. *Neuropsychopharmacology* 1999; **20**: 612–27.

Lechin F, van der Dijs B, Gómez F, et al. On the use of clonidine and thioproperazine in a woman with Gilles de la Tourette's disease. *Biol Psychiatry* 1982; **17**: 103–8.

Leckman JF, Doinansky ES, Hardin M, et al. The perinatal factors in the expression of Tourette's syndrome. *J Am Acad Child Adolesc Psychiatry* 1990; **29**: 220–6.

Leckman JF, Hardin MT, Riddle MA, et al. Clonidine treatment of Gilles de la Tourette's syndrome. *Arch Gen Psychiatry* 1991; **48**: 24–8.

Leckman JF, Pauls DL, Peterson BS, et al. Pathogenesis of Tourette's syndrome: clues of the clinical phenotype and natural history. *Adv Neurol* 1992; **58**: 15–24.

Leckman JF, de Lotbiniere AJ, Marek K, et al. Severe disturbances in speech, swallowing, and gait following stereotactic infrathalamic lesions in Gilles de la Tourette's syndrome. *Neurology* 1993; **43**: 890–4.

Leckman JF, Cohen DJ. Tic disorders. In: Rutter M, Taylor E, Hersov L, eds. *Child and Adolescent Psychiatry – modern approaches*, 3rd edn. London: Blackwell Scientific Publications; 1994: 455–66.

Leckman JF, Peterson BS, Anderson GM, et al. Pathogenesis of Tourette's syndrome. *J Child Psychol Psychiatry* 1997a; **38**: 119–42.

Leckman JF, Peterson BS, Pauls DL, Cohen DJ. Tic disorders. *Psychiatr Clin North Am* 1997b; **20**: 839–62.

Leckman JF, Grice DE, Boardman J, et al. Symptoms of obsessive-compulsive disorder. *Am J Psychiatry* 1997c; **154**: 911–17.

Leckman JF, Peterson BS, Pauls DL, et al. Tic disorder. *Psychiatr Clin North Am* 1997a; **20**: 691–962.

Leckman JF, Pauls DL, Zhang H, et al. Obsessive-compulsive symptom dimensions in affected sibling pairs diagnosed with Gilles de la Tourette syndrome. *Am J Med Genet* 2003; **1**: 60–8.

Lipcsey A. Gilles de la Tourette's disease. *Sem Hop* 1983; **59**: 695–6.

Lipinski JF, Sallee FR, Jackson C, et al. Dopamine agonist treatment of Tourette disorder in children: results of an open-label trial of pergolide. *Mov Disord* 1997; **12**: 402–7.

Lombroso PJ, Scahill L, King RA, et al. Risperidone treatment of children and adolescents with chronic tic disorders: a preliminary report. *J Am Acad Child Adolesc Psychiatry* 1995; **34**: 1147–52. (Erratum in: *J Am Acad Child Adolesc Psychiatry* 1996; **35**: 394.)

Lucas AR, Kauffman PE, Morris EM. Gilles de la Tourette's disease. A clinical study of fifteen cases. *J Am Acad Child Psychiatry* 1967; **6**: 700–22.

Lucas Taracena MT, Montanes Rada F. Olanzapine in Tourette's syndrome: a report of three cases. *Actas Esp Psiquiatr* 2002; **30**: 129–32.

McKeith IG, Willians A, Nicol AR. Clonidine in Tourette's syndrome. *Lancet* 1981; **1**: 270–1.

McMahon WM, van de Wetering BJM, Filloux F, et al. Bilineal transmission and phenotypic variation of Tourette's disorder in a large pedigree. *J Am Acad Child Adolesc Psychiatry* 1996; **35**: 672–80.

Malison RT, McDougle CJ, van Dyck CH, et al. [123I]-βCIT SPECT imaging demonstrates increased striatal dopamine transporter binding in Tourette's syndrome. *Am J Psychiatry* 1995; **152**: 1359–61.

Mataix-Cols D, do Rosário-Campos MC, Leckman JF. A multidimensional model of obsessive-compulsive disorder. *Am J Psychiatry* 2005; **162**: 228–38.

Matur Z, Ucok A. Quetiapine treatment in a patient with Tourette's syndrome, obsessive-compulsive disorder and drug-induced mania. *Isr J Psychiatry Relat Sci* 2003; **40**: 150–2.

Meisel A, Winter C, Zschenderlein R, et al. Tourette syndrome: efficient treatment with ziprasidone and normalization of body weight in a patient with excessive weight gain under tiapride. *Mov Disord* 2004; **19**: 991–2.

Mérette C, Brassard A, Potvin A, et al. Significant linkage for Tourette syndrome in a large French Canadian family. *Am J Hum Genet* 2000; **67**: 1008–13.

Merikangas JR, Merikangas KR, Kopp U, et al. Blood choline and response to clonazepam and haloperidol in Tourette's syndrome. *Acta Psychiatr Scand* 1985; **72**: 395–9.

Mercadante MT, Filho GB, Lombroso PJ, et al. Rheumatic fever and co-morbid psychiatric disorders. *Am J Psychiatry* 2000; **157**: 2036–8.

Messiha FS. Biochemical pharmacology of Gilles de la Tourette's syndrome. *Neurosci Biobehav Rev* 1988; **12**: 295–305.

Meuldijk R, Colon EJ. Methadone treatment of Tourette's disorder. *Am J Psychiatry* 1992; **149**: 139–40.

Micheli F, Gatto M, Lekhuniec E, et al. Treatment of Tourette's syndrome with calcium antagonists. *Clin Neuropharmacol* 1990; **13**: 77–83.

Miguel EC, Coffey BJ, Baer L, et al. Phenomenology of intentional repetitive behaviors in obsessive-compulsive disorder and Tourette's syndrome. *J Clin Psychiatry* 1995; **56**: 420–30.

Miguel EC, Baer L, Coffey BJ, et al. Phenomenological differences appearing with repetitive behaviours in obsessive-compulsive disorder and Gilles de la Tourette syndrome. *Br J Psychiatry* 1997; **170**: 140–5.

Miguel EC, do Rosário-Campos MC, Silva Prado H, et al. Sensory phenomena in patients with obsessive-compulsive disorder (OCD) and/or Gilles de la Tourette syndrome (TS). *J Clin Psychiatry* 2000; **61**: 150–6.

Miltenberger RG, Fuqua RW, Woods DW. Applying behavior analysis to clinical problems: review and analysis of habit reversal. *J Appl Behav Anal* 1998; **31**: 447–69.

Montgomery MA, Clayton PJ, Friedhoff AJ. Psychiatric illness in Tourette syndrome patients and first-degree relatives. In: Friedhoff AJ, Chase TN, eds. *Gilles de la Tourette syndrome*. New York: Raven Press; 1982: 335–9.

Morphew JA, Sim M. Gilles de la Tourette's syndrome: a clinical and psychopathological study. *Br J Med Psychol* 1969; **42**: 293–301.

Mukaddes NM, Abali O. Quetiapine treatment of children and adolescents with Tourette's disorder. *J Child Adolesc Psychopharmacol* 2003; **13**: 295–9.

Muller N, Kroll B, Schwarz MJ, et al. Increased titers of antibodies against streptococcal M12 and M19 proteins in patients with Tourette's syndrome. *Psychiatry Res* 2001; **101**: 187–93.

Muller-Vahl KR, Schneider U, Koblenz A, et al. Treatment of Tourette's syndrome with delta 9-tetrahydrocannabinol (THC): a randomized crossover trial. *Pharmacopsychiatry* 2002; **35**: 57–61.

Muller-Vahl KR, Schneider U, Prevedel H, et al. Delta 9-tetrahydrocannabinol (THC) is effective in the treatment of tics in Tourette syndrome: a 6-week randomized trial. *J Clin Psychiatry* 2003; **64**: 459–65.

Nadvornik P, Sramka M, Lisy L, Svicka I. Experiences with dentatotomy. *Confin Neurol* 1972; **34**: 320–4.

Nee LE, Caine ED, Polinsky RJ, Eldridge R, Ebert MH. Gilles de la Tourette syndrome: clinical and family study of 50 cases. *Ann Neurol* 1980; **7**: 41–9.

Nee LE, Polinsky RJ, Ebert MH. Tourette syndrome: clinical and family studies. In: Friedhoff AJ, Chase TN, eds. *Gilles de la Tourette syndrome*. New York: Raven Press; 1982: 291–5.

Nöthen MM, Chichon S, Hemmer S, et al. Human dopamine D4 receptor gene: frequent occurrence of a null allele and observation of homozygosity. *Hum Mol Genet* 1994a; **3**: 2207–12.

Nöthen MM, Hebebrand J, Knapp H, et al. Association analysis of the dopamine D2 receptor gene in Tourette's syndrome using the haplotype relative risk method. *Am J Med Genet* 1994b; **54**: 249–52.

Onofrj M, Paci C, D'Andreamatteo G, et al. Olanzapine in severe Gilles de la Tourette syndrome: a 52-week double-blind cross-over study vs. low-dose pimozide. *J Neurol* 2000; **247**: 443–6.

Paolucci S, Buttinelli C, Fiume S, et al. Treatment of Gilles de la Tourette syndrome with depot neuroleptics. *Acta Neurol (Napoli)* 1984; **6**: 222–4.

Parraga HC, Woodward RL. Quetiapine for Tourette's syndrome. *J Am Acad Child Adolesc Psychiatry* 2001; **40**: 389–91.

Paschou P, Feng Y, Pakstis AJ, et al. Indications of linkage and association of Gilles de la Tourette syndrome in two independent family samples: 17q25 is a putative susceptibility region. *Am J Hum Genet* 2004; **75**: 545–60.

Pauls DL, Leckman JF. The inheritance of Gilles de la Tourette's syndrome and associated behaviors: evidence for autosomal dominant transmission. *N Engl J Med* 1986; **315**: 993–7.

Pauls DL, Kruger SD, Leckman JF, Cohen DJ, Kidd KK. The risk of Tourette Syndrome (TS) and Chronic Multiple Tics (CMT) among relatives of TS patients: obtained by direct interview. *J Am Acad Child Psychiatry* 1984; **23**: 134–7.

Pauls DL, Towbin KE, Leckman JF, Zahner GEP, Cohen DJ. Gilles de la Tourette syndrome and obsessive compulsive disorder: evidence supporting an etiological relationship. *Arch Gen Psychiatry* 1986; **43**: 1180–2.

Pauls DL, Pakstis AJ, Kurlan R, et al. Segregation and linkage analyses of Gilles de la Tourette's syndrome and related disorders. *J Am Acad Child Adolesc Psychiatry* 1990; **29**: 195–203.

Pauls DL, Raymond CL, Leckman JF, Stevenson JM. A family study of Tourette's syndrome. *Am J Hum Genet* 1991; **48**: 154–63.

Pauls DL, Alsobrook JP 2nd, Goodman W, Rasmussen S, Leckman JF. A family study of obsessive-compulsive disorder. *Am J Psychiatry* 1995; **152**: 76–84.

Perera HV. Two cases of Gilles de la Tourette's syndrome treated with haloperidol. *Br J Psychiatry* 1975; **127**: 324–6.

Perlmutter SJ, Leitman SF, Garvey MA. Therapeutic plasma exchange and intravenous immunoglobulin for obsessive-compulsive disorder and tic disorders in childhood. *Lancet* 1999; **354**: 1153–8.

Petek E, Windpassinger C, Vincent JB, et al. Disruption of a novel gene (IMMP2L) by a breakpoint in 7q31 associated with Tourette syndrome. *Am J Hum Genet* 2001; **68**: 848–58.

Peterson BS, Cohen DJ. The treatment of Tourette's syndrome: multimodal, developmental intervention. *J Clin Psychiatry* 1998a; **59**: 62–72.

Peterson B, Riddle MA, Cohen DJ, et al. Reduced basal ganglia volumes in Tourette's syndrome using three-dimensional reconstruction techniques from magnetic resonance images. *Neurology* 1993; **43**: 941–9.

Peterson BS, Skudlarski P, Anderson AW, et al. A functional magnetic resonance imaging study of tic suppression in Tourette syndrome. *Arch Gen Psychiatry* 1998a; **55**: 326–33.

Peterson BS, Zhang H, Anderson GM, et al. A double-blind, placebo-controlled, crossover trial of an antiandrogen in the treatment of Tourette's syndrome. *J Clin Psychopharmacol* 1998b; **18**: 324–31.

Peterson BS, Staib L, Scahill L, et al. Regional brain and ventricular volumes in Tourette syndrome. *Arch Gen Psychiatry* 2001; **58**: 427–40.

Peterson BS, Thomas P, Kane MJ, et al. Basal ganglia volumes in patients with Gilles de la Tourette syndrome. *Arch Gen Psychiatry* 2003; **60**: 415–24.

Pitman RK, Green RC, Jenike MA, Mesulam MM. Clinical comparison of Tourette's disorder and obsessive-compulsive disorder. *Am J Psychiatry* 1987; **144**: 1166–71.

Polites DJ, Kruger D, Stevenson I. Sequential treatments in a case of Gilles de la Tourette's syndrome. *Br J Med Psychol* 1965; **38**: 43–52.

Prabhakaran N. A case of Gilles de la Tourette's syndrome with some observations on aetiology and treatment. *Br J Psychiatry* 1970; **116**: 539–41.

Price RA, Kidd KK, Cohen DJ, Pauls DL, Leckman JF. A twin study of Tourette syndrome. *Arch Gen Psychiatry* 1985; **42**: 815–20.

Price RA, Pauls DL, Kruger SD, Caine ED. Family data support a dominant major gene for Tourette syndrome. *Psychiatry Res* 1988; **24**: 251–61.

Rauch SL, Baer L, Cosgrove GR, Jenike MA. Neurosurgical treatment of Tourette's syndrome: a critical review. *Compr Psychiatry* 1995; **36**: 141–56.

Redmond DE Jr. Alterations in the function of the nucleus locus ceruleus: a possible model for studies of anxiety. In: Hanin I, Usdin E, eds. *Animal models in psychiatry and neurology.* New York: Pergamon Press; 1977: 293–304.

Regeur L, Pakkenberg B, Fog R, et al. Clinical features and long-term treatment with pimozide in 65 patients with Gilles de la Tourette's syndrome. *J Neurol Neurosurg Psychiatry* 1986; **49**: 791–5.

Reynolds JEF, ed. *Martindale: the extra pharmacopoeia,* 31st edn. London: Pharmaceutical Press, 1996.

Riddle MA, Rasmusson AM, Woods SW, et al. SPECT imaging of cerebral blood flow in Tourette syndrome. *Adv Neurol* 1992; **58**: 207–11.

Robertson MM. The Gilles de la Tourette syndrome: the current status. *Br J Psychiatry* 1989; **154**: 147–69.

Robertson MM. Annotation: Gilles de la Tourette syndrome – an update. *J Child Psychol Psychiatry* 1994; **35**: 597–611.

Robertson MM. Tourette syndrome: associated conditions and the complexities of treatment. *Brain* 2000; **123**: 425–62.

Robertson MM. Diagnosing Tourette syndrome: is it a common disorder? *J Psychosom Res* 2003; **55**: 3–6.

Robertson MM, Trimble MR, Lees AJ. The psychopathology of the Gilles de la Tourette: a phenomenological analysis. *Br J Psychiatry* 1988; **52**: 383–90.

Robertson MM, Schnieden V, Lees AJ. Management of Gilles de la Tourette syndrome using sulpiride. *Clin Neuropharmacol* 1990a; **13**: 229–35.

Robertson M, Doran M, Trimble M, Lees AJ. The treatment of Gilles de la Tourette syndrome by limbic leucotomy. *J Neurol Neurosurg Psychiatry* 1990b; **53**: 691–4.

Ross MS, Moldofsky H. Comparison of pimozide with haloperidol in Gilles de la Tourette's syndrome (letter). *Lancet* 1977; **1**: 103.

Ross MS, Moldofsky H. A comparison of pimozide and haloperidol in the treatment of Gilles de la Tourette's syndrome. *Am J Psychiatry* 1978; **135**: 585–7.

Sallee FR, Nesbitt L, Jackson C, et al. Relative efficacy of haloperidol and pimozide in children and adolescents with Tourette's disorder. *Am J Psychiatry* 1997; **154**: 1057–62.

Sallee FR, Sethuraman G, Rock CM. Effects of pimozide on cognition in children with Tourette syndrome: interaction with comorbid attention deficit hyperactivity disorder. *Acta Psychiatr Scand* 1994; **90**: 4–9.

Sallee FR, Kurlan R, Goetz CG, et al. Ziprasidone treatment of children and adolescents with Tourette's syndrome: a pilot study. *J Am Acad Child Adolesc Psychiatry* 2000; **39**: 292–9.

Sandor P, Musisi S, Moldofsky H, et al. Tourette syndrome: a follow-up study. *J Clin Psychopharmacol* 1990; **10**: 197–9.

Sandor P, Singal S, Angus C. Remoxipride vs. haloperidol treatment of Tourette's syndrome. *Mov Disord* 1996; **11**: 248.

Scahill L, King RA, Leckman JF, et al. Contemporary approaches to the treatment of tics in Tourette syndrome. *Rev Bras Psiquiatr* 2000; 2.

Scahill L, Leckman JF, Schultz RT, et al. A placebo-controlled trial of risperidone in Tourette syndrome. *Neurology* 2003; **60**: 1130–5.

Schaller JL, Behar D. Quetiapine treatment of adolescent and child tic disorders. Two case reports. *Eur Child Adolesc Psychiatry* 2002; **11**: 196–7.

Seuchter SA, Hebebrand J, Klug B, et al. Complex segregation analysis of families ascertained through Gilles de la Tourette syndrome. *Genet Epidemiol* 2000; **18**: 33–47.

Shapira NA, McConville BJ, Pagnucco ML, et al. Novel use of tramadol hydrochloride in the treatment of Tourette's syndrome. *J Clin Psychiatry* 1997; **58**: 174–5.

Shapiro AK, Shapiro E. Treatment of Gilles de la Tourette's syndrome with haloperidol. *Br J Psychiatry* 1968; **114**: 345–50.

Shapiro AK, Shapiro E, Wayne H. Treatment of Tourette's syndrome with haloperidol: review of 34 cases. *Arch Gen Psychiatry* 1973; **28**: 92–7.

Shapiro ES, Shapiro AK, Sweet RD, et al. The diagnosis, etiology and treatment of Gilles de la Tourette's syndrome. In: Sankar DVS, ed. *Mental health in children. Vol I. Genetics, family and community studies*. Westbury, NY: PJD Publication; 1975: 167–73.

Shapiro AK, Shapiro ES, Bruun RD, et al. *Gilles de la Tourette syndrome*. New York: Raven Press; 1978: 1–9.

Shapiro AK. Remarks at the tenth anniversary membership meeting of the Tourette Syndrome Association. 22 May 1982. Mt Sinai Hospital, New York City. *TSA Newsletter* 1982a; **9**: 1–2.

Shapiro AK, Shapiro E. Clinical efficacy of haloperidol, pimozide, penfluridol, and clonidine in the treatment of Tourette syndrome. *Adv Neurol* 1982b; **35**: 383–6.

Shapiro AK, Shapiro E, Eisenkraft GJ. Treatment of Gilles de la Tourette's syndrome with clonidine and neuroleptics. *Arch Gen Psychiatry* 1983; **4**: 1235–40.

Shapiro AK, Shapiro ES, Young JG, et al. *Gilles de la Tourette syndrome*, 2nd edn. New York: Raven Press; 1988.

Shapiro E, Shapiro AK, Fulop G, et al. Related articles, links controlled study of haloperidol, pimozide and placebo for the treatment of Gilles de la Tourette's syndrome. *Arch Gen Psychiatry* 1989; **46**: 722–30.

Silver AA, Shytle RD, Sheehan KH, et al. Multicenter, double-blind, placebo-controlled study of mecamylamine monotherapy for Tourette's disorder. *J Am Acad Child Adolesc Psychiatry* 2001; **40**: 1103–10.

Simonic I, Gericke GS, Ott J, Weber JL. Identification of genetic markers associated with Gilles de la Tourette syndrome in an Afrikaner population. *Am J Hum Genet* 1998; **63**: 839–46.

Singer HS. PANDAS and immunomodulatory therapy. *Lancet* 1999; **354**: 1137–8.

Singer HS, Butler IJ, Tune LE, et al. Dopaminergic dysfunction in Tourette syndrome. *Ann Neurol* 1982; **12**: 361–6.

Singer HS. Current issues in Tourette syndrome. *Movement Disord* 2000; **15**: 1051–63.

Singer HS, Gammon K, Quaskey S. Haloperidol, fluphenazine and clonidine in Tourette syndrome: controversies in treatment. *Pediatr Neurosci* 1986; **12**: 71–4.

Singer HS, Wong DF, Brown JE, et al. Positron emission tomography evaluation of dopamine D-2 receptors in adults with Tourette syndrome. *Adv Neurol* 1992; **58**: 233–9.

Singer HS, Reiss AL, Brown JE, et al. Volumetric MRI changes in basal ganglia of children with Tourette's syndrome. *Neurology* 1993; **43**: 950–6.

Singer HS, Wendlandt J, Krieger M, et al. Baclofen treatment in Tourette syndrome: a double-blind, placebo-controlled, crossover trial. *Neurology* 2001; **56**: 599–604.

Stahl SM, Thornton JE, Simpson ML, et al. Gamma-vinyl-GABA treatment of tardive dyskinesia and other movement disorders. *Biol Psychiatry* 1985; **20**: 888–93.

Staley D, Wand R, Shady G. Tourette disorder: a cross-cultural review. *Compr Psychiatry* 1997; **38**: 6–16.

Stamenkovic M, Schindler SD, Aschauer HN, et al. Effective open-label treatment of Tourette's disorder with olanzapine. *Int Clin Psychopharmacol* 2000; **15**: 23–8.

Stanciu E, Csiky K, Csiky C. On a case of tics (Gilles de la Tourette's disease) treated with haloperidol. *Neurol Psihiatr Neurochir* 1972; **17**: 43–8.

State MW, Lombroso PJ, Pauls DL, Leckman JF. The genetics of childhood psychiatric disorders: a decade of progress. *J Am Acad Child Adolesc Psychiatry* 2000; **39**: 946–62.

State MW, Greally JM, Cuker A, et al. Epigenetic abnormalities associated with a chromosome 18(q21–q22) inversion and a Gilles de la Tourette syndrome phenotype. *Proc Natl Acad Sci USA* 2003; **100**: 4684–9.

Stefl ME. Mental health needs associated with Tourette syndrome. *Am J Public Health* 1984; **74**: 1310–13.

Stephens RJ, Bassel C, Sandor P. Olanzapine in the treatment of aggression and tics in children with Tourette's syndrome: a pilot study. *J Child Adolesc Psychopharmacol* 2004; **14**: 255–66.

Stevens H. The syndrome of Gilles de la Tourette and its treatment. *Med Ann District Columbia* 1964; **36**: 277–9.

Stevens JR, Blachly PH. Successful treatment of the maladie des tics. Gilles de la Tourette's syndrome. *Am J Dis Child* 1966; **112**: 541–5.

Swedo SE. Sydenham's chorea: a model for childhood autoimmune neuropsychiatric disorders. *JAMA* 1994; **272**: 1788–91.

Swedo SE, Leonard HL, Schapiro MB, et al. Sydenham's chorea: physical and psychological symptoms of St Vitus dance. *Pediatrics* 1993; **91**: 706–13.

Swedo SE, Leonard HL, Mittleman BB, et al. Identification of children with pediatric autoimmune neuropsychiatric disorders associated with streptococcal infections by a marker associated with rheumatic fever. *Am J Psychiatry* 1997; **154**: 110–12.

Swedo SE, Leonard HL, Garvey M, et al. Pediatric autoimmune neuropsychiatric disorders associated with streptococcal infections (PANDAS): a clinical description of the first fifty cases. *Am J Psychiatry* 1998; **155**: 264–71.

Taranta A, Stollerman GH. Relationship of Sydenham's chorea to infection with Group A streptococci. *Am J Med* 1956; **20**: 170–5.

Temel Y, Visser-Vandewalle V. Surgery in Tourette syndrome. *Mov Dis* 2004; **91**: 3–14.

The Tourette Syndrome Association International Consortium for Genetics. A complete genome screen in sib pairs affected by Gilles de la Tourette syndrome. *Am J Hum Genet* 1999; **65**: 1428–36.

The Tourette Syndrome Classification Study Group. Definitions and classification of tic disorders. *Arch Neurol* 1993; **50**: 1013–16.

Thompson M, Comings DE, Feder L, George SR, O'Dowd BF. Mutation screening of the dopamine D1 receptor gene in Tourette's syndrome and alcohol dependent patients. *Am J Med Genet* 1998; **81**: 241–4.

Toren P, Laor N, Cohen DJ, et al. Ondansetron treatment in patients with Tourette's syndrome. *Int Clin Psychopharmacol* 1999; **14**: 373–6.

Tourette GG. Étude sur une affection nerveuse caractérisée par de l'incoordination motrice accompagnée d'écholalie et de coprolalie (jumping, latah, and myriachit). *Arch Neurol* 1885; 9: 19–42,158–200.

Trillet M, Moreau T, Dalery J, et al. Treatment of Gilles de la Tourette's disease with amisulpride (letter). *Presse Med* 1990; 19: 175.

Turjanski N, Sawle GV, Playford ED, et al. PET studies of the presynaptic and postsynaptic dopaminergic system in Tourette's syndrome. *J Neurol Neurosurg Psychiatry* 1994; 57: 688–92.

Van der Linden C, Bruggeman R, van Woerkom TC. Serotonin–dopamine antagonist and Gilles de la Tourette's syndrome: an open pilot dose-titration study with risperidone. *Mov Disord* 1994; 9: 687–8.

Vandewalle V, van der Linden C, Groenewegen HJ, Caemaert J. Stereotactic treatment of Gilles de la Tourette syndrome by high frequency stimulation of thalamus. *Lancet* 1999; 353: 724.

van Wattum PJ, Chappell PB, Zelterman D, Scahill LD, Leckman JF. Patterns of response to acute naloxone infusion in Tourette's syndrome. *Mov Disord* 2000; 15: 1252–4.

Wagaman JR, Miltenberger RG, Willians DE. Treatment of a vocal tic by differential reinforcement. *J Behav Ther Exp Psychiatry* 1995; 26: 35–9.

Walkup JT, Leckman JF, Price RA, et al. The relationship between Tourette syndrome and obsessive compulsive disorder: a twin study. *Psychopharmacol Bull* 1988; 24: 375–9.

Walkup JT, Scahill LD, Riddle MA. Disruptive behavior, hyperactivity, and learning disabilities in children with Tourette's syndrome. *Adv Neurol* 1995; 65: 259–72.

Walkup JT, LaBuda MC, Singer HS, et al. Family study and segregation analysis of Tourette syndrome: evidence for a mixed model of inheritance. *Am J Hum Genet* 1996; 59: 684–93.

Wertheim J. A 10th anniversary message: who we are, how we help. *TSA Newsletter* 1982; 9: 1–2.

Wilhelm S, Deckersbach T, Coffey BJ, et al. Habit reversal versus supportive psychotherapy for Tourette's disorder: a randomized controlled trial. *Am J Psychiatry* 2003; 1670: 1175–7.

Witelson SF. Hand and sex differences in the isthmus and genu of the human corpus callosum. *Brain* 1989; 112: 779–835.

Wolf SS, Jones DW, Knable MB, et al. Tourette syndrome: prediction of phenotypic variation in monozygotic twins by caudate nucleus D2 receptor binding. *Science* 1996; 273: 1225–7.

Woods DW, Miltenberger RG, Lumley VA. Sequential application of major habit-reversal components to treat motor tics in children. *J Appl Behav Anal* 1996; 29: 483–93.

World Health Organization. *The ICD-10 – Classification of mental and behavioral disorders: clinical descriptions and diagnostic guidelines*. Geneva; 1992.

Wright S, Peet M. Gilles de la Tourette's syndrome. Amelioration following acute akinesia during lorazepam withdrawal. *Br J Psychiatry* 1989; 154: 257–9.

Yaryura-Tobias JA, Neziroglu F, Howard S, Fuller B. Clinical aspects of Gilles de la Tourette syndrome. *Orthomolec Psychiatry* 1981; 10: 263–8.

Young JG, Cohen DJ, Hattox SE, et al. Plasma free MHPG and neuroendocrine responses to challenge doses of clonidine in Tourette's syndrome: preliminary report. *Life Sci* 1981; 29: 1467–75.

Yvonneau M, Bezard P. Apropos of a case of Gilles de la Tourette's disease blocked by sulpiride: psycho-biological study. *Encephale* 1970; 59: 439–59.

Zhang H, Leckman JF, Pauls DL, et al. Tourette Syndrome Association International Consortium for Genetics. Genomewide scan of hoarding in sib pairs in which both sibs have Gilles de la Tourette syndrome. *Am J Hum Genet* 2002; 70: 896–904.

Appendix: Examples of coaching sessions for TS patients

Example 1

Behavior: a 25-year-old young adult has a vocal tic. She keeps saying, "Rape me! Raaaaaape, raaaaape, raaape, rape me!"

Statement: *Oh, I feel awful because I have to do this so many times that my throat usually aches! What bothers me more are these words, its meaning! People stare at me, probably thinking I'm out of my mind!*

Sensory phenomena: energy that builds up, muscle-skeletal physical sensation.

Therapist/coach: Do you have any special feeling or a sensation that precedes this tic?

Yes … something happens inside of my body. Try to be more specific. *It is like a volcano in my body.* Where in your body? *… It is like an extra energy that begins from nowhere and by the time it reaches my throat I feel my vocal cords striking like a string of a guitar.* Yes, anything else? *Yes! I'm figuring out … when I say these words, specially the "A", I produce a "counter vibration" that nulls the original vibes!* Anything more? *No … isn't that enough? I'm so tired … I don't laugh anymore, I just want to go to bed … when I'm sleeping I don't have tics!! I'm out of problems!*

We should usually work with an interdisciplinary team. In this case, I suggested phonologic help to help the patient find special phonemes or some exercises that may result in the same "counter vibration" and help in making a strategy for the habit reversal. Besides, psychiatric consultation to treat comorbid depression is warranted.

Example 2

Behavior: a 12-year-old girl sometimes says "no! no! no!" three times and sometimes she takes several deep breaths and screams " ahhh, ahhh, ahhh, … ahhh".

Statement: *my friends in school call me "Nonoahhh" and I get so upset … and I can't handle … I know that a girl shouldn't do this and I'm so ashamed and nobody knows how I feel … No one has ever asked me why this happens to me …*

Sensory phenomena: "Just right" feeling/perception triggered by auditory stimuli.

Therapist/coach: Is there any difference in saying "no! no! no!" and "ahhh, ahhh, ahhh … ahhh"? *Yes! They are completely different! As a matter of fact I say "no! no! no!" because I have a thought, a bad thought, that comes to my mind … and I have to say "no" exactly three times to "clean up" this bad thought! People think that it is a tic but it's not. I get embarrassed about my thinking so it is easier to be this way … a "tic". The "ahhh, ahhh, ahhh … ahhh" is really a tic … is like having too much air inside but when I begin to do it I only can finish it when it sounds "just right."* If I understood correctly the "no, no, no" is a *tic-like compulsion*? You do this to calm down your anxiety about your bad thoughts? *Yes, but I'm not going to say my thoughts!!! Don't ask me!*

(Continued)

(Continued)

OK, don't worry ... which one is worst? The one you just say three times or the other that you might keep saying it several times? *Well ... this is very hard to answer because I feel so guilty about my thoughts ... and usually the real tics come just after the tic-like compulsion ...* This thought that you have is intrusive? *Yes!* Does it happen frequently? *Sure! Most of the time! I can't stop them!* Have you ever told somebody about those thoughts before? *No ... I'm so ashamed of them ... and as I said, nobody ever asked me before about these feelings ... My friends tease me, my parents get upset, they say that I don't try hard enough and they always get embarrassed when we go out together.* Have you been diagnosed with obsessive-compulsive disorder? *No. Just TS.* Well, it seems to me that you might have OCD plus TS. I think we should take care, first of all, of your OCD because it is distressing you so much and this may be influencing the frequency and severity of your TS. Would you like to stop being called Nonoahhh? *Yes!* So we are going to explain to your parents that you also may have OCD and should consult a psychiatrist and, if the diagnosis is confirmed, you will probably have to take some medicine that will improve this awful thinking. *OK, but I'm not going to tell my thoughts!* Ok, you'll do that only when you feel comfortable to talk about them, ok? *Yes ...*

TS with comorbid OCD is very common. Sometimes, treating OCD symptoms secondarily reduces tic severity through the improvement of anxiety. Nevertheless, we still may need to approach tics by choosing together with the patient the best strategy to deal with the tic behavior.

Example 3

Behavior: a 16-year-old adolescent shakes his head lightly.

Statement: *I don't care about this! It doesn't bother me at all! I just came here 'cause my parents wanted to. They are stressed about my tic! I'm not! I'm ok. I'm doing fine. I don't feel anything about my tics. I just do it! My parents need help, not me!*

Sensory phenomena: none. No "just right," no urges, absence of subjective experiences.

Therapist/coach: Good, that's good. We will talk with your parents and invite them to participate in the family group coaching.

chapter 8

Pharmacotherapy of psychotic disorders in children and adolescents

Gabriele Masi

Clinical features of psychotic disorders

Introduction

Even though psychotic symptoms can be part of the clinical picture of different psychiatric disorders, including mood disorders, according to the restrictive definition of DSM-IV psychotic disorders are defined by a gross impairment of reality testing and a loss of ego boundaries. The prototypical pictures of this section are schizophrenia and schizophreniform disorder. Other disorders included in this chapter are the schizoaffective disorder, the brief psychotic disorder, the delusional disorder, and the shared psychotic disorder. Finally, psychotic disorders due to a general medical condition and to substances (drugs of abuse, medication, or toxins) are also included. Schizophrenic and schizophreniform disorders will be briefly summarized in the following section.

Schizophrenia in subjects younger than 13 years is defined as very early-onset schizophrenia (VEOS). When the onset of the disorder is between 13 and 18 years, the term of early-onset schizophrenia (EOS) is used. The diagnosis is made using the same diagnostic criteria of adults. These disorders are rare before the age of 10 (fewer than 20% of the VEOS subjects are in the prepubertal age range), while their incidence increases during adolescence and reaches its peak in early adulthood. A continuity is supposed among these different forms of schizophrenia, even though presenting clinical features may be different according to age at onset. Like other early-onset forms of multifactorial disorders, VEOS and EOS are associated with a greater disease severity than the adult form of schizophrenia, and may be also associated with greater heritability (Asarnow et al, 1994).

Definition

Signs and symptoms of schizophrenia can be attributed to two broad domains, positive and negative symptoms. Positive symptoms reflect an excess or a distortion of a normal function, while negative symptoms reflect a diminution or a loss of a normal function.

Positive symptoms are delusions, that is distortions or exaggerations of inferential thinking, hallucinations, that is distortions or exaggerations of perception, disorganized speech, that is a distortion or exaggeration of language and communication, and disorganized or catatonic behavior, that is a distortion or exaggeration of the behavioral control. Positive symptoms may be in turn attributed to two different dimensions, the "psychotic" dimension, including delusions and hallucinations, and the "disorganization" dimension, including the disorganized speech and behavior.

Negative symptoms include affective flattening, that is a diminution or loss of the range and intensity of emotional expression, alogia, that is a diminution or loss of the fluency and productivity of thought and speech, and avolition, that is a diminution or loss of goal-directed behavior.

In order to make a diagnosis of schizophrenia, at least two of the five characteristic symptoms of schizophrenia (delusions, hallucinations, disorganized speech, disorganized or catatonic behavior, and negative symptoms) must be present concurrently for at least one month, even though bizarre delusions or hallucinations including "voices commenting" or "voices conversing" allow for a diagnosis per se.

Premorbid and prodromal phases

Premorbid developmental impairments are extremely frequent in earlier-onset forms of schizophrenia (Nicolson et al, 2000; McClellan et al, 2003). In about one third of the subjects, IQ is below 70. Premorbid impairments include social withdrawal and isolation, motor and language impairments, disruptive behavior disorder, and scholastic difficulties. Notably, an onset of schizophrenia before age 13 is associated with a significantly greater incidence of premorbid language delays and difficulties than onset later in adolescent. The prepsychotic developmental data from 49 consecutive children with VEOS from the USA National Institute of Mental Health study on childhood-onset schizophrenia (Nicolson et al, 2000) support these findings: 55% had language abnormalities, 57% had motor abnormalities, and 55% had social abnormalities years before the onset of psychotic symptoms. Sixty-three percent of the patients had either failed a grade or required placement in a special education setting before the onset of their illness.

McClellan and colleagues (2003) found that premorbid social withdrawal and isolation were significantly correlated with ratings of negative symptoms (e.g. flat affect, lack of motivation and of social interest), which are particularly frequent in VEOS. In addition, 34% of the NIMH childhood-onset schizophrenia sample demonstrated transient symptoms of pervasive developmental disorder, such as flapping and echolalia, during the premorbid period (Alaghband-Rad et al, 1995); such symptoms have not been reported in the premorbid history of later-onset schizophrenia. The nature of these premorbid conditions is still under discussion. Since the landmark studies of Kolvin (1971), a differentiation between pervasive developmental disorders and childhood schizophrenia has been established. However, a premorbid social impairment is the most commonly reported feature, being present in 50–80% of VEOS. The diagnosis of pervasive developmental disorder is not rarely raised in the first phase of development of VEOS cases, even though most studies found that risk of schizophrenic development in autistic patients is not higher than in the general population (Volkmar and Cohen, 1991; Mouridsen et al, 1999). Furthermore, subjects with VEOS and a lifetime diagnosis of pervasive developmental disorders were not found to be different from VEOS without pervasive developmental disorders with respect to age at onset, IQ, response to medications, and rates of familial schizotypy (Sporn et al, 2004). These findings suggest that premorbid social withdrawal and isolation may represent early manifestations of a liability to schizophrenia or an exaggeration of neurodevelopmental abnormalities seen in adulthood schizophrenia, and stem from whatever pathophysiologic processes ultimately are manifested as negative symptoms (McClellan et al, 2003).

These findings argue for a more severe early disruption of brain development in childhood-onset schizophrenia than for adult-onset. This group of patients with greater disruption of premorbid development also has a greater familial vulnerability for schizophrenia, indicating that their earlier age of onset may be due, in part, to more aberrant neurodevelopment secondary to a higher level of familial loading for schizophrenia (Nicolson and Rapoport, 1999).

Those patients who develop a schizophrenic disorder enter into a prodromal phase with a further gradual decline in social and cognitive functioning that precedes the onset of the psychotic symptoms. This decline includes social withdrawal, worsening of school performance, odd behaviors, deteriorating self-care skills, bizarre hygiene and eating behaviors, eccentric interests, changes in affect, impulse dyscontrol, hostility and aggression, poor thought and speech, blunting affects and thought (tangentiality), and anergia. These changes may occur abruptly, during days or weeks, or, more frequently (namely in VEOS) insidiously, during months or one year, especially when they represent a worsening of premorbid personality features.

Clinical picture

The onset of symptoms is usually insidious in children, while in adolescents both acute and insidious onset can occur. Given the high rate of premorbid problems, it is often difficult to distinguish between premorbid personality, cognitive abnormalities, and the onset of the disorder. The full clinical picture generally resembles that of adult patients, namely with hallucinations and delusions, bizarre behavior or rituals, flat or inappropriate affect, deterioration of function, avolition, and alogia.

The negative symptom dimension is particularly represented in VEOS, as well as disorganized behavior and hallucinations, while delusions are more rare, and usually poorly systematized and not readily ascertainable in younger children. Auditory hallucinations are more frequently reported, while less common are somatic or visual hallucinations. Delusions are less frequent, they are often difficult to assess in younger patients and they are usually centered around parents, fantasy figures, and animals. Formal thought disorders include magical or irrational thinking and loosening of associations, but frequently these features are not so severe as to meet diagnostic criteria, mainly in the first phase of the disorder (Caplan, 1994). Furthermore, they may be difficult to detect in younger or more impaired children. Incoherence or loosening of association, illogicality, and alogia can be more evident as the illness worsens. Negative symptoms are more clearly associated with a poorer premorbid functioning, with an increased familial risk of schizophrenia and with a poorer adult outcome. This phase usually lasts 1 to 6 months.

Different subtypes of schizophrenia have been described in adult patients, including paranoid, disorganized, catatonic, undifferentiated, and residual. The undifferentiated subtype is the most frequent in VEOS and EOS.

About one out of five children and adolescents with EOS have mental retardation. It is not clear whether the low intelligence may precede the onset of psychotic symptoms and represent a risk factor, or whether it is due to the impact of the illness.

The earliest onset of the disorder is still under discussion. In the majority of the reported cases the age of 5–6 years seems to be the earliest onset, even though in most cases the onset is assessed by history, as the diagnosis is made after several years of insidious symptomatology. However, frequency of schizophrenia in school-age children is very rare. During and after puberty the frequency raises and reaches its peak between late adolescence and early adulthood (21–22 years).

Generally, the clinical picture is markedly impairing. The dysfunction is not only expressed by deterioration in multiple areas, but in younger children by a failure to achieve the expected level of interpersonal, academic, and social achievement.

A dimensional approach to schizophrenia

Liability to schizophrenia stems from the multi-gene model, which assumes that multiple genes combine with one another and with the environment, and the resulting genetic liability is distributed on a continuum in the population. Individuals with the higher loading of risk factors may present the full-blown schizophrenia, while subjects with the lower risk may show clinical markers of liability, in terms of schizotypal personality disorder, negative symptoms, and cognitive impairment. The schizotypal personality disorder may be considered a milder version of schizophrenia, with disturbances of perception and thinking. The term schizotaxia, firstly introduced in early 1960s by

Meehl to describe an unexpressed genetic liability to schizophrenia, has been more recently revisited (Tsuang et al, 2000) to describe patients with mild negative symptoms, cognitive impairment in executive functions, and brain abnormalities. In this perspective, schizotaxia is on a continuum, including at the extreme manifestations a full-blown schizophrenia. Even though up to 20–50% of relatives of patients with schizophrenia have features of schizotaxia, only about 10% will become psychotic. According to this dimensional view, the biologic risk for schizophrenia may be expressed as part of a broader phenotype and this phenotype may be present before the onset of the full-blown psychosis as an impairment of social and cognitive functioning. This view may have important implications in treatment planning, even though a preventive pharmacological treatment in adult patients with prodromic mild symptoms is still debatable (Tsuang et al, 1999; Cannon et al, 2002; McGorry et al, 2002; Koenigsberg et al, 2003; Woods et al, 2003). The concept of schizotaxia, and more generally of a broader schizophrenia spectrum, is still not well explored in children and adolescents and may have interesting diagnostic and preventive implications, which will be considered in the following chapters.

Outcome

A cyclic pattern is typical of the majority of schizophrenic adult patients after the first episode, with increasing deterioration after every cycle. Eventually, a chronic state with residual symptoms determines a stable impairment, with different degrees of severity. It is not clear whether this natural history can occur in VEOS and EOS; however, an incomplete recovery is present in about 80% of young patients with more than one cycle (Werry and Taylor, 1994). Only 10–15% of patients have a full symptomatic recovery from the first episode, compared to the 50% in the affective psychoses (psychotic depression, bipolar disorder with psychotic symptoms). The course is even poorer in the earlier forms of the disorder. This finding is confirmed by Remschmidt et al (1991), according to whom only 14% of adolescent patients with schizophrenia had a complete remission during the index hospitalization. Other reports (Werry et al, 1991; McClellan et al, 1993) confirm that only a minority of patients show a complete recovery, the majority of the affected adolescents presenting a moderate to severe impairment at the outcome.

In Maziade et al's study (1996), 40 subjects with EOS were followed up for a mean of 14.8 years. Only two subjects had a complete recovery, while 70% had moderate to severe impairment. Eggers and Bunk (1997) followed up 44 patients with childhood-onset schizophrenia with a 42-year long-term follow-up. Overall, 50% were significantly impaired at outcome, 25% had a partial remission, and 25% had a complete remission. The subjects with "schizoaffective disorder" had the best outcome, patients with onset of symptoms before age 10 had the worst prognosis (Eggers, 1989). A chronic, insidious onset was more frequent before age 12, and it was associated with the worst prognosis (none of these patients remitted completely).

Data from Asarnow et al's UCLA sample of schizophrenic children (2004), evaluated originally between 7 and 14 years of age, are similar to those observed in Eggers' sample. Over the course of a 3- to 7-year follow-up, 67% showed continuing schizophrenia or schizoaffective disorder. There was considerable variability in global adjustment, with 56% of the sample showing improvement in functioning over the course of follow-up, and the other 44% showing minimal improvement or deteriorating course.

Hollis (2000) evaluated the predictive validity of a DSM-III-R diagnosis of schizophrenia in childhood and early adolescence after an 11.5-year follow-up, revealing a high level of predictive validity for the DSM-III-R diagnosis (positive predictive value 80%), similar to affective psychoses, suggesting an etiologic continuity with adult schizophrenia. Moreover, when compared to non-schizophrenic psychoses, schizophrenia with onset in childhood and adolescence was associated with significantly poorer symptomatic and social outcome, with a chronic illness course and severe impairments in social relationships and independent living.

During the recovery phase, lasting several months, there is a shift from positive to negative symptoms (flattening affect, social withdrawal, avolition), and depression may also occur, with an improvement in deterioration of functioning. Some patients do not recover, but they have a persisting deterioration with negative symptoms between acute phases.

A chronic course with schizophrenic symptoms over years can occur in the most severely impaired patients despite adequate and intensive treatments. More recent psychopharmachologic approaches (i.e. atypical antipsychotics) have improved the prognosis of these patients.

Premorbid and intellectual functioning are the best prognostic predictors (Eggers, 1989; McClellan et al, 1993; Maziade et al, 1996). The high mortality (suicide or accidental death) of these patients is noteworthy, at least 5% (Eggers et al, 1989; Werry et al, 1991).

Diagnostic challenges

Accurate diagnosis of schizophrenia can be difficult when the onset is insidious, and the premorbid phase is characterized by cognitive, social, and behavioral abnormalities, which may overshadow the psychotic change. This is particularly true in children with VEOS, when the disorder is rare, the onset is usually chronic, developmental delays are often in continuity with the prodromal phase, and symptoms can be erroneously attributed to other psychiatric domains, which are much more frequent in school-age children. In the Schaffer and Ross study (2002) a diagnosis of schizophrenia or schizoaffective disorder was made 2 ± 2 years after the onset of psychotic symptoms, and 4.5 ± 2.4 years after the onset of the first presenting symptoms. Before the correct diagnosis, the 17 patients received 43 other diagnoses, the most frequent being pervasive developmental disorders (PDD) (52.9%), attention deficit hyperactivity disorder (ADHD) (47.1%), bipolar disorder (41.2%), depression (23.5%), and obsessive-compulsive disorder (OCD) (17.6%). These findings support the notion that families are seeking help several years before the diagnosis of childhood-onset schizophrenia.

On the other hand, the diagnosis of schizophrenia can be inappropriately made for children with psychotic symptoms associated with other primary disorders, which do not meet diagnostic criteria for schizophrenia when clinical interviews or other structured diagnostic instruments are used. In an ongoing National Institute of Mental Health (NIMH) project, 1300 children were referred as possible VEOS cases, and only 215 were considered putative cases after telephone screening and chart reviews. The 215 children and their parents were interviewed using the K-SADS, and only 64 met diagnostic criteria for VEOS according to the DSM-III-R or DSM-IV criteria for schizophrenia (Calderoni et al, 2001).

Non-psychotic hallucinations and delusions

Psychotic-like symptoms may be misleading, as their presence usually suggests a diagnosis of psychotic disorder NOS, or schizophrenia, although they have been described in different psychiatric disorders. When hallucinations and/or delusions are specifically investigated, their prevalence in the general population before age 21 is estimated to be about 3–5% or even higher (McGee et al, 2000). Auditory hallucinations are the most frequent psychotic symptom, whereas in prepubertal children delusions are less frequent and usually poorly elaborated, as a function of cognitive development.

Hallucinations have been described in a variety of childhood mental disorders, including psychotic affective disorders (both depression and bipolar disorder), post-traumatic stress disorder, other abuse-related disorders, and severe social and psychologic deprivation, bereavement, dissociative disorders, personality disorders (namely schizotypal and borderline), and in organic processes, including neurologic illness such as epilepsy (namely temporal lobe epilepsy) and migraine.

An epidemiologic study from New Zealand (McGee et al, 2000) considered a birth cohort of children born beween 1972 and 1973. According to a diagnostic interview at age 11, 8% of the children ($n=788$) reported at least sometimes experiencing hallucinatory phenomena, most of them non-pathologic. The children reporting hallucinations did not differ in many psychopathological respects from the children not reporting hallucinations. It has been proposed that the term hallucination should be limited to only the phenomena related to a mental or physical illness. Non-psychotic children who hallucinate differ from psychotic children in several ways: they are more rarely delusional, do not present disturbances in language production, do not exhibit decreased motor activity or incongruous mood, and do not present bizarre behavior or social withdrawal. However, there may be a subgroup of children for which these experiences are predictive of a psychopathology later in life (Fennig et al, 1997).

Mood disorders

A major challenge is the differentiation between schizophrenia and mood disorders, which may also co-occur with a schizophrenic disorder. In these patients mania can be confused with disorganization and depressive symptoms can be erroneously interpreted as negative symptoms. Children and adolescents with depression may present hallucinations, or, more rarely, delusions (Chambers et al, 1982; Ulloa et al, 2000; Calderoni et al, 2001). Psychotic symptoms are even more frequent in mania, more frequently with a rapid-cycling course

(Geller et al, 1995). Typical features of psychotic depression are a chronic and severe course, with psychotic symptoms usually congruent with the mood (Calderoni et al, 2001). However, the grossly disorganized behavior or speech is usually absent, as well as a deterioration of functioning. Hallucinations (prevalently auditory) are much more frequent (80%), while delusions (prevalently reference, "read my mind" or "hear my thoughts") (22%) and, even more, thought disorders (sentence incoherence, looseness of associations, illogical thinking) are not frequent symptoms of early affective psychoses. The psychotic symptoms in major depression are associated with a higher family loading of bipolar disorder and with a higher risk of developing a bipolar disorder.

In the seminal study of Werry et al (1991), while all the subjects aged 7 to 17 years first diagnosed as schizophrenic resulted in a correct diagnosis at follow-up, over half of the bipolar patients first received a diagnosis of schizophrenia, and only at follow-up was the mislabeled diagnosis changed. Even though diagnostic accuracy has probably increased in the last decade, parallel to an increased knowledge of the early-onset bipolar phenotype (Masi et al, in press), this diagnostic mistake is still not rare, mainly when psychotic symptoms co-occur.

Compared with bipolar patients, schizophrenic patients have more premorbid abnormal and odd personalities and developmental disabilities, while the most frequent antecedent of a bipolar disorder is an ADHD. From a phenomenologic point of view, schizophrenic patients have more frequently an insidious onset, more delusions, and, particularly, a flattened mood. The distinction between mood-congruent and mood-incongruent hallucinations and delusions, even if not pathognomonic, may be of interest in the differential diagnosis. The outcome is markedly worse in schizophrenic patients, with a greater persistence of psychotic symptoms, and a poorer prognosis, in terms of additional episodes or chronicity, and of recovery from the index episode. Depressed or manic mood is more frequent in bipolar patients, even though a depressive episode can occur during a schizophrenic illness. Family history of a bipolar disorder can be a helpful indicator of an affective disorder, even though a history of both depression and bipolar disorder is often reported in relatives of schizophrenic children and adolescents. The follow-up is often the best aid for avoiding a misdiagnosis, which may lead to an unnecessary use of antipsychotic medications.

Post-traumatic stress disorder

After a traumatic experience children are very distressed and in shock. They can have repetitive thoughts, or vivid recollections or even flashbacks, triggered by reminders in the environment, during which the children report that they are re-experiencing the frightening event. In these cases psychotic-like symptoms represent dissociative and/or anxiety phenomena, including intrusive thoughts, derealization, or depersonalization. This is a sort of dissociative experience. Cognitive changes (attention, memory), increased alertness, and suspiciousness can be prominent, as well as a behavioral change such as irritability or aggression, with increased impulsivity and temper tantrums. Acute fears, and sleep disturbances with nightmares, are associated. Physiologic arousal is usually increased, with startle reactions. All these symptoms can be misleading, and can suggest a diagnosis of acute psychosis when an adequate knowledge about the traumatic experience is not available. However, it must be remembered that a true psychotic disorder can be triggered by a traumatic experience, or it can occur as a part of a chronic post-traumatic stress disorder (PTSD) in 15% of the children (Famularo et al, 1996). When they occur within a PTSD, disturbances of the reality testing are more frequently brief and recall the trauma, while classical thought disorders of paranoia, illogicality, flat affect, and bizarre delusions are not usually associated with PTSD, at least in children and adolescents.

Personality disorders

Some personality disorders may present psychotic-like symptoms, which may lead to a misdiagnosis of childhood or adolescent schizophrenia. Schizotypal personality disorder is characterized by marked abnormalities in social and interpersonal behavior, associated to cognitive and perceptual distortions, behavior oddities, usually evident in early adulthood, with possible transient psychotic-like symptoms. Subclinical levels of thought disorder in children have been reported, even though the concept of schizotypal personality disorder in children has not been adequately explored to date. According to Asarnow et al (1994), only one out of 12 youths with schizotypal personality disorder developed schizophrenia during a 3-year follow-up, but 80% showed continuing schizophrenia spectrum disorders and 20% had a schizoaffective disorder. After a 7-year follow-up, 25% of the subjects had a bipolar spectrum disorder.

Schizoid personality disorder is characterized by a pervasive pattern of detachment from social relationships and a restricted range of expression of emotions. Only sparse data are reported on the phenomenology of this condition in children, which includes increased sensitivity and paranoid ideas, an unusual style of communication, which strongly resembles that of the schizotypal personality disorder, and a continuity with the schizotypal personality disorder in adolescent and adult life (Wolff, 1991).

Borderline personality disorder has been more frequently studied in children, although developmentally adapted clinical features are even more unclear, and the construct lacks a clear diagnostic specificity. These children often exhibited brief episodes of frankly psychotic behavior and thinking during childhood, associated with many affective features. The typical "adult-like" clinical picture includes instability of interpersonal relationships, self-identity, emotions, and impulse control (namely self-injurious behaviors). Different studies have related this unstable pattern to early traumatic life experiences, resulting in emotional dysregulation and failure of reflective function. The clinical picture of borderline personality disorder has also been strictly related to the multiple complex developmental disorder (MCDD) (see later) (Towbin et al, 1993).

Obsessive-compulsive disorder

The relationship between obsessive-compulsive disorder (OCD) and schizophrenia is more subtle than has previously been reported, in terms of both comorbidity and differential diagnosis. A co-occurrence between schizophrenia and OCD has been reported in 26% of 50 consecutive adolescents with schizophrenia (Nechmad et al, 2003). This comorbid subgroup showed higher rates of affective flattening and blunting and may represent a subtype among patients with schizophrenia.

A major issue is the possible diagnostic confusion between severe, bizarre, and pervasive obsessions and compulsions without insight of a severe OCD, and a psychotic delusion of the schizophrenic spectrum. In school-age children or young adolescents, the ego dystonicity of obsessions and compulsions may be lacking, and the content of the obsessions may be bizarre. Children may present intrusive thoughts and repetitive behaviors which may resemble a psychotic disorder. Even though OCD patients do recognize that their symptoms are unreasonable and are the product of their mind, this may not be the case in younger children. Sometimes children describe their intrusive thoughts as an inner or external "voice," and this report may lead to a misinterpretation of a hallucination.

Pervasive developmental disorders

Pervasive developmental disorders (PDD) are usually well separated from schizophrenia, from a clinical and nosologic point of view (Kolvin, 1971). The earlier onset and the absence of a normal period are discriminant features in PDD spectrum disorders. However, it is not rare that the history of children with VEOS is characterized by developmental delays, including language, motor, and social development, which allow for a diagnosis of PDD-NOS. However, long-term follow-up studies of children with autism do not support the notion that autism is a risk factor for schizophrenia (Volkmar and Cohen, 1991; Mouridsen et al, 1999).

In children who will develop a VEOS, as well as in children with multidimensional impairment (MDI) and MCDD (see later), the PDD is usually not as severe and pervasive as in autistic children. The clinical features of the PDD spectrum can progressively improve or, more rarely, they can persist, with less severity, and psychotic symptoms can superimpose. In these conditions both PDD and schizophrenia can be diagnosed.

Several possible explanations for a high PDD spectrum diagnosis in VEOS are possible. This association may be only phenomenic, and PDD features may be an exaggeration of non-specific developmental delays. In other words, the same underlying pathology presents differently at different phases of life: with early delays in the developmental course (motor, language), with PDD-like disorders, with non-specific attentional and behavioral dysfunction, with more subtle thought disorders, and finally with the full-blown psychotic syndrome.

The continuity between this PDD-like or schizoid-like dimension and the negative symptoms which are often prominent in the VEOS may suggest a possible developmental continuity. It has been proposed that impaired premorbid sociability may be a precursor of negative symptom dimension rather than of schizophrenia, as a longitudinal syndrome of social impairment (Hollis, 2003).

Alternatively, subjects with preschizophrenic PDD features may represent a specific subtype with specific clinical earlier onset of psychotic symptoms (greater severity of illness, poorer response to antipsychotic medications, poorer outcome) and biologic features (shared by PDD and schizophrenia). Sporn and colleagues (2004) screened their 75 children with VEOS for PDD and autism, and 19 (25%) had a lifetime diagnosis of PDD (16 PDD-NOS, 2 Asperger's disorder, and 1 autism). VEOS children with or without PDD comorbidity did not differ according to age at onset of psychotic symptoms, baseline and 2- to 6-year outcome, response to clozapine, and brain abnormalities, even though the PDD-schizophrenic patients had a more rapid gray matter loss.

On the borders of childhood schizophrenia

Some atypical children can hardly be classified in the conventional clinical categories, including the psychotic disorders, and new labels have been proposed in the last decade, such as the MID (McKenna et al, 1994; Kumra et al, 1998a), more related to the schizophrenic spectrum, and the multiple complex developmental disorder (MCDD) (Towbin et al, 1993), more related to the PDD spectrum.

Multidimensionally impaired disorder

Data from the NIMH study of childhood schizophrenia have shown that about one fifth of children with putative VEOS do not strictly meet the diagnostic criteria for the disorder, even though psychotic symptoms are prominent (McKenna et al, 1994; Kumra et al, 1998a). These psychotic symptoms (both hallucinations and delusions) are transitory, namely under stress conditions, and may occur a few times a month, without clear evidence of a thought disorder. These symptoms are associated with a significant mood instability and emotional and behavioral outbursts, which often are the most important reasons of concern for parents and teachers. These children usually present deficits in social strategies, but without a clear isolation or withdrawal, and even with distress after peer rejection. This clinical picture has been interpreted as an atypical psychosis, or a psychotic disorder NOS, and called "multidimensional impairment." These subjects share some symptoms of several different diagnostic categories, such as borderline personality disorder, conduct disorder, and schizotypal personality disorder, and most of them have symptoms of ADHD, but this diagnosis does not account for the whole clinical picture. However, the ADHD comorbidity (85%, versus 31% in schizophrenic children in the McKenna et al (1994) study) significantly distinguished MDI children from schizophrenic children.

The onset of difficulties in development or behavior is reported earlier in the MDI patients than in VEOS patients (1.5±2 years, versus 4.6±3.4 years). Similarly, the onset of psychosis is significantly earlier in MDI than in VEOS (7.9±2.1 years versus 10.3±2 years). Prevalent features of MDI are a poor ability to distinguish reality from fantasy, with mild psychotic symptoms (delusions of reference, perceptual disturbances), mood lability, impaired interpersonal relationships, deficits in information processing, and absence of formal thought disorders. Compared with the children with schizophrenia, children with MDI have much more rarely thought disorders (9.5% versus 84.5% in McKenna et al's sample), negative symptoms (9.5% versus 89.5%) and flat affect (9.5% versus 94.7%). The high percentage of grandiose delusions (38.1%), affective instability (100% in MDI versus 52.2% in schizophrenic children), and aggression (90.5% versus 42.1%) is noteworthy. The interpersonal relationship is described as "immature" in 95.2% of the MDI children (and in 5.3% of the schizophrenic children), while a deficit in interpersonal relatedness is much more rare (42.9% versus 84.2% in schizophrenic children). Transient features of PDD are more frequent in MDI than in VEOS, even though these features are not enduring at the moment of the psychotic symptomatology, and at least a partial remission is usual. Solitariness, gross impairment in ability to make peer friends, obsessive preoccupations, abnormalities in the forms or content of speech, inability to initiate or sustain a conversation are not rare in MDI patients. Fifty percent of MDI patients and 28.6% of the VEOS patients had a parent with a schizotypal or paranoid personality disorder.

The diagnostic stability of the MDI subjects remains unclear. At a 2-year follow-up, despite recurrent brief psychotic episodes, no progression to schizophrenia was reported, suggesting that MDI is not a prodrome of VEOS. Seventy-two percent of the probands remained stable or improved, while 27% developed a more severe and chronic schizoaffective disorder (bipolar type), with a progression of the duration, severity, and overlap of psychotic and affective symptoms (McKenna et al, 1994; Kumra et al, 1998a). Clinical outcome assessed

2 to 8 years after the initial evaluation shows that children may fall into two general groups: half of the sample developed more specific mental disorders (schizoaffective, bipolar, major depressive), all involving mood episodes; the other half of the sample was characterized by disruptive behavior disorders, with most showing remission of psychotic symptoms (Nicolson et al, 2001). More recent findings confirm the developmental link between MDI and mood disorder. Stayer and colleagues (2005) have found that at the end of the follow-up (mean 4.0 ± 1.3 years) of 32 children with MDI, 38% of the patients met criteria for bipolar disorder type I, 12% for major depressive disorder, and 3% for schizoaffective disorder. The remaining 47% of the patients were divided into two groups, on the basis of whether they were in remission and not assuming antipsychotics, or still severely impaired regardless of pharmacotherapy. The best predictor of a good outcome was a lower severity and a higher level of functioning at the baseline.

Despite the earlier onset of cognitive, behavioral, and psychotic symptoms, the outcome of MDI and the social impairment are significantly better than that of VEOS. It may represent a variant, milder form, with an affective component (schizoaffective development in one quarter of the children).

In summary, the development of the syndrome is characterized by transient features of pervasive developmental disorder, attention deficit hyperactivity disorder, then transitory psychotic symptoms (namely auditory hallucinations and grandiose delusions), aggressive-impulsive behavior, disturbed distinction between reality and fantasy, mood disturbances, very low rates of thought disorder and negative symptoms, and immature rather than reduced relatedness.

Multiple complex developmental disorder

As stated by McKenna and colleagues (1994), the MDI diagnosis is close to the DSM-IV borderline personality disorder. However, an exploration around the conceptualizations of childhood borderline personality disorder of childhood and childhood schizophrenia has led Towbin and colleagues (1993) to describe a syndrome, called multiple complex developmental disorder (MCDD), which presents striking similarities with the MDI, in terms of both clinical expression and premorbid natural history, even though it is more close to the PDD spectrum.

The MCDD is characterized by an impairment in the regulation of affective state (intense anxiety and tension, unusual fears, recurrent panic episodes, transient episodes of behavioral disorganization, with aggressive or self-injurious behaviors), impairment of social behavior and sensitivity (from social disinterest and withdrawal to superficial and apparently friendly attachments, inability to maintain peer relationships, limitations in the capacity of empathy), and impaired cognitive processing, confusion between reality and fantasy life, perplexity and/or confusion, transitory delusions, including fantasies of omnipotence, overengagement with fantasy figures, paranoid preoccupations, and referential ideation (Buitelaar and Van der Gaag, 1998). In Towbin et al's study (1993), the 30 children diagnosed as having MCDD had previously received the following diagnoses: schizophrenia or psychotic disorder NOS (50%), ADHD (37%), PDD-NOS (33%), conduct disorder (30%), dysthymia (27%), borderline personality (13%), and schizotypal personality (7%). A crucial element is the early onset of the social deficits, usually before the age of 5 years, which often results in a first diagnosis within the PDD of the non-autistic variety (PDD-NOS). A typical feature of the syndrome is the marked fluctuation in affect regulation, thought, and relatedness, which are grossly different from the stability in functioning of the PDD autistic children. Compared with children with typical PDD, these children are less disturbed in social interaction, communication, and stereotyped and rigid behavior, whereas they exhibit affective symptoms, thought disorders, anxiety, and aggression. Episodes of regression to more immature levels of functioning may occur under stress and last from hours to weeks, intermixed with periods of higher functioning when environmental stressors are reduced. These fluctuations can be more or less dramatic among different individuals.

The affective dysregulation is expressed by marked mood instability, high levels of anxiety, odd phobias or fears, and rage reactions which are exaggerated and overwhelming. Social impairment can include social deficits in reciprocity, but in some of these children social abnormalities are more subtle, inconsistent, odd, immature, and constricted. Thought disorder is qualitatively and quantitatively different from that of schizophrenic children, with mild slippages and distortions, sometimes psychotic symptoms (hallucinations, delusions), and only rarely are contamination, incoherence, and neologism present. Under stress these symptoms may become more severe or frequent.

According to Van der Gaag and colleagues (1995), a five-factor cluster principal-component analysis was found for MCDD, with psychotic thinking/anxiety (that is thought disorder and dysregulation of affective states, and primitive anxieties), aggression (with hyperactive and impulsive behavior), deficient interaction, stereotyped/rigid behavior, and suspiciousness/odd interaction (which resembles the schizotypal personality disorder).

VEOS is a possible differential diagnosis for these children, even though delusions and/or hallucinations are not a prominent feature. However, it was hypothesized that at least some of these children may eventually develop schizophrenia (Towbin et al, 1993), and it has been supported by a follow-up study (Buitelaar and Van der Gaag, 1998). A possible use of low-dose antipsychotic medications has been postulated as well (Towbin et al, 1993), especially when thought disorder, oddities in relatedness, and affective dysregulation are prominent.

Biological basis of pharmacotherapy of schizophrenia

The efficacy of antipsychotic medications in schizophrenia is well established in adult populations. All the antipsychotic agents share a blocking effect on dopaminergic transmission. For this reason the neurotransmitter dopamine is considered to play a central role in the pathophysiology of schizophrenia. More recently other neurotransmitter systems (namely glutamatergic system) have been (not alternatively) involved in the pathophysiology of schizophrenia, generating new potential pathways of pharmacologic treatment. However, dopamine neurotransmission still remains the cornerstone of the pharmacotherapy of schizophrenia (Stahl, 2000).

Four dopamine pathways can be described, which project from the brainstem, namely the ventral tegmental area and the substantia nigra, to different areas of the CNS. The first pathway is the mesolimbic, which projects from the ventral tegmental area to part of the limbic area, namely the nucleus accumbens. This pathway has an important role in the regulation of emotions. It is supposed that hyperactivity of this pathway may mediate the emergence of positive psychotic symptoms, such as hallucinations, delusions, and thought disorders, and it may also be involved in aggressive and hostile behavior. The therapeutic effect of antipsychotic medication on positive psychotic symptoms may be related to blocking of the dopaminergic transmission in this pathway.

The second pathway is the mesocortical, which projects from the ventral tegmental area of the brainstem to the cerebral cortex, especially the limbic cortex and prefrontal cortex. This pathway is involved in higher cognitive functions, and in schizophrenic patients it is thought to mediate negative and cognitive symptoms, through a deficit in dopaminergic neurotransmission, possibly secondary to an excitotoxic effect of the glutamate system. This toxic effect may produce a progressive degenerative process in this pathway, thus increasing the negative symptoms and worsening the deficit state, as the schizophrenic illness progresses. A deficit in this pathway may be worsened by blockade of dopaminergic neurotransmission by antipsychotic medication. A potentiation of the dopaminergic transmission in this pathway may thus improve some cognitive and negative symptoms of schizophrenia.

The third pathway is from the substantia nigra of the brainstem to the basal ganglia. This pathway, called the nigro-striatal, plays a crucial role in motor control, as part of the extrapyramidal system. When the dopaminergic transmission in this pathway is blocked, i.e. during a pharmacologic treatment with antipsychotics, extrapyramidal side-effects (EPS) can result, such as dystonias, akathisia, and parkinsonism (rigidity, bradykinesia, tremor). A chronic blockade of dopaminergic receptors during antipsychotic treatment may result in a hyperkinetic disorder called tardive dyskinesia (see later).

The fourth pathway is called tuberoinfundibular, which projects from the hypothalamus to the anterior pituitary. This pathway normally inhibits prolactin release. During the postpartum period, the activity of this pathway is reduced, and the increase in prolactin release favors lactation. If the dopaminergic activity of this pathway is blocked by an antipsychotic treatment, an increase in prolactin levels can cause amenorrhea, gynecomastia, galactorrhea, and possibly sexual dysfunction.

Conventional antipsychotics

The first effective treatments for psychotic disorders and schizophrenia were found during serendipitous clinical observations with an antihistamine compound, chlorpromazine. Only thereafter was it found that the antipsychotic action of chlorpromazine and other antipsychotic agents was mediated by blockade of the dopamine receptors, namely the D2 receptor. In experimental animals these agents caused extreme slowness or inhibition of motor activity, called neurolepsis, and for this reason these agents were called neuroleptics.

The antipsychotic effect was shown to be mainly mediated by the blocking effect on the mesolimbic dopaminergic pathway, which mediates the positive psychotic symptoms. However, the blocking effect is equally distributed among all the dopaminergic pathways, including the mesocortical, nigro-striatal, and tuberoinfundibular pathways. This blocking effect is responsible for some of the most disturbing side-effects. When a conventional antipsychotic blocks the mesocortical pathway, which is already deficient, a worsening of negative and cognitive symptoms may occur, determining a neuroleptic-induced negative syndrome. Furthermore, blockade of dopaminergic transmission in the nigro-striatal pathway causes dystonias, parkinsonism, and akathisia. In long-term treatment a tardive dyskinesia may occur, with facial and tongue movements, such as chewing, tongue protrusion, facial grimacing, and sometimes involuntary limb movements, determined by irreversible changes in the D2 dopamine receptors in the nigro-striatal pathway. About 5% of patients develop a tardive dyskinesia every year of treatment, and this is a particularly worrying side-effect in a chronic disorder such as schizophrenia. Finally, a neuroleptic-induced chronic blockade of the tuberoinfundibular pathway may result in hyperprolactinemia. This may be particularly troublesome in females, causing amenorrhea, galactorrhea, and interfering with sexual functioning and fertility.

Besides the clinical effects of the dopamine blockade, additional effects in patients treated with conventional antipsychotics may arise from their ability to block the cholinergic receptors. Dry mouth, blurred vision, constipation, and cognitive blunting can be associated with this pharmacologic activity, as well as a lesser ability to cause EPS.

Furthermore, blockade of the alpha-1 adrenergic receptors can determine cardiovascular side-effects, namely orthostatic hypotension. Finally, blockade of the histamine 1 receptor is associated with increased appetite and weight gain, and sedation. These pharmacologic actions can be inequally distributed among the different conventional antipsychotics.

According to the affinity for D2 dopamine receptors and the degree of dopamine receptor blockade, typical antipsychotics can be divided into low-potency neuroleptics, such as phenothiazines (chlorpromazine,

promazine, levomepromazine) or thioridazine, and high-potency neuroleptics, such as the buthyrophenones (haloperidol). The antipsychotic effects require a striatal D2 receptor occupancy of at least 65–70%, but an occupancy greater than 80% significantly increases the risk of EPS. High-potency agents have a higher risk of producing EPS, whereas low-potency neuroleptics have more anticholinergic effects, including sedation and memory deficits.

Even though typical neuroleptics vary in their tolerability profile, little evidence is available in adult patients that they differ in their efficacy. However, a patient may fail to respond to one neuroleptic and respond to another. The main limitations in the use of typical neuroleptics are the risk of EPS (even greater in younger populations), the treatment resistance in at least one third of the patients and the partial response in about 50% of the patients, and the low efficacy on negative and cognitive symptoms, which can even be worsened by treatment with a neuroleptic. Thus treatment with a typical neuroleptic may result in a lower clinical improvement and a lower tolerability, that is a lower quality of life.

Atypical antipsychotics

For many years there was a deeply rooted view that every antipsychotic medication should also induce EPS. The availability of clozapine, and then of other antipsychotics called "atypical," has changed this notion. The pharmacologic basis of atypicality is still not clear, other than the clinical definition of an antipsychotic effect with a lower risk of extrapyramidal side-effects and hyperprolactinemia. Clozapine was first marketed in 1958, but its development was arrested or strongly limited by serious concerns about lethal side-effects, namely agranulocytosis. In the 1990s a renaissance of clozapine was promoted by the evidence of its efficacy in treatment-refractory schizophrenia. This renaissance stimulated the development of a second generation of atypical antipsychotics, with a similar efficacy to clozapine, but with lower side-effects and easier management. Several other compounds have been marketed, including risperidone, olanzapine, quetiapine, and ziprasidone. From a clinical point of view, these medications have been proposed as having a lower risk of EPS, a lower risk of hyperprolactinemia, a greater efficacy on both negative and cognitive symptoms of schizophrenia, and a greater efficacy in patients who failed to respond to conventional antipsychotics. From a pharmacologic point of view, all these compounds share a combined dopamine– serotonin antagonism, and a lower affinity for dopamine receptors. One or both of these characteristics may account for the above reported clinical properties, through a less radical blockade of dopaminergic transmission, namely in the fronto-striatal, nigro-striatal, and tuberoinfundibular pathways. If these pharmacologic properties are common to all the compounds of this class, other pharmacologic actions (not completely understood) on the different naurotransmitter systems account for differential clinical characteristics (in terms of efficacy and side-effects) of the various atypical antipsychotics, and for the differential responses in individual patients. These pharmacologic properties are beyond the aims of this handbook.

More recently, a new antipsychotic has been marketed, aripiprazole, which has a more specific mechanism, as a partial dopamine agonist. It acts as an antagonist at dopamine D2 receptors in hyperdopaminergic conditions, and displays agonist properties under hypodopaminergic conditions. It has been hypothesized that aripiprazole may be able to stabilize the dopaminergic system without inducing a hypodopaminergic state, reducing the risk of side-effects associated with pure blockade of dopamine receptors, such as negative symptoms, movement disorders, and elevated prolactin levels. Furthermore, aripiprazole acts as a partial agonist at some serotonin receptor subtypes and as an antagonist at others.

It must be remembered that even though more recent meta-analyses limit the differences between typical and atypical antipsychotics (Davis et al, 2003), many guidelines all around the world suggest that atypical antipsychotics are at least as effective as typical antipsychotics, and better tolerated and safe, namely in long-term treatment. Clozapine, the first marketed atypical antipsychotic, is also proven to be more effective than conventional antipsychotics in treatment-refractory cases.

Review of the literature on pharmacotherapy of childhood and adolescent schizophrenia

The core treatment in the psychotic disorders is pharmacologic, and the antipsychotic medications are the first-line choice, in adults as well as in children and adolescents. However, given the rarity of early-onset disorders, clinical evidence from empirical studies is still quite limited, in terms of both efficacy and safety. A critical review of the available literature will be described in the following sections.

Typical antipsychotics

The efficacy and safety of conventional neuroleptics are explored by open or retrospective studies considering small samples of affected children and adolescents with VEOS and EOS. Only a few controlled studies suggest efficacy of these older medications. Pool and colleagues (1976) explored the efficacy of loxapine (87.5 mg/day), haloperidol (9.8 mg/day), and placebo in 75 adolescents aged 13 to 18 years with acute schizophrenia or chronic schizophrenia with acute exacerbation. Both loxapine and haloperidol were superior to placebo for most of the measures considered for the outcome. It is noteworthy that loxapine, a congener of clozapine with a high affinity for serotonin receptors, was superior to haloperidol in some measures, including hallucinations, social interest, and manifest psychosis at 2 weeks.

Realmuto and coworkers (1984) compared the high-potency neuroleptic thiothixene (0.3 mg/kg per day) and the low-potency neuroleptic thioridazine (3.3 mg/kg per day, mean 178 mg/day) in 21 inpatient adolescents with schizophrenia (aged 11.75 to 18.75 years). Nine out of 21 subjects responded to both treatments, even though both were very sedating.

The efficacy of typical antipsychotics, namely haloperidol, is supported by a randomized, double-blind, placebo-controlled cross-over study with appropriate assessment instruments (Spencer et al, 1992). This study showed that 12 hospitalized children (aged 5.5 to 11.75 years) responded to haloperidol (optimal dose 0.5–3.5 mg/day, mean 1.92 mg/day) significantly better than to placebo. Delusions, hallucinations, ideas of reference, and thought disorders significantly improved in the patients receiving haloperidol, even though sedation, severe dystonic reactions, and parkinsonism were the most frequently reported side-effects in the haloperidol group. In an expansion of the study, considering 16 children, all the patients had a good response to haloperidol: 12 showed marked improvement, and 4 showed mild or moderate improvement (Spencer et al, 1994). Response to haloperidol was inversely related to the duration of illness and positively related to age and level of intellectual functioning of the 16 children. Older children, those with higher IQs and later onset schizophrenia showed greater response to haloperidol in this sample. These findings were confirmed at the completion of the study, when the sample was enlarged to 24 children and the same design and measures were used. A double-blind study comparing subjects treated with haloperidol, risperidone and olanzapine (Sikich et al, 2004) will be described in the following pages.

Atypical antipsychotics

Clozapine

Clozapine is the first marketed atypical antipsychotic, and it can be considered the prototypical agent in this class of medications. It is associated with extremely rare EPS or tardive dyskinesia, and it does not cause hyperprolactinemia. Furthermore, it is the first-line medication in adults who are refractory to treatment with typical neuroleptics and other atypical neuroleptics, and it appears to present a greater efficacy in both negative and cognitive symptoms. It is also particularly effective when hostile and aggressive behaviors are prominent. Finally, it is associated with a reduced risk of suicidal behavior. The major concerns in the use of clozapine are the risk of agranulocytosis and the convulsant effect. The risk of agranulocytosis is about 0.5–1%, and it is not dose-dependent (Alvir et al, 1993), while the risk of seizures is dose-dependent, and increases up to 5% when dosage is over 400 mg/day. EEG modifications are frequent during clozapine treatment (ranging from 10 to 44%) (Frazier et al, 1994; Kumra et al, 1996), but they are not necessarily predictive of a seizure risk, when they are not excessively severe. Much more concerning are pretreatment seizures, and/or EEG abnormalities, and/or brain lesions.

The pharmacologic bases of these quite specific clinical properties, above all the efficacy in treatment-refractory patients and the life-threatening side-effects, are still unclear. Clozapine is currently not considered a first-line treatment in schizophrenic patients, but it becomes a first choice in treatment-resistant patients, namely when extrapyramidal side-effects, and/or negative symptoms, and/or hostility/aggressiveness, and/or suicidality are present.

Most of the findings rely on retrospective chart reviews. As many as 270 children and adolescents treated with clozapine have been described in the literature, prevalently in open-label, efficacy studies for treatment-resistant schizophrenia or "psychotic disorders" (Toren et al, 1998).

A double-blind, placebo-controlled study assessed efficacy and safety of clozapine and haloperidol in 21 patients with VEOS (mean age 14±2.3 years), who failed to respond to typical neuroleptics (Kumra et al, 1996). These subjects were randomized to haloperidol (16±8 mg/day) or clozapine (178±149 mg/day) for 6 weeks. Clozapine was superior for all the measures of psychosis, both positive and negative. On the basis of the CGI-Improvement (CGI-I) score, 13 out of 21 subjects were considered much or very much improved (61.9%), two of them being very much improved (one of them had a complete remission of the symptoms). Particularly important was the effect of clozapine on primary negative symptoms. It is interesting that, according to monthly contacts and a 2-year follow-up, the maximum clozapine effect occurred after 6–9 month of treatment, as reported in adults.

Serious side-effects occurred during the study in the clozapine group. Five patients had a fall in the neutrophil count to below 1500/mm³, 3 of them normalized spontaneously and 2 dropped out. Both the latter two patients were receiving concomitant antibiotic medication (amoxacilline and penicillin). This finding suggests the need for careful monitoring when these medications are associated. Two patients without pre-existing epilepsy had seizures during the treatment while they were receiving 400 mg/day of clozapine. Clozapine was reduced and an anticonvulsant treatment was started, but the EEG remained abnormal, leading to a discontinuation of clozapine. In three additional subjects a clinical deterioration was evident during the treatment, in parallel to EEG abnormalities. Clozapine dosage was reduced, and a cotreatment with valproate was started. Two of these patients improved, whereas the third patient had facial myoclonus and a worsening of EEG, and clozapine was discontinued. It is noteworthy that, despite the short term of the study, the two best responders in the study were also the patients who gained the most weight during the trial.

It should be considered that the mean clozapine dosage in the controlled study was particularly high, and this may have increased the rate of adverse events other than neutropenia, namely seizures and EEG abnormalities. According to the review by Freedman and colleagues (1994), three out of 80 adolescents who received clozapine (4%) experienced seizures, and 32 out of 53 (60%) had epileptiform changes in their EEG. Some patients whose EEG clinical status worsens may improve after cotherapy with valproate.

Several earlier naturalistic studies from Germany are consistent with the placebo-controlled study. Blanz and Schmidt (1993) reported on a sample of 57 adolescents, "prevalently schizophrenics," treated with clozapine (mean dosage 285mg/day, with a wide range of

75–800 mg/day), with a significant improvement in 67% and a partial improvement in 21% of the subjects. The safety profile in this sample was particularly favorable, as only 5% of the patients discontinued the medication because of side-effects. Remschmidt et al (1994) reported a significant improvement in 75% of 36 schizophrenic adolescents who were resistant to previous treatments. Seventeen percent of the patients discontinued the treatment due to side-effects, and only 8% did not show any improvement after clozapine. The dosage was quite high (mean 330 mg/day, but ranging from 50 to 800 mg/day). These early studies indicate a high rate of responders, with a positive effect on both positive and, to a lesser degree, on negative symptoms.

A study from Israel (Turetz et al, 1997) described the open-label clozapine treatment (227 ± 34 mg/day) of 11 schizophrenic children younger than 13 years who were resistant to previous neuroleptic treatment. A significant reduction in all the measures, including the Brief Psychiatric Rating Scale (BPRS), Positive and Negative Symptoms Scale (PANSS), and CGI, was reported with a peak of efficacy between the sixth and eighth weeks. Drooling and somnolence were the most frequently reported symptoms.

A study from the USA, during a NIMH ongoing study on childhood schizophrenia (Frazier et al, 1994) described 11 adolescents (mean age 14 years) who were resistant to a previous treatment with conventional antipsychotics, and who were included in on open-label study with clozapine (mean dose at the sixth week 370.5mg/day, range 125–825mg/day). Eighty-two percent of the patients presented an improvement of at least 30% of the BPRS total score during clozapine treatment.

The efficacy of clozapine has been confirmed in a brief report on an adolescent with acute catatonia, who was refractory to a previous treatment with haloperidol, but responded after 3 weeks of clozapine treatment, at a dosage of 150 mg/day (Masi et al, 2002), without significant side-effects.

More recently, Kranzler and colleagues (2005) assessed the efficacy of clozapine treatment in controlling aggressive behavior in 20 treatment-refractory schizophrenic adolescents (476 ± 119 mg/day). A significant clinical improvement, naturalistically assessed according to the frequency of administration of emergency oral and/or injectable medications and the frequency of seclusion, was found during weeks 12 to 24 of treatment.

In summary, despite the above reported risks, clozapine is an effective treatment for treatment-refractory VEOS and EOS. It should be mentioned that childhood schizophrenia is an extremely severe disorder, and when it does not improve after a treatment with atypical antipsychotics, the social and cognitive development is pervasively and persistently impaired. Negative symptoms grossly increase the social disability and the risk for long-term outcome. In these selected conditions clozapine may lead to meaningful improvements, and sometimes can induce real "awakenings" from thought disorders and negative psychotic symptoms. The advantages of clozapine in schizophrenic children include the antipsychotic efficacy in the acute phase, the efficacy on chronic and negative symptoms, fewer EPS, and low risk of elevation of prolactin levels.

Risperidone

A double-blind study and several open-label studies and case reports are available on risperidone in schizophrenic children and adolescents, with 86 recruited subjects.

Sikich and colleagues (2004) blindly randomized 50 psychotic children and adolescents (age range 8–19 years) with schizophrenic and/or affective psychoses and prominent positive symptoms, into a risperidone group (19 subjects, mean dose 4 ± 1.2 mg/day), olanzapine group (16 subjects, mean dose 12.3 ± 3.5 mg/day), and haloperidol group (15 subjects, mean dose 5 ± 2 mg/day). The efficacy and tolerability of these treatments were assessed during an 8-week trial. All the treatments were shown to be effective, with a similar magnitude of improvement. The number of responders, according to a CGI-I 1 or 2 (much or very much improved) and a reduction in the BPRS for Children of at least 20%, was 88% with olanzapine, 74% with risperidone, and 53% with haloperidol. The most frequent side-effect was sedation (about 90% of the subjects in all the groups), which tended to improve with time, mainly in the risperidone group. Extrapyramidal side-effects (53–67%) and weight gain (ranging from 3.5 ± 3.7 kg to 7.1 ± 4.1 kg) did not differ among the three groups, and were more frequent and severe than in adult patients. The differences in the diagnoses of the participants, as well as the high frequency of polypharmacy, limit the interpretation of these findings. The role of the pubertal status was not reported.

After several case reports, the first small study on risperidone treatment in schizophrenic children and adolescents described four adolescents (age range 12 to 17 years) treated with risperidone (4–5 mg/day) with a positive response in three of the patients (Quintana and Keshevan, 1995). A significant improvement was specifically reported in negative symptoms. Mandoki (1995) described a case series of 10 patients, 8 of them younger than 12 years, with "psychosis" and/or bipolar disorder. Risperidone resulted in the psychotic symptoms, but four out of these seven prepubertal children presented EPS and two a significant weight gain. The rapid titration is probably responsible for the high rate of EPS. Another retrospective study assessed efficacy and tolerability of risperidone (mean dose 5.9 mg/day, range 2–10 mg) in 16 children and adolescents (age range 9 to 20 years) with a psychotic disorder (Grcevich et al, 1996). Fifteen out of the 16 patients were responders according to the BPRS and CGI scores. The BPRS total score and the BPRS Negative Symptoms score were significantly decreased from the baseline, as was the CGI score. The medication was well tolerated, but three patients presented EPS.

A third study openly assessed the efficacy of risperidone (starting dose 2 mg/day, with further 1 mg/day increases every 2 days, mean dose 6.6 mg/day, range 4 to 10 mg/day) in 10 schizophrenic adolescents (age range 11–18 years) (Armenteros et al, 1997). A significant improvement was noted in the BPRS scale, Positive and Negative Symptoms Scale, and CGI. In 60% of the patients a decrease of at least 20% at the PANSS was found, and the clinical improvement was evident from the first week of treatment. Major adverse events were not reported, however three subjects presented parkinsonism and oro-facial dyskinesias.

Kumra and colleagues (1997b) screened, for hepatotoxicity and weight gain, the charts of 13 psychotic children treated with risperidone (6–8 mg/day) in the previous 3 years. Two patients presented obesity, liver enzyme abnormalities, and evidence of a fatty liver, which reversed after risperidone discontinuation, and related weight loss. The authors recommended periodic monitoring of hepatic function during risperidone treatment, especially when weight gain is associated.

Long-acting intramuscular risperidone is the first atypical antipsychotic available in a formulation which offers a sustained, steady release of drug and is thus an attractive, new option in the treatment of patients with schizophrenia. This novel, intramuscular formulation has shown efficacy in the treatment of adult patients with schizophrenia, but data on children and adolescents are still not available. It is an aqueous suspension of microspheres, which begin to release risperidone 3 weeks after the first injection. Long-acting risperidone 25, 37.5, or 50 mg every 2 weeks demonstrated significantly greater antipsychotic efficacy than placebo and equivalent efficacy to oral risperidone 2–6 mg/day in randomized, double-blind, 12-week trials of patients with schizophrenia. According to one study on adult schizophrenic patients, switching treatment from oral antipsychotics to long-acting risperidone was associated with a further clinical improvement in stable patients with schizophrenia (Lindenmayer et al, 2004).

In summary, even though data supporting the efficacy of risperidone in schizophrenic children and adolescents are fewer than for clozapine, the greater ease of management, without a mandatory blood cell count, suggests risperidone to be among the first-line pharmacologic treatments of VEOS and EOS. However, some "poorly atypical" features of risperidone should be kept in mind during the treatment, particularly EPS, which can occur more frequently when emergency interventions require a rapid titration. Elevated levels of prolactin resulting in amenorrhea are not rarely a disturbing side-effect in adolescent girls, especially when high dosages are needed to control the psychotic symptomatology.

Olanzapine

One double-blind study, several open-label and case reports studies have assessed the efficacy and tolerability of olanzapine in a total of 112 children and adolescents.

Data on the double-blind study comparing olanzapine, risperidone, and haloperidol have been reported above (Sikich et al, 2004).

In one of the first open studies, Mandoki (1997) assessed the efficacy of olanzapine (5–20 mg/day) in eight children and adolescents previously treated with clozapine; the switch to olanzapine did not affect the clinical status of the patients.

Kumra et al (1998b) reported on their clinical experience with olanzapine in schizophrenic adolescents, suggesting a moderate efficacy of olanzapine. Eight adolescents (mean age 15.2±2.3 years) with onset of schizophrenic disorder before age 12 (mean 10.5±2.4 years) and a mean duration of illness of 4.6±2.4 years received an olanzapine trial, at a dose of 17.5±2.3 mg/day (range 12.5–20 mg/day). At week 8 a 17%

improvement in the BPRS total score, a 27% improvement in the Scale for the Assessment of Negative Symptoms (SANS), and a 1% improvement in the Scale for the Assessment of Positive Symptoms (SAPS) were registered. The authors compared these results with those registered in a parallel, double-blind, placebo-controlled study on clozapine. Improvement in the clozapine group at week 6 was greater than that of the olanzapine groups at week 8. Furthermore, in the four patients who received both clozapine and olanzapine, clozapine was significantly superior, according to the improvement in the BPRS total score. According to a responders' criterion of a reduction in BPRS total score of more than 20%, a post-treatment CGI-S of 3 or less, or a BPRS total score of 35 or less, two out of the eight patients in the olanzapine group were considered full responders, and one a partial responder.

Other more recent studies suggest that olanzapine may be effective in schizophrenic children and adolescents. Sholevar et al (2000) naturalistically treated 15 schizophrenic children (age range 6–13 years) with olanzapine. The first five enrolled children started olanzapine 5 mg at bedtime, and all presented morning sedation and lethargy. The other 12 children were started on 2.5 mg at bedtime, with increase to 5 mg if no adverse effects were noted. Only one child received 2.5 mg, all the other had a final dosage of 5 mg/day. Five patients presented a marked improvement in psychotic symptoms, five a moderate improvement, and three a slight improvement. The only two patients with no improvement were the oldest (13-year-olds). A better response was found in the younger patients, and age explained the 53% of the variance. Sedation was the most common side-effect; the length of initial sedation was positively correlated with improvement in psychosis. These findings are based on the observation during the hospitalization, which lasted a mean of 11.3 days. Data on follow-up are not available, namely on weight gain.

Findling and colleagues (2003) openly treated 16 adolescents (12–17 years) with psychotic disorder with olanzapine (2.5–20 mg/day) for 8 weeks. A significant improvement was found in the PANSS, CGI-S, and CGAS scores. Olanzapine was effective on both positive and negative symptoms. Weight gain and sedation were the most frequently reported side-effects, and two subjects presented extrapyramidal side-effects.

Ross and coworkers (2003) followed up for one year 20 children and adolescents (age range 6–15 years) with childhood-onset schizophrenia naturalistically treated with olanzapine, using as outcome measures the BPRS, SAPS, and SANS. Seventy-four percent of the patients were responders according to a reduction in the BPRS total score of at least 20% and a mild to great improvement. The subscales of thought disturbance and psychomotor excitation of the BPRS and the SAPS significantly improved at the sixth week of treatment, while the anxiety scale of the BPRS and the SANS significantly improved only after 1-year follow-up. All the patients presented weight gain, and this side-effect was responsible for four out of the five medication discontinuations during the 12 months of treatment. The apparent greater efficacy of olanzapine in the Ross et al study, compared with the Kumra et al (1998a) study may be accounted for by differences in the sample selection (older children who had failed two previous trials of typical neuroleptics in the Kumra study, prevalently medication-naïve younger children in the Ross et al study) and the longer follow up (6 weeks in the Kumra study, 1 year in Ross's study), suggesting that greater benefits are evident after a longer duration of treatment.

Mozes et al (2003) examined the efficacy of olanzapine in nine children who were refractory to two other antipsychotic treatments. Patients received olanzapine at a maximum dosage of 20 mg/day for 12 weeks. A reduction in all the psychiatric measures was found at the 12th week, without EPS and significant side-effects, including blood chemistry, but with a significant weight gain (6.1 ± 3.2 kg). The improvement was more evident from weeks 4 to 12, at the therapeutic doses. Eight patients maintained the clinical improvement at a 1 year follow-up.

Ercan et al (2004) treated eight schizophrenic adolescents with olanzapine, followed up for 17.5 weeks (range 4–26 weeks). According to the CGI-I, three of the patients were much or very much improved, while three were mildly improved. The treatment was well tolerated, but a significant weight gain was reported.

A study from NIMH reported on the pharmacokinetics of olanzapine (2.5–20 mg/day) in eight schizophrenic children and adolescents (age range 10 to 18 years, mean age 13.8 ± 1.5 years) after an 8-week treatment (Grothe et al, 2000). Plasma concentrations were similar to those found in non-smoking adult schizophrenic patients. The mean elimination half-life was 37.2 ± 5.1 hours. On the basis of the pharmacokinetic findings, the authors recommended a once daily 5–10 mg dose of olanzapine, with a target dose of 10 mg for most adolescents with psychosis. Intramuscular olanzapine will be described in a following section (acute treatment).

In summary, the available literature suggests that olanzapine can be considered among the first-line treatments in EOS and VEOS. It is relatively safe and well tolerated, in terms of EPS risk and prolactin levels, even when a more rapid titration is needed. Reasons for concern are the marked weight gain, and the possible effect on glucose metabolism. These aspects should be carefully monitored during treatment.

Quetiapine

Only some open-label studies and case reports support the efficacy of quetiapine in schizophrenic children and adolescents.

McConville et al (2000) assessed the pharmacokinetics, efficacy, and tolerability of quetiapine in 10 adolescents (12.3–15.9 years) with psychotic disorder. The patients received increasing doses of quetiapine, starting from 25 mg bid, up to 400 mg bid after 3 weeks. The pharmacokinetics were dose proportional and similar to those reported in adult patients. A positive effect was found on both positive and negative symptoms, according to the BPRS, CGI-S, and a specific scale for the assessment of negative symptoms. The medication was well tolerated, and only postural tachycardia and insomnia were noted. Extrapyramidal side-effects improved from the baseline.

Shaw and colleagues (2001) studied the efficacy of quetiapine (300–800 mg/day, mean 467 mg/day) in 15 adolescents, aged 13 to 17 years, with psychotic disorder, using multiple measures (BPRS, CGI, PANSS, and Young Mania Rating Scale (YMRS)). Psychotic symptomatology improved according to all these measures. A weight gain was reported in the patients after treatment (mean 4.1 kg after 8 weeks). Somnolence, agitation, drowsiness, and headache were the most frequently reported side-effects.

In an open-label extension of the previous study, McConville et al (2003) further explored the efficacy and safety of quetiapine in an 88-week open-label study. According to a flexible dose titration, the 10 adolescents received different doses of quetiapine (up to 800mg/day), possibly associated with other medications. The BPRS, CGI, and SANS improved significantly during the trial. Quetiapine was well tolerated in the long term with no EPS and weight gain at week 64.

In summary, to date, fewer data support the efficacy of quetiapine in children and adolescernts with schizophrenia, compared with the above described atypical antipsychotics. Quetiapine, at the standard dosages, is better tolerated than clozapine, risperidone, and olanzapine, in terms of weight gain and glucose metabolism, as well as in terms of prolactin elevation and EPS. For this reason, it may represent a good choice when risperidone and olanzapine are effective, but result in intolerable side-effects (namely weight gain).

Ziprasidone

Ziprasidone is a recently marketed atypical antipsychotic, with a lower effect on appetite and weight gain, but with more concerns about a possible prolongation of the QTc interval of the ECG (Blair et al, 2005).

Only two studies have explored to date the efficacy of ziprasidone in psychotic children and adolescents. Patel and colleagues (2002) have described their clinical experience with 13 children and adolescents (13–18 years) with different psychiatric disorders, including four schizophrenics, four depressed with psychotic symptoms, three bipolar, and two psychotic NOS. The mean endpoint dose was 52.3 ± 25.2 mg/day. Nine patients were improved or much improved at the CGI. Nine patients received a baseline ECG and four of them were followed up; one of them had an increase in the QTc interval. Akathisia and agitation were the most frequent side-effects.

Meighen et al (2004) successfully treated with ziprasidone two psychotic adolescents with severe psychosis, hallucinations, and grossly disorganized speech and behavior, who failed to improve after treatment with other atypical antipsychotics. Ziprasidone treatment (40 mg bid) resulted in a significant improvement in both positive and negative symptoms, including social relatedness and flow of conversation. One patient experienced mild EPS, but weight gain and ECG abnormalities were not found. Intramuscular ziprasidone will be described in the following paragraphs.

Aripiprazole

To date, only a single case report of a 16-year-old adolescent with mental retardation and schizophrenia treated with aripiprazole, with a starting dose of 10 mg once a day, who developed a severe extrapyramidal symptomatology, is available (Lindsey et al, 2003). The patient had experienced EPS during previous treatments with antipsychotics, and this hypersensitivity, possibly related to brain lesions, and the co-occurring treatments (quetiapine, chlorpromazine), may have favored the EPS.

Practical guidelines of pharmacotherapy

The treatment of schizophrenia always needs both pharmacologic and non-pharmacologic interventions. Non-pharmacologic interventions include counseling for the patients and the family, psychologic support, behavioral treatments, social and cognitive rehabilitation, assistance in social and scholastic activities, enhancement of social skills, and family support.

Pharmacologic treatment is necessary, in order to obtain a remission and to control positive and negative symptoms. Furthermore, a proper pharmacotherapy can greatly increase the efficacy of psychosocial interventions. The setting of the treatment should be as outpatient, even though hospitalization can be necessary during the acute phases.

Pharmacotherapy can be gradually started in psychotic disorders with an insidious onset, while an acute presentation of the symptomatology usually represents a psychiatric emergency which needs a rapid intervention.

Antipsychotic medications are the first-line treatment of pychotic disorders. Atypical antipsychotics should be preferred to older neuroleptics, as they show at least the same efficacy and a better tolerance. Risperidone and olanzapine are the medications more supported by empirical studies, while quetiapine and ziprasidone present a more favorable profile of side-effects, namely weight gain, but there are fewer available data. Data on aripiprazole in childhood schizophrenia are still not available, even though it appears a promising treatment according to adult studies.

When a treatment with an atypical antipsychotic is started, a good practical principle is to search for the lowest effective dose. While excessive low doses can determine dose-unrelated side-effects, with modest clinical benefits, excessively high doses do not increase efficacy, but can determine dose-related side-effects (included sedation and iatrogenic negative and cognitive symptoms). When the symptomatology is relatively stable, a gradual increase in the doses is preferred. Risperidone can be started at a dose of 0.5 mg/day in prepubertal children and 1 mg/day in adolescents, with increases every 2 or 3 days, up to a first level of 1.5–2 mg/day in prepubertal children and 3–4 mg/day in adolescents. A faster titration significantly increases the risk of EPS. Olanzapine can be started at a dose of 2.5 mg/day in prepubertal children and 5 mg/day in adolescents, with increases every 2 or 3 days up to 5–7.5 mg/day in prepubertal children and 10–15 mg in adolescents. Quetiapine can be started at a dose of 25–50 mg in children and 50 mg in adolescents, with increases of 25–50 mg every 2 or 3 days, up to 100–150 mg/day in children and 200–300 mg/day in adolescents. Ziprasidone can be started at a dose of 20 mg, with a mean dose of 40–60 mg/day. Aripiprazole can be started in adolescent patients at a dose of 5 mg/day, with increases of 5 mg every 3–4 days up to 15–20 mg/day. Further increases in the dosage should be considered after 3 or 4 weeks of treatment.

During the first weeks of treatment side-effects as well as efficacy should be monitored, with an intensive follow-up and using standardized measures (BPRS, SAPS, SANS, Abnormal Involuntary Movement Scale (AIMS), and specific checklists for side-effects for each atypical antipsychotic).

Clinical response to an antipsychotic treatment may vary among individuals. At least 6 weeks are needed to assess treatment refractoriness, which, if present, should suggest switching to another antipsychotic.

A higher response of both positive and negative symptoms is reported in first-episode samples during the first year of antipsychotic treatment, even though residual symptoms are not infrequent (Lieberman et al, 1993). However, drug-naive patients are more sensitive to side-effects, including EPS. The issue of the effective management of psychotic symptoms in the first psychotic episode is particularly important, as it is recognized that an early and effective treatment at the onset of the disorder can positively affect the subsequent course, according to a model of the neurotoxicity of untreated psychosis (Loebel et al, 1992).

Extrapyramidal side-effects are not frequent with the above proposed treatment schedule and when atypical antipsychotics are used. If EPS appear (risperidone is more frequently associated with dystonic reactions, tremors, and akathisia), a slowing of the rate of dosage increase should be considered before starting with an anticholinergic medication. When the EPS persist, an anticholinergic can be administered for at least 8 weeks. After this period, a gradual withdrawal should be considered, over 3 or 4 weeks. A sparing use of anticholinergic medications is warranted, given the possible impairing side-effects of these compounds.

Treatment of the patient with acute symptomatology

An acute administration may be needed when severe psychotic symptoms and/or aggressive, agitated, or hostile behavior represent a real danger for the patient and/or others. In these cases hospitalization is usually needed during the first period of pharmacotherapy, with an adequate involvement and collaboration of the family and, whenever possible, of the patient. In the acute treatment, the definition of an optimal dose is more difficult and the risk of overdosing and of severe side-effects is greater. These side-effects will reduce the compliance of the patients in the subsequent phases of treatment.

The atypical antipsychotics described before can be effectively used in the acute phase, when the patient is relatively compliant. The rate of titration may be faster, even though it can increase the risk of EPS, particularly with risperidone. Olanzapine can more rapidly reach its target dose with a lower risk of EPS, and may be considered first. A liquid formulation of risperidone or Velotab preparation of olanzapine are more indicated in less compliant patients. Only when the patient is totally refusing pharmacotherapy, should an injected medication be considered.

Very sparse literature is available on acute injection treatments of psychotic children and adolescents in the emergency room, and empirical studies describe clinical experience with adult patients, with positive outcome, but increased risk for EPS and cardiotoxicity. More recent reports have underlined the advantages of using atypical intramuscular injection of olanzapine or ziprasidone in adults with acute psychosis or agitation. The atypical antipsychotics in the acute phase offer an opportunity for a pharmacologic continuum by transferring the patients to oral maintenance once the acute symptoms have ameliorated (Yildiz et al, 2003). Unfortunately, they have not been adequately assessed for their use in adolescents, and they should be used only by highly experienced clinicians.

A single case of treatment by olanzapine injection in an acutely agitated 10-year-old child has been described (Scheikh and Ahmed, 2002). More information is available on ziprasidone injections in a case series of 49 agitated children and adolescents, two of them with psychosis, at doses of 10 or 20 mg (Staller, 2004). Ziprasidone was effective and well tolerated. The treatment of another three non-psychotic adolescents, with acute aggression, with intramuscular ziprasidone has been described (Hazaray et al, 2004); doses of 10 mg were used, with good efficacy, but one patient developed a transitory syncopal episode 90 minutes after a ziprasidone injection.

Alternative injection medications are the typical antipsychotics, high-potency neuroleptics (haloperidol), or low-potency neuroleptics (phenothiazines, such as chlorpromazine). In this case a "sedative" management of the acute phase with typical antipsychotics should be followed by a "treatment" phase with atypical antipsychotics, with an undesiderable dichotomy in the treatment strategy and an increased length of the treatment plan.

The adult literature is centered on haloperidol, in monotherapy or associated with benzodiazepines (BDZs). Data from the literature suggest that haloperidol, 5–10 mg, alone or combined with a BDZ (e.g. lorazepam 2 mg) in the same syringe, is usually an effective approach to rapid tranquilization. An alternative strategy is with a low-potency neuroleptic, such as chlorpromazine, which can allow for a more rapid sedation with a relatively lower risk of EPS. The cotherapy with a BDZ is usually a safe and effective procedure, even though the risk exists for a worsening of dyscontrol in about 15–20% of younger patients. Whenever typical neuroleptics are used in the acute phase, it is important to consider the risk of akathisia, which may further worsen the agitation, and that is often misinterpreted as a non-response to treatment.

During the treatment with a high-potency neuroleptic EPS may occur. Only in this event should an anticholinergic compound be started.

When it is decided to switch from a typical neuroleptic to an atypical antipsychotic, the first should be tapered during the titration of the second, with an intermediate phase of combined treatment. Alternatively, in the most severe patients, the atypical antipsychotic should be titrated to the target dose before the typical antipsychotic is slowly tapered, in order to reduce the risk of a relapse during the switch. The tapering of the typical neuroleptic should be gradual, in order to minimize the risk of withdrawal dyskinesias. The anticholinergic medication, when needed, should be continued for 2 or 3 weeks after the discontinuation of the neuroleptic.

Management of negative symptoms

Negative symptoms are often the most debilitating part of the schizophrenic disorder. They can be present since the onset of the disorder, in continuity with a premorbid condition, namely in VEOS, or they can represent a sequela of the acute phase, during which positive symptoms are prevalent. Negative symptoms are usually more resistant to pharmacotherapy, and they are considered a negative predictor of treatment efficacy and clinical outcome.

Typical antipsychotics, particularly at the highest doses, can induce a negative-like symptomatology, through a blockade of the dopaminergic fronto-striatal pathway. This iatrogenic manifestation can be ameliorated by a reduction in the dosage of the neuroleptic. Iatrogenic negative symptoms are less evident during treatment with atypical antipsychotics, which are thus even more the first-choice medications when negative symptoms are the predominant clinical feature. However, even though atypical antipsychotics seem to present a higher efficacy in treating negative symptoms, the improvement is frequently quite modest (Zuddas et al, 1996).

When negative symptoms persist during a treatment with an atypical antipsychotic, a trial with clozapine monotherapy may be recommended, as this medication is probably the most effective in the treatment of negative symptoms, even in EOS and VEOS (Kumra et al, 1996). An alternative treatment, not yet tested in children and adolescents, is aripiprazole, which can further enhance the fronto-striatal dopaminergic transmission.

When a combined pharmacotherapy is selected to treat negative symptoms, different options are available, but none of them has been tested in children and adolescents. For this reason these strategies should be used only in severely ill and treatment-refractory patients, and managed by expert clinicians.

A selective serotonin re-uptake inhibitor (SSRI) may be added to the atypical antipsychotic, on the basis of empirical studies. Fluoxetine, fluvoxamine, sertraline, and paroxetine are, to date, the best studied SSRI agents in adult patients, prevalently combined with typical neuroleptics (Evins and Goff, 1996; Jockers-Scherubl et al, 2005). Careful monitoring of these combined therapies is needed, given the possible pharmacologic interactions between SSRIs (particularly fluvoxamine) and typical and atypical antipsychotics (especially clozapine).

Antagonism of serotonergic 5HT2A receptors has been hypothesized to enhance the effect of typical and atypical antipsychotics on negative symptoms and depressed mood, by increasing the firing of midbrain dopaminergic neurons. Mirtazapine and nefazodone (as 5HT2A blockers) may be used. However, the available atypical antipsychotics are yet strong antagonists of 5HT2A receptors, thus the efficacy of this strategy is at least questionable. It is possible that some negative-like symptoms may be unrecognized depressive symptoms, which are particularly frequent during the course of a psychotic disorder and may improve during treatment with antidepressant medications.

Glutamatergic agents (e.g. glycine, cyclo-serine) have been proposed in adult patients with negative psychotic symptoms, according to a glutamatergic model of schizophrenia. Unfortunately, data on younger patients are not available to date. Significant improvements with the addition to conventional antipsychotics of agonists of the glycine site of the NMDA receptor have been reported in controlled studies with adult patients. The full agonist, glycine, at a dose of 60 g/day, has shown a positive effect in adult patients on both negative symptoms (30%) and cognitive functioning (Heresco-Levy et al, 1999). Another full agonist, D-serine, at a dose of 30 mg/kg per day, was associated with a significant improvement in negative, positive, and cognitive symptoms, when added to risperidone in adult patirents (Tsai et al, 1999). Significantly, these agents did not improve negative symptoms when added to clozapine, confirming the specific activity of this atypical antipsychotic on negative symptomatology (Evins et al, 2000).

Dopaminergic agents have been proposed in association with typical antipsychotics, i.e. amphetamine, methylphenidate, and buproprion, but findings supporting these strategies in adult populations are still scarce (Sanfilippo et al, 1996). More recently the dopaminergic antiparkinsonian selegiline, a selective MAO inhibitor ($MAOI_B$) has been shown to be effective at a dose of 5 mg bid in a controlled trial (Bodkin et al, 2005).

The addition of anticholinergic compounds to typical neuroleptics has been proven to improve some negative symptoms, in some studies, but not in others, probably through an improvement in the psychomotor side-effects of typical neuroleptics, even though a specific cholinergic/dopaminergic interaction has been proposed in schizophrenic patients (Tandon and Grenden 1989). There are no studies exploring the effect of anticholinergic agents in patients treated with atypical antipsychotics, which have per se an anticholinergic activity. In summary, evidence for a positive effect of anticholinergic compounds is poorly supported, while the negative effects of these medications on cognitive functioning are well known (Strauss et al, 1990).

Management of treatment-resistant psychotic disorder

About 30% of schizophrenic children and adolescents do not present a satisfying clinical response to treatment. It is important to remind clinicians that the first approach in treatment-resistant patients is to enhance the non-pharmacologic interventions, with effective psychosocial, psychotherapeutic, behavioral treatments, social and cognitive rehabilitation, social skills training, and family support.

When the diagnosis is correct, the medication is taken in the appropriate dosage, for the appropriate length of time, and in the appropiate way; when the treatment resistance is not an iatrogenic effect (i.e. negative symptoms, akathisia), and when the patient is still taking a conventional antipsychotic, the first step is to switch to an atypical antipsychotic. When the patient is already taking an atypical antipsychotic, an increase in the dosage is recommended, in order to evaluate, in the next few weeks, the clinical effect and the tolerability (dose-dependent side-effects). When this strategy is ineffective, a switch to another atypical antipsychotic different from clozapine is possible. Which is the most effective among these atypical antipsychotics in treating treatment refractoriness is not clear, the results still being inconsistent. It is likely that different refractory patients respond differently to different atypical antipsychotics, and thus a single strategy is not feasible.

When two atypical antipsychotics have been ineffective, a switch to clozapine is recommended, this medication being the only antipsychotic with documented efficacy for psychotic symptoms in treatment-refractory patients. Clozapine monotherapy is currently the best-supported strategy for treatment resistance; however, given the complexity of the management (i.e. white blood cell monitoring) and the possible side-effects (i.e. seizures), other atypical antipsychotics should be assessed before a clozapine trial. The management of clozapine treatment in children and adolescents will be described later in more detail.

A still debated issue is related to the possible combination of an atypical antipsychotic and a neuroleptic, when monotherapy with an atypical antipsychotic is ineffective. Even though this procedure should usually be avoided, clinical practice shows that positive symptoms (namely delusions) may sometimes persist, even after adequate treatment with an atypical antipsychotic. In these cases the addition of a low-dose, high-potency neuroleptic (haloperidol) can give a better control of positive symptoms, through a more extensive D2 receptor blockade. After 2 or 3 months of stable improvement of psychotic symptoms, a gradual tapering of the typical neuroleptic should be considered, while monitoring a possible worsening of the delusions or hallucinations. Careful monitoring of side-effects is even more warranted in these selected cases.

Another strategy explored in adult non-responders is to combine two atypical antipsychotics (Lerner et al, 2004). Clozapine augmentation of an antipsychotic treatment has been critically revised (Chong and Remington, 2000), but data on efficacy and safety are still very scarce, even in adults. Even though controlled evidence is scarce, some clinicians report significant improvements during the phase of switching from one medication to another, when both are combined. Risperidone has been openly added to clozapine (Morera and Barrero, 1999); other combinations of risperidone and olanzapine, as well as risperidone or olanzapine with quetiapine, are not infrequently used in clinical practice (Lerner et al, 2004). The rationale for these combinations is still rather obscure, since all these medications have a maximal D2 and 5HT2A occupancy. However, the review by Lerner et al (2004) suggests that an improvement in positive symptoms, and occasionally in negative symptoms, can occur in refractory cases. Controlled studies are needed to confirm the efficacy of these combinations even in adults, and above all their tolerability in younger patients.

Adjunctive treatment has been proposed in refractory patients. Lithium augmentation has been supported by open, but not by controlled studies. This augmentation has a specific indication in patients with affective symptoms, or with aggression and impulsivity. An increased risk of neuroleptic malignant syndrome has been reported in combined antipsychotic–lithium treatment. Carbamazepine should be used more cautiously, as it can determine an enzymatic induction which lowers the blood levels of the antipsychotics. The carbamazepine–clozapine combination should be avoided, given the negative effect of both these medications on white blood cells. The addition of BDZ can improve anxiety and agitation in the short term, but the initially hypothesized positive effect mediated by the GABAergic modulation of dopaminergic transmission has not been confirmed.

Clozapine in children and adolescents

The management of clozapine in children and adolescents is particularly complex, given the risk of agranulocytosis and seizures. Before the onset of treatment physical and laboratory assessments must be undertaken, including medical history, neurologic and physical examinations, complete blood cell count, and electroencephalogram (EEG) while awake and asleep. When abnormalities in the EEG are present before treatment, clozapine should be avoided, or a clozapine–valproic acid combined treatment should be considered. In contrast, mild EEG abnormalities are frequent during treatment (up to 40%), and they are not strongly predictive of a seizure risk, if they are not severe.

The clozapine dosage should be individualized in each patient, and adapted according to the side-effects. A possible schedule of titration of clozapine in adolescents is to start with 25 mg/day, with increases of 25 mg every first or second day (based on clinical severity) up to 75–100 mg as the first target dose. Some patients show a positive clinical response even with very low doses of clozapine, and this possibility should be explored before titration to higher doses. After a first evaluation of efficacy and tolerability during the next 2 or 3 weeks, an increase to 125–150 mg/day, and then possibly to 250–300 mg/day is recommended. Further increases can be evaluated with more caution, given the risk of seizures with increasing dosage. It should be remembered that the risk of seizures is particularly high (5%) when dosage is higher than 400 mg/day.

When clozapine is used in prepubertal children, a much more prudent approach is needed, with a starting dose of 12.5 mg and increases of 12.5 mg every 2 or 3 days, with target doses of 50–75 mg/day, and further increases of 12.5 mg up to 125–150 mg.

When the target dose is reached, the patient should be maintained at that level, as the full effect is evident in the following 4–6 weeks, even though further improvements can occur during the following 6–8 months.

Common side-effects which can necessitate a slower titration are sedation, drooling, hypotension, and mild fever. Major, even if relatively uncommon, adverse effects are agranulocytosis and seizures. In order to minimize the risk of agranulocytosis, monitoring of white blood cells is needed in the drug guidelines, which are specific in different countries. Given that the risk is higher in the early phases of the treatment, a weekly white blood cell count is warranted for the first 12 weeks, then monthly, and one month after the discontinuation of clozapine. When white blood cells are significantly reduced from the previous control, or when they are between 3500 and 3000/mm^3 (and neutrophils are between 1500 and 2000/mm^3) biweekly monitoring is recommended. When white blood cells are between 3000 and 2000/mm^3 (and/or neutrophils are below 1500/mm^3) clozapine should be immediately discontinued, the white blood cells should be checked every 2 days, and screening for possible infection should be undertaken. When the white blood cells are below 2000/mm^3, immediate discontinuation of the medication and hospitalization in hematologic unit is mandatory. A combined treatment with lithium has been suggested in order to improve the hematologic situation (Sporn et al, 2003). Following recovery from agranulocytosis, clozapine should not be restarted if possible, and an alternative medication should be used.

Seizure risk is dose-related and periodic EEG should monitor this risk at least every 3 months. When EEG abnormalities are particularly evident, dosage may be reduced, or the possibility of a concurrent treatment with valproic acid should be considered.

The risk of EPS and parkinsonism, as well as of hyperprolactinemia, is particularly low.

Management of complicating problems

Some additional problems can further complicate the clinical picture of a psychotic disorder, particularly in adolescents. In adolescents with a violent or aggressive behavior, clozapine may be particularly indicated. Alternatively, lithium may be added to one of the other atypical antipsychotics (risperidone, olanzapine). The risk of neuroleptic malignant syndrome should be carefully considered in these patients.

When the risk of suicidal behavior is particularly high, clozapine is the most effective treatment, according to the adult literature. Alternatively, lithium may be added to another atypical antipsychotic (risperidone, olanzapine). An SSRI may be another second-line medication in add-on with atypical antipsychotics, with careful monitoring for a possible increase in agitation or suicidality during the first weeks of treatment (see Chapter 4).

When a patient has positively responded to an atypical antipsychotic, but with a great increase in weight and obesity, a gradual and careful switch to another antipsychotic with less weight gain liability should be considered (quetiapine, ziprasidone, aripiprazole). If the antipsychotic is clozapine, and the patient was refractory to other treatments, clozapine should be maintained, and other nutritional and exercise counseling should be provided. Lowering the dosage is rarely effective, since weight gain is often not a dose-related effect. Concurrent medications to reduce appetite are poorly explored in children and adolescents. Trials with sibutramine, amantadine, orlistat, metformin, nizatidine, and topiramate have been reported in the literature on adult patients, but only topiramate has been tested anecdotally in children and adolescents (Lessing et al, 2001; Pavuluri et al, 2002).

The management of affective symptoms

In adult schizophrenic patients, affective symptoms, particularly depressive symptoms, occur in at least 25–30% during the first psychotic episode, and in up to 50% in the chronic course, even if the severity of psychotic symptoms often overshadows this important comorbidity. Data on the prevalence of depressive symptoms in schizophrenic children and adolescents are not available, but it may account for at least a part of the risk of suicide after puberty. Depressive symptoms can more frequently occur or worsen during treatment with typical antipsychotics. In contrast, the atypical antipsychotics clozapine, risperidone, olanzapine, and quetiapine have been proven to have mood stabilizing properties, and they can be effective in controlling both depressive and manic symptoms. Data on the management of depression in schizophrenic patients rely on adult studies, and prevalently on adjunctive treatments with tricyclic antidepressants, which are poorly effective in childhood and adolescent depression. SSRIs have been scarcely explored as antidepressant agents in adults with schizophrenia, while they have been studied primarily in the treatment of negative symptoms.

When a child or an adolescent shows evident features of depression during treatment with atypical antipsychotics, an SSRI should be cautiously added, monitoring for possible worsening of impulsive, aggressive, and hostile behaviors, or self-harm behaviors, or suicidality. A differential diagnosis of bipolar disorder is particularly important before starting a treatment with an antidepressant medication, in order to prevent a manic or mixed switch.

Alternatively, a mood stabilizer (valproic acid in prepubertal children, lithium in adolescents) may be added to the atypical antipsychotic, especially when dysphoria, irritability, and manic-like symptoms are present. Typical neuroleptics should be avoided, as they can worsen the depressive symptomatology.

Long-term strategy

There is still poor consensus on how best to define the long-term recovery. The level of positive symptoms is usually considered the single most important indicator of remission. Second-line indicators are the levels of cognitive/disorganized behavior and of negative symptoms. The improvements should be maintained for at least 3 months in patients in remission and at least 1 year in patients in recovery.

In patients at the first psychotic episode, the treatment strategy is related to the typology of the episode. When the onset of the psychotic symptoms was acute, the premorbid functioning (including IQ) was good, symptoms were predominantly positive, and they rapidly improved after antipsychotic treatment, the medication should be maintained for at least 12 months after remission. The dosage should be the lowest effective in the acute phase, and it should be decreased only when side-effects are significantly impairing. Every lowering of the dosage, however small, should be carefully monitored for the risk of relapse or worsening of symptoms. After 1 year in the symptom-free condition, a tapering of the medication (by a reduction in the medication not exceeding one quarter of the dose every month) and then a medication-free period can be tried. However, the risk of relapse should always be considered, and worsening of the symptomatology requires an immediate restoration of the treatment.

When symptomatology persists, even partially, the treatment should be maintained at the lowest effective dosage.

Depot antipsychotics have not been well studied in pediatric patients, and their use increases the risk of EPS. Their use should thus be limited to adolescents with chronic symptomatology and persistent problems of compliance. A promising option in maintenance drug treatment is the only long-acting atypical antipsychotic available, long-acting risperidone, administered at a dose of 25 mg once every 2 weeks (Knox and Stimmel, 2004). No data have been published to date on the use of long-acting risperidone in adolescents.

Side-effects

Extrapyramidal side-effects

Extrapyramidal side-effects are more frequent with typical antipsychotics, but they can also occur during treatment with atypical antipsychotics (more frequently with risperidone), in particularly sensitive subjects or when titration is too fast (Mandoki, 1995).

Even though EPS more frequently occur with higher doses, they can also appear with small doses of antipsychotics. They are more frequent in children and adolescents, in patients with mental retardation or CNS damage, and in drug-naive subjects. A specific sensitivity to EPS may be reported in other members of the same family.

Anticholinergic agents are usually the first-line medications, including benztropine, biperiden, and triexhyphenidyl. Dyphenidramine has an anticholinergic effect, even if it is primarily an anti-histaminic agent, and for this reason it has a more sedating effect. Other agents used in EPS in adult patients are medications with a central dopaminergic action, such as L-DOPA, bromocriptine, and amantadine. However, these compounds can worsen the psychotic symptomatology, as well as the agitation. Amantadine seems to present the lowest risk for inducing psychotic symptoms.

Dystonias more frequently occur in the first phases of the treatment, and they can range from mild to severe manifestations, for example laryngospasm, which can compromise respiration. More frequent manifestations are cramping and pain, usually involving the head, neck, and back musculature, and oculogyric crises are not uncommon as well. They usually respond to anticholinergic medications, intramuscular and/or per os. After the acute intervention, a decrease in the dose or a switch to another antipsychotic should be considered, before adding regular doses of an anticholinergic agent. When an anticholinergic medication is added, the real need for this combination should be periodically reconsidered after the acute phase of treatment, or when the antipsychotic dosage is lowered, and at least every 8–12 weeks, because many patients no longer need this treatment.

Withdrawal dyskinesias can occur when the medication is tapered too fast, even though they can also appear during a slow tapering, in particularly sensitive patients or after a long treatment, or during an irregular intake of the medication in non-compliant patients. A slowing of the tapering should be considered before starting an anticholinergic medication.

Drug-induced parkinsonism can be manifested by different symptoms, such as tremors, decreased body movements, slowed body movements, less facial expression, less prosodic speech, and stiff walking without the normal pendulum-like arm movements. These symptoms can occur even at small doses, while more severe manifestations, such as bradykinesia, akinesia, shuffling gait, and mask-like facies, occur at the higher doses and after a longer treatment. Parkinsonism can be treated with anticholinergic medications, but their efficacy is lower, particularly when symptomatology is severe. A dopaminergic agent can be useful, but careful monitoring of psychotic symptoms is needed.

Akathisia is an important side-effect of antipsychotic treatment, and it is frequently unrecognized or incorrectly interpreted. It is a subjective or objective restlessness, with a need for movement and sometimes a worsening of the agitation, which can in turn induce the clinician to increase the antipsychotic dosage, with further worsening of the akathisia. Akathisia is poorly responsive to medications. A decrease in the antipsychotic dose can sometimes improve the restlessness. Anticholinergic medications are poorly effective, while low-dose clonazepam (0.5–2 mg/day), propanolol (10–30 mg/day), or dyphenhidramine (100–200 mg/day) can sometimes be effective. The antipsychotic clozapine can also reduce the symptomatology in severe and resistant cases.

Tardive dyskinesia is one of the most severe extrapyramidal sequelae of an antipsychotic treatment. Even though it can occur in the first phases of the treatment, the risk increases with longer treatments (5% every year of treatment, that is, after a 10-year treatment half of the patients will have a tardive dyskinesia), which is the rule rather the exception in severe and chronic psychotic disorders. Typical manifestations of tardive dyskinesia are rhythmic movements of the tongue, mouth, and jaws, but the upper limbs and trunk can also be involved. It is important to remember that, during long antipsychotic treatment, transitory manifestations (1 or 2 weeks) of a dyskinetic disorder can occur, and then spontaneously disappear. This possibility should be considered before starting treatments of tardive dyskinesia, which unfortunately are poorly effective. The first step is an early detection of the disorder, which can lead, when possible, to a decrease in the antipsychotic dose. Some cases of tardive dyskinesia can improve with treatment by dopamine agonists, such as L-DOPA or amantadine. There is some evidence that clozapine can be effective in the treatment of tardive dyskinesias, and a switch to this medication should be considered in the more severe and refractory forms of this impairing side-effect.

Neuroleptic malignant syndrome

This is a potentially life-threatening side-effect of uncertain origin during treatment with antipsychotics. The rate of this condition is still under discussion, ranging between 0.5 and 1.5% of the patients exposed to neuroleptics. The prevalence in children and adolescents is still uncertain, but clear descriptions of neuroleptic malignant syndrome in children have been reported (Ty and Rothner, 2004). It is characterized by hyperthermia, muscular rigidity, tachycardia, hyper- or hypotension, autonomic instability, mionecrosis, and altered mental status. When unrecognized and untreated, this condition can progress to a loss of consciousness and death. Possible diagnostic errors are catatonia, EPS, or infectious disease. An elevation of creatine phosphokinase (CPK) and leukocytosis can occur, but these findings are not always present, and thus their absence may be misleading and may induce a delay in treatment. Furthermore, mild elevations of CPK are not infrequent in agitated patients receiving im injections of sedative agents. In summary, the following four symptoms, fever, muscular rigidity, altered level of consciousness, and autonomic dysregulation, should be considered as alarming signs. Higher doses of antipsychotics and polypharmacy (particularly with lithium) have been considered as increasing the risk of neuroleptic malignant syndrome.

When this severe condition is suspected, the antipsychotic and anticholinergic agent should be immediately stopped and all the vegetative functions should be supported, including respiratory, cardiac, and renal functions, together with management of hyperthermia (hydration and cooling), and monitoring of electrolytes and fluids. The peripheral muscle relaxant dantrolene (0.8–2.5 mg/kg intravenously every 6 hours) can improve rigidity, mionecrosis, and tachycardia through a peripheral action on muscles. The dopamine agonist bromocriptine (5–7.5 µg three times a day) can improve mental status and rigidity through a central dopaminergic stimulation. These two medications can be administered simultaneously, and they can improve the efficacy of supportive interventions.

The mortality of adult cases of neuroleptic malignant syndrome is estimated to be about 10–20%, with a reduction in recent decades, in parallel with better recognition and treatment. The most negative predictors of outcome are myoglobinuria and renal failure. In a review considering mortality in the available case reports of children and adolescents from 1973 to 1998 (Ty and Rothner, 2004), the percentage was 44% (4/9) from 1973 to 1980, 5.5% (1/19) from 1981 to 1990, and no mortality from 1991 to 1998. These findings may be accounted for by the increasing awareness and early recognition of the syndrome, with a timely intervention and prevention of complications.

Weight gain

Weight gain is the most significant side-effect in all the studies on the atypical antipsychotics risperidone, olanzapine, and clozapine (Theisen et al, 2001; Baptista et al, 2002). Ratzoni et al (2002) conducted a prospective study of 50 adolescents with schizophrenia ($n=46$), schizoaffective disorder ($n=2$), and conduct disorder ($n=2$), who were treated with risperidone, olanzapine, and haloperidol. During the 12 weeks of follow-up, 19 of the 21 (90.5%) patients treated with olanzapine and 9 of the 21 (42.9%) patients treated with risperidone showed at least a 7% increase in weight. The mean weight gain was 11.1 ± 7.8% with olanzapine, and 6.6 ± 8.6% with risperidone, while the average weight of the haloperidol group did not change.

Quetiapine, ziprasidone, and aripiprazole are reported to have a lower incidence of weight gain. This side-effect cannot be disregarded, given the increased morbidity and mortality in subjects with obesity. Furthermore, the difficult management of food craving in patients with psychotic disorder adds further conflict in the families, reducing the compliance with treatment. Dietary recommendations and psychoeducational counseling are needed at the beginning of the treatment. Careful monitoring of weight gain, parallel to monitoring of liver functioning and glycemia, is highly recommended in all these patients.

As reported above, pharmacologic management of increased appetite and weight gain is poorly supported by empirical evidence, even in adult patients. A trial with topiramate, or alternatively with sibutramine, amantadine, orlistat, metformin, or nizatidine, can be cautiously attempted in adolescents (Lessing et al, 2001; Pavuluri et al, 2002).

Sedation

The sedative effects of antipsychotics may be particularly deleterious to the pediatric population because drowsiness can impair attention and learning at school. However, the sedation is usually transient and does not lead to drug withdrawal.

Sedation is a common adverse effect observed with clozapine, risperidone, olanzapine, quetiapine, and ziprasidone (Findling et al, 2000) and it can be minimized by using gradual dose escalation. Treatment with olanzapine is more likely to produce sedation in children and adolescents than in adults (Woods et al, 2002). Gothelf and coworkers (2003), in an open-label comparative trial of risperidone, olanzapine, and haloperidol, found that fatiguability occurred with all three drugs, though to a lesser extent with risperidone (11.8% for risperidone vs 42.1% for olanzapine and 71.4% for haloperidol); a similar pattern was observed for sedation. Armenteros et al (1997) described mild sedation in eight of ten risperidone-treated patients, which subsided after 2 weeks. Sedation was reported in six of the eight patients treated with olanzapine in the study of Kumra et al (1998a), in 11 of 15 olanzapine-treated patients in the study of Sholevar et al (2000) and in nine of 16 olanzapine-treated patients in he study of Findling et al (2003a). Sedation is also common with clozapine, occurring in 90% of patients in the studies of Kumra et al (1996) and Turetz et al (1997), and it was the most common adverse effect related to quetiapine treatment in adolescents (Shaw et al, 2001; McConville et al, 2003).

Hyperprolactinemia

Although hyperprolactinemia is a common side-effect of antipsychotics in adult patients, a growing literature shows that this side-effect can be of clinical significance in children and adolescents as well. All the typical neuroleptics can induce hyperprolactinemia, and risperidone has the highest risk among the atypical antipsychotics (Wudarski et al, 1999; Masi et al, 2001; Findling et al, 2003b). Usually serum prolactin levels tend to rise and peak within the first 2 months, then they can progressively decline during the next 6 months, but they can also persist at the higher levels, as well as their negative consequences.

Clinical implications of asymptomatic antipsychotic-induced hyperprolactinemia in children are not clear. Data from children with prolactinomas suggest that growth arrest, osteopenia, and delayed pubertal development may be determined by enduring high levels of prolactin. These data should be considered cautiously because prolactin levels in these patients are many times higher than those normally found in children treated with antipsychotics; furthermore, symptoms may be affected by the effect of a prolactinoma on pituitary function. Due to the lack of clear guidelines, monitoring of serum prolactin levels during treatment, namely with risperidone is warranted. In the case of high levels of prolactin associated with a good efficacy of treatment, a careful consideration of the risk–benefit ratio should include the switch to another atypical antipsychotic.

In adolescent girls the effects of hyperprolactinemia can be more evident and impairing, mainly due to amenorrhea and other menstrual cycle disorders. Gynecomastia is a rare side-effect in adolescent males. Galactorrhea can occur in both males and females. Sexual side-effects are rare, but possible effects in adolescents are decreased libido, anorgasmia, erectile difficulties, and ejaculatory problems. All these problems should be investigated during antipsychotic treatment, even when they are not spontaneously reported by the patients.

Management of these problems begins with an attempt to reduce the antipsychotic dosage. When this step is ineffective, or when it is associated with a worsening of the psychotic symptoms, a switch to another antipsychotic with a lesser effect on prolactin levels (olanzapine, quetiapine) is recommended. Cohen and Biederman (2001) have reported on efficacy and safety of a co-treatment with a dopamino-agonist, cabergoline, at a dose of 2.13 ± 0.09 mg/week (mean duration of treatment 523.5 ± 129.7 days) in 4 children (6–11 years) with risperidone-induced hyperprolactinemia. An alternative dopamine agonists is bromocriptine.

Hyperglycemia and hyperlipidemia

Both typical and atypical antipsychotics, particularly clozapine and olanzapine, are associated with higher glucose and lipid levels (Newcomer, 2004). Specific data on children and adolescents are scarce. Koller et al (2001) found hyperglycemia in 11 adolescents (aged 13 to 18) treated with clozapine (100–1000 mg/day). Bloch and colleagues (2003) reported on five adolescents who developed an overt diabetes (two subjects) or glucose dysregulation (three subjects) during olanzapine treatment. Saito and Kafantaris (2002) described two patients aged 13 and 17 who developed diabetes mellitus after combined treatment with risperidone and valproate semisodium.

Martin and L'Ecuyer (2002) found no significant changes in serum triglyceride or cholesterol levels in a sample of 22 children and adolescents treated with risperidone. A regular metabolic follow-up including fasting blood glucose is recommended in healthy children and adolescents receiving olanzapine and clozapine treatment.

Hematologic side-effects

All the antipsychotics can induce a leukopenia, usually mild and without clinical relevance. The higher risk of agranulocytosis is associated with clozapine treatment, and monitoring of white blood cells is needed, according to the guidelines of the drug (Alvir et al, 1993). However, agranulocytosis and granulocytopenia are seldom reported during treatment with other typical and atypical antipsychotics (Kodesh et al, 2001; Ruhe et al, 2001). A blood cell count is warranted when clinical indices of leukopenia are suspected (i.e. recurrent infections).

Even though neutropenia usually occurs during the first weeks of treatment, late-onset neutropenias have been reported, thus such a possibility should be kept in mind during every antipsychotic treatment.

When an antipsychotic-induced neutropenia has occurred, a rechallenge with the same antipsychotic should be avoided, even though experts' opinions on the issues are not totally consistent. The successful management of clozapine-induced neutropenia with adjunctive lithium carbonate (0.8–1.1 μg/ml) has been recently reported in a schizophrenic child (Sporn et al, 2004), and it may represent a possible alternative to discontinuation in treatment-refractory children.

Hepatotoxicity

Antipsychotic-induced hepatotoxicity, which may, in part, be related to weight gain in long-term use of this drug, has also been reported. Liver enzyme abnormalities (elevated serum aminotransferase levels) and fatty infiltration evidenced by abdominal ultrasound can be detected (Kumra et al, 1997b; Woods et al, 2002). Szighety and colleagues (1999) reviewed the charts of 38 children and adolescents aged 5 to 17 years with a variety of psychiatric diagnoses who received risperidone (mean 2.5 mg/day) for a mean of 15.2 months. Thirty-seven out of the 38 subjects did not present liver enzyme abnormalities at the end of the study and only one patient had a mild and clinically non-relevant increase of the alanine aminotransferase (7 U/I above the upper normal limit). Liver function should be monitored in children who are taking atypical antipsychotics, particularly in obese children or in those with rapid weight gain.

Seizures

Even though atypical antipsychotics produce EEG abnormalities, the higher risk of dose-dependent epileptic seizures is associated with clozapine treatment, while the risk is milder with risperidone and quetiapine (Centorrino et al, 2002). According to Freedman and colleagues' review (1994), three out of 80 adolescents who received clozapine (4%) experienced seizures, and 32 out of 53 (60%) had epileptiform changes in their EEGs. Two of the ten clozapine-treated subjects of the double-blind clozapine–haloperidol study (Kumra et al, 1996) had seizures during the treatment. In one patient, myoclonus and tonic-clonic seizures occurred at a dose of 400 mg/day. Clozapine was reduced and an anticonvulsant treatment was started; no further seizures occurred, but the EEG remained abnormal, prompting discontinuation of the clozapine. The other patient had tonic-clonic seizures at a dose of 275 mg/day and discontinued treatment.

Cardiovascular effects

Cardiac side-effects are more rarely reported in children and adolescents than in adult patients. Ziprasidone has the potential to cause QTc prolongation in adults and therefore concerns have been raised regarding this cardiac risk in children and adolescents. Very few reports on ziprasidone treatment in young patients are available, and no significant cardiovascular effects have been reported in these studies. Only one patient in the series of Patel and colleagues (2002) had a slight prolongation (19 msec) of the QTc during the ECG follow-up. More recently, Blair and colleagues (2005) have assessed the ECG safety profile of low-dose ziprasidone (less than 40 mg/day) in pediatric outpatients treated for up to 6 months. Statistically significant changes from baseline in heart rate, PR, and QTc intervals were found, and the QTc prolongation did not correlate to dose. The mean QTc prolongation was 28 ± 26 ms, but one subject had a 114-ms prolongation. These findings suggest careful ECG monitoring during ziprasidone treatment in children and adolescents, even with low doses.

Cardiac side-effects are more evident with low-potency neuroleptics, and include orthostatic hypotension, increased heart rate, dizziness, and ECG changes (longer QT and PR intervals, reduced ST). Hypotension can occur during treatment with phenotiazines, and should be managed by changing the antipsychotic. More severe cardiac effects can occur during acute im or iv administration of antipsychotics in agitated patients. In these conditions cardiac function should be carefully monitored.

Cardiac symptoms (usually a transient increase in heart rate) with no relevant clinical significance have been reported in young children during risperidone treatment. An ECG at baseline and as part of routine monitoring is recommended in younger patients (Masi et al, 2003).

Anticholinergic effects

Anticholinergic effects can be disturbing side-effects which can reduce the compliance with treatment, even in children and adolescents. They include dry mouth, constipation, blurry vision, nausea, mydriasis, and urinary difficulties. Some anticholinergic agents can worsen these symptoms, as well as other agents with anticholinergic effects, such as tricyclic antidepressants. The management of the anticholinergic symptoms is by decreasing or discontinuing the combined anticholinergic agent, and/or reducing the dose of the antipsychotic.

References

Alaghband-Rad J, McKenna K, Gordon CT, et al. Childhood-onset schizophrenia: the severity of premorbid course. *J Am Acad Child Adolesc Psychiatry* 1995; **34**: 1273–83.

Alvir JM, Lieberman JA, Safferman AZ, et al. Clozapine-induced agranulocytosis. Incidence and risk factors in the United States. *N Engl J Med* 1993; **329**: 162–7.

Armenteros JL, Withaker AH, Welikson M, et al. Risperidone in adolescents with schizophrenia: an open pilot study. *J Am Acad Child Adolesc Psychiatry* 1997; **36**: 694–700.

Asarnow JR, Tompson MC, Goldstein MJ. Childhood-onset schizophrenia: a follow-up study. *Schizophr Bull* 1994; **20**: 599–617.

Asarnow JR, Tompson MC, McGrath E. Annotation: childhood-onset schizophrenia: clinical and treatment issues. *J Child Psychol Psychiatry* 2004; **45**: 180–94.

Baptista T, Kin NM, Beaulieu S, deBaptista EA. Obesity and related metabolic abnormalities during antipsychotic drug administration: mechanism, management and research perspectives. *Pharmacopsychiatry* 2002; **35**: 205–19.

Blair J, Scahill L, State M, Martin A. Electrocardiographic changes in children and adolescents treated with ziprasidone: a prospective study. *J Am Acad Child Adolesc Psychiatry* 2005; **44**: 73–9.

Blanz B, Schmidt M. Clozapine for schizophrenia. *J Am Acad Child Adolesc Psychiatry* 1993; **32**: 223–4.

Bloch Y, Vardi O, Mendlovic S, et al. Hyperglicemia from olanzapine treatment in adolescents. *J Child Adolesc Psychopharmacol* 2003; **13**: 97–102.

Bodkin JA, Siris SG, Bermanzohn PC, et al. Double-blind, placebo-controlled, multi-center trial of selegiline augmentation of antipsychotic medication to treat negative symptoms in outpatients with schizophrenia. *Am J Psychiatry* 2005; **162**: 388–90.

Buitelaar JK, Van der Gaag RJ. Diagnostic rules for children with PDD-NOS and multiple complex developmental disorder. *J Child Psychol Psychiatry* 1998; **39**: 911–19.

Calderoni D, Wudarsky M, Bhangoo R, et al. Differentiating childhood onset schizophrenia from psychotic mood disorders. *J Am Acad Child Adolesc Psychiatry* 2001; **40**: 1190–6.

Cannon TD, Huttunen MO, Dahlstrom HD, et al. Antipsychotic drug treatment in the prodromal phase of schizophrenia. *Am J Psychiatry* 2002; **159**: 1230–2.

Caplan R. Thought disorder in children. *J Am Acad Child Adolesc Psychiatry* 1994; **33**: 605–15.

Centorrino F, Price BH, Tuttle M, et al. EEG abnormalities during treatment with typical and atypical antipsychotics. *Am J Psychiatry* 2002; **159**: 109–15.

Chambers WJ, Puig-Antich J, Tabrizi MA, Davis M. Psychotic symptoms in prepubertal major depressive disorder. *Arch Gen Psychiatry* 1982; **39**: 921–7.

Chong SA, Remington G. Clozapine augmentation: safety and efficacy. *Schizophr Bull* 2000; **26**: 421–40.

Cohen LG, Biederman J. Treatment of risperidone-induced hyperprolactinemia with a dopamine agonist in children. *J Child Adolesc Psychopharmacol* 2001; **11**: 435–40.

Davis JM, Chen N, Glick ID. A meta-analysis of the efficacy of second-generation antipsychotics. *Arch Gen Psychiatry* 2003; **60**: 553–64.

Eggers C. Schizoaffective psychosis in childhood: a follow-up study. *J Autism Dev Disord* 1989; **19**: 327–34.

Eggers C, Bunk D. The long-term course of childhood-onset schizophrenia: a 42-year follow-up. *Schizophren Bull* 1997; **23**: 105–17.

Ercan ES, Kutlu A, Varon A, et al. Olanzapine treatment of eight adolescent patients with psychosis. *Hum Psychopharmacol* 2004; **19**: 53–6.

Evins A, Goff D. Adjunctive antidepressant drug therapies in the treatment of negative symptoms of schizophrenia. *CNS Drugs* 1996; **6**: 130–47.

Evins AE, Fitzgerald SM, Wine L, et al. Placebo-controlled trial of glycine in added to clozapine in schizophrenia. *Am J Psychiatry* 2000; **157**: 826–8.

Famularo R, Fenton T, Kinscherff R, Augustyn M. Psychiatric comorbidity in childhood post-traumatic stress disorder. *Child Abuse Negl* 1996; **20**: 953–61.

Fennig S, Susser ES, Pilowsky DJ, et al. Childhood hallucinations preceding the first psychotic episode. *J Nerv Ment Dis* 1997; **185**: 115–17.

Findling RL, McNamara NK, Gracious BL. Pediatric uses of atypical antipsychotic. *Expert Opin Pharmacother* 2000; **62**: 967–74.

Findling RL, McNamara NK, Youngstrom EA, et al. A prospective, open-label trial of olanzapine in adolescents with schizophrenia. *J Am Acad Child Adolesc Psychiatry* 2003(a); **42**: 170–5.

Findling RL, Kusumakar V, Daneman D, et al. Prolactin levels during long-term risperidone treatment in children and adolescents. *J Clin Psychiatry* 2003(b); **64**: 1362–9.

Frazier A, Gordon CT, McKenna K, et al. An open trial of clozapine in 11 adolescents with childhood-onset schizophrenia. *J Am Acad Child Adolesc Psychiatry* 1994; **33**: 658–63.

Freedman J, Wirshing W, Russel A, Bray M, Unitzer J. Absence status seizures after successful long-term clozapine treatment of an adolescent with schizophrenia. *J Child Adolesc Psychopharmacol* 1994; **4**: 53–62.

Geller B, Sun K, Zimerman B, et al. Complex and rapid-cycling in bipolar children and adolescents: a preliminary study. *J Affect Disord* 1995; **34**: 259–68.

Gothelf D, Apter A, Reidman J, et al. Olanzapine, risperidone and haloperidol in the treatment of adolescent patients with schizophrenia. *J Neural Trans* 2003; **110**: 545–60.

Grcevich SJ, Findling RL, Rowane WA, et al. Risperidone in the treatment of children and adolescents with schizophrenia: a retrospective study. *J Child Adolesc Psychopharmacol* 1996; **6**: 251–7.

Grothe DR, Calis KA, Jacobsen L, et al. Olanzapine pharmacokinetics in pediatric and adolescent inpatients with childhood-onset schizophrenia. *J Clin Psychopharmacol* 2000; **20**: 220–5.

Hazaray E, Ehret J, Posey DJ, et al. Intramuscular ziprasidone for acute agitation in adolescents. *J Child Adolesc Psychopharmacol* 2004; **14**: 464–70.

Heresco-Levy U, Javitt DC, Ermilov M, et al. Efficacy of high-dose glycine in the treatment of enduring negative symptoms of schizophrenia. *Arch Gen Psychiatry* 1999; **56**: 29–36.

Hollis C. Adult outcomes of child- and adolescent-onset schizophrenia: diagnostic stability and predictive validity. *Am J Psychiatry* 2000; **157**: 1652–9.

Hollis C. Developmental precursors of child- and adolescent-onset schizophrenia and affective psychoses: diagnostic specificity and continuity with symptom dimensions. *Br J Psychiatry* 2003; **182**: 327–44.

Jockers-Scherubl MC, Bauer A, Godemann F, et al. Negative symptoms of schizophrenia are improved by the addition of paroxetine to neuroleptics: a double-blind placebo-controlled study. *Int Clin Psychopharmacol* 2005; **20**: 27–31.

Knox ED, Stimmel GL. Clinical review of a long-acting, injectable formulation of risperidone. *Clin Ther* 2004; **26**: 1994–2002.

Kodesh A, Finkel B, Lerner AG, et al. Dose-dependent olanzapine-associated leukopenia: three case reports. *Int Clin Psychopharmacol* 2001; **16**: 117–19.

Koenigsberg HW, Reynolds P, Goodman M, et al. Risperidone in the treatment of schizotypal personality disorder. *J Clin Psychiatry* 2003; **64**: 628–34.

Koller E, Malozowski S, Doraiswamy PM. Atypical antipsychotic drugs and hyperglycemia in adolescents. JAMA 2001; **286**: 2547–8.

Kolvin I. Studies in childhood psychoses. I. Diagnostic criteria and classification. *Br J Psychiatry* 1971; **118**: 81–4.

Kranzler H, Roofeh D, Gerbino-Rosen G, et al. Clozapine: its impact on aggressive behavior among children and adolescents with schizophrenia. *J Am Acad Child Adolesc Psychiatry* 2005; **44**: 55–63.

Kumra S, Frazier J, Jacobsen LK, et al. Childhood onset schizophrenia: a double-blind clozapine haloperidol comparison. *Arch Gen Psychiatry* 1996; **53**: 1090–7.

Kumra S, Jacobsen LK, Lenane M, et al. Case series: spectrum of neuroleptic-induced movement disorders and extrapyramidal side-effects in childhood-onset schizophrenia. *J Am Acad Child Adolesc Psychiatry* 1997a; **37**: 221–7.

Kumra S, Herion D, Jacobsen LK, et al. Case study: Risperidone-induced hepatotoxicity in pediatric patients. *J Am Acad Child Adolesc Psychiatry* 1997b; **36**: 701–5.

Kumra S, Jacobsen LK, Lenane M, et al. "Multidimensionally Impaired Disorder": is it a variant of very early onset schizophrenia? *J Am Acad Child Adolesc Psychiatry* 1998a; **37**: 91–9.

Kumra S, Jacobsen LK, Lenane M, et al. Childhood-onset schizophrenia: an open label study of olanzapine in adolescents. *J Am Acad Child Adolesc Psychiatry* 1998b; **37**: 377–85.

Lerner V, Libov I, Kptler M, Strous RD. Combination of atypical antipsychotic medication in the management of treatment-resistant schizophrenia and schizoaffective disorder. *Prog Neuropsychopharmacol Biol Psychiatry* 2004; **28**: 89–98.

Lessing MC, Shapira NA, Murphy TK. Topiramate for reversing atypical antipsychotic weight gain. *J Am Acad Child Adolesc Psychiatry* 2001; **40**: 1364.

Lieberman J, Jody D, Geisler S, et al. Time course and biological correlates of treatment response in first episode schizophrenia. *Arch Gen Psychiatry* 1993; **50**: 369–76.

Lindenmayer JP, Eerdekens E, Berry SA, Eerdekens M. Safety and efficacy of long-acting risperidone in schizophrenia: a 12-week, multicenter, open-label study in stable patients switched from typical and atypical oral antipsychotics. *J Clin Psychiatry* 2005; **66**: 656–7.

Lindsey RL, Kaplan D, Koliatsos V. Aripiprazole and extrapyramidal symptoms. *J Am Acad Child Adolesc Psychiatry* 2003; **42**: 1268–9.

Loebel AD, Lieberman JA, Alvir JMJ, et al. Duration of pychosis and outcome in first-episode schizophrenia. Am J Psychiatry 1992; **149**: 1183–8.

McClellan JM, Werry JS, Ham M. A follow-up study of early-onset psychosis: comparison between outcome diagnoses of schizophrenia, mood disorders and personality disorders. *J Autism Dev Disord* 1993; **23**: 243–62.

McClellan J, Breiger D, McCurry C, Hlastala SA. Premorbid functioningt in early-onset psychotic disorders. *J Am Acad Child Adolesc Psychiatry* 2003; **42**: 666–72.

McConville BJ, Arvanitis LA, Thyrum PT, et al. Pharmacokinetics, tolerability, and clinical effectiveness of quetiapine fumarate: an open-label trial in adolescents with psychotic disorders. *J Clin Psychiatry* 2000; **61**: 252–60.

McConville B, Carrero L, Sweitzer D, et al. Long-term safety, tolerability, and clinical efficacy of quetiapine in adolescents: an open-label extension trial. *J Child Adolesc Psychopharmacol* 2003; **13**: 75–82.

McGee R, Williams S, Poulton R. Hallucinations in nonpsychotic children. *J Am Acad Child Adolesc Psychiatry* 2000; **39**: 12–13.

McGorry PD, Yung AR, Phillips LJ, et al. Randomized controlled trials of interventions designed to reduce the risk of progression to the first episode of psychosis in a clinical sample with subthreshold symptoms. *Arch Gen Psychiatry* 2002; **59**: 921–8.

McKenna K, Gordon CT, Lenane M, et al. Looking for childood-onset schizophrenia; the first 71 cases screened. *J Am Acad Child Adolesc Psychiatry* 1994; **33**: 636–44.

Mandoki MW. Risperidone treatment of children and adolescents: increased risk of extrapyramidal side-effects? *J Child Adolesc Psychopharmacol* 1995; **5**: 49–67.

Mandoki M. Olanzapine in the treatment of early-onset schizophrenia: an open label study of olanzapine in adolescents. *Biol Psychiatry* 1997; **41**: 22S.

Martin A, L'Ecuyer S. Triglyceride, cholesterol and weight changes among risperidone-treated youths: a retrospective study. *Eur Child Adolesc Psychiatry* 2002; **11**: 129–33.

Masi G, Cosenza A, Mucci M. Prolactin levels in preschool autistic children during risperidone treatment. *J Child Adolesc Psychopharmacol* 2001; **11**: 389–94.

Masi G, Mucci M, Floriani C. Catatonic episode after first and single dose of ecstasy. *J Am Acad Child Adolesc Psychiatry* 2002; **41**: 892.

Masi G, Cosenza A, Brovedani P, Mucci M. A three-year naturalistic study of 53 preschool children with pervasive developmental disorder treated with risperidone. *J Clin Psychiatry* 2003; **64**: 1039–47.

Masi G, Perugi G, Toni C, et al. The clinical phenotypes of juvenile bipolar disorder: toward a validation of the episodic-chronic distinction. *Biol Psychiatry*, in press.

Maziade M, Bouchard SD, Gingras N, et al. Long-term stability of diagnosis and symptoms dimensions in a systematic sample of patients with onset of schizophrenia in childhood and early adolescence, I: nosology, sex and age at onset. *Br J Psychiatry* 1996a; **169**: 361–70.

Maziade M, Bouchard SD, Gingras N, et al. Long-term stability of diagnosis and symptom dimensions in a systematic sample of patients with onset of schizophrenia in childhood and early adolescence, II: postive/negative distinction and childhood predictors of adult outcome. *Br J Psychiatry* 1996b; **169**: 371–8.

Meighen KG, Shelton HM, McDougle CJ. Ziprasidone treatment of two adolescents with psychosis. *J Child Adolesc Psychopharmacol* 2004; **14**: 137–42.

Morera AL, Barrero PJL. Risperidone and clozapine combination for the treatment of refractory schizophrenia. *Acta Psychiatr Scand* 1999; **99**: 305–6.

Mouridsen SE, Rich B, Isager T. Psychiatric morbidity in disintegrative psychosis and infantile autism: a long-term follow-up study. *Psychopathology* 1999; **32**: 177–83.

Mozes T, Greenberg Y, Spivak B, et al. Olanzapine treatment in chronic drug-resistant childhood onset schizophrenia: an open label study. *J Child Adolesc Psychopharmacol* 2003; **13**: 311–17.

Nechmad A, Ratzoni G, Poyurovsky M, et al. Obsessive-compulsive disorder in adolescent schizophrenia patients. *Am J Psychiatry* 2003; **160**: 1002–4.

Newcomer JW. Abnormalities of glucose metabolism associated with atypical antipsychotic drugs. *J Clin Psychiatry* 2004; **65**: 36–46.

Nicolson R, Rapoport JL. Childhood-onset schizophrenia: rare, but worth studying. *Biol Psychiatry* 1999; **46**: 1418–28.

Nicolson R, Lenane M, Singaracharlu S, et al. Premorbid speech and language impairments in childhood-onset schizophrenia: association with risk factors. *Am J Psychiatry* 2000; **157**: 794–800.

Nicolson R, Lenane M, Brookner F, et al. Children and adolescents with psychotic disorder not otherwise specified: a 2- to 8-year follow-up study. *Compr Psychiatry* 2001; **42**: 319–25.

Patel NC, Sierk P, Dorson PG, et al. Experience with ziprasidone. *J Am Acad Child Adolesc Psychiatry* 2002; **41**: 495.

Pavuluri MN, Janicak PG, Carbray J. Topiramate plus risperidone for controlling weight gain and symptoms in preschool mania. *J Child Adolesc Psychopharmacol* 2002; **12**: 271–3.

Pool D, Bloom W, Mielle DH, et al. A controlled evaluation of loxitane in seventy-five adolescent schizophrenic patients. *Curr Ther Res Clin Exp* 1976; **19**: 99–104.

Quintana H, Keshavan M. Case study: risperidone in children and adolescents with schizophrenia. *J Am Acad Child Adolesc Psychiatry* 1995; **34**: 1292–6.

Ratzoni G, Gothelf D, Brand-Gothelf A, et al. Weight gain associated with olanzapine and risperidone in adolescent patients: a comparative prospective study. *J Am Acad Child Adolesc Psychiatry* 2002; **41**: 337–43.

Realmuto GM, Erickson WD, Yellin AM, et al. Clinical comparison of thiothixene and thioridazine in schizophrenic adolescents. *Am J Psychiatry* 1984; **141**: 440–2.

Remschmidt H, Martin M, Schulz E, Gutenbrunner C, Fleischhaker C. The concept of positive and negative schizophrenia in child and adolescent psychiatry. In: Marneros A, Andreasen NC, Tsuang MT, eds. *Positive versus negative schizophrenia*. Springer-Verlag: Berlin 1991: 219–42.

Remschmidt H, Schiltz E, Martin M. An open trial of clozapine in thirty-six adolescents with schizophrenia. *J Child Adolesc Psychopharmacol* 1994; **4**: 31–41.

Ross RG, Novins D, Farley GK, et al. A 1-year open-label trial of olanzapine in school-age children with schizophrenia. *J Child Adolesc Psychopharmacol* 2003; **13**: 301–9.

Ruhe HG, Becker HE, Jessum P, et al. Agranulocytosis and granulocytopenia associated with quetiapine. *Acta Psychiatr Scand* 2001; **104**: 311–13.

Saito E, Kafantaris V. Can diabetes mellitus be induced by medication? *J Child Adolesc Psychopharmacol* 2002; **12**: 231–6.

Sanfilippo M, Wolkin A, Angrist B, et al. Amphetamine and negative symptoms of schizophrenia. *Psychopharmacology* 1996; **123**: 211–14.

Schaffer JL, Ross RG. Childhood-onset schizophrenia: premorbid and prodromal diagnostic and treatment histories. *J Am Acad Child Adolesc Psychiatry* 2002; **41**: 538–45.

Scheikh R, Ahmed K. The efficacy of olanzapine, as needed, to treat acute agitation in juveniles. *J Child Adolesc Psychopharmacol* 2002; **12**: 71–3.

Shaw JA, Lewis JE, Pascal S, et al. A study of quetiapine: efficacy and tolerability in psychotic adolescents. *J Child Adolesc Psychopharmacol* 2001; **11**: 415–24.

Sholevar EH, Baron DA, Hardie TL. Treatment of childhood-onset schizophrenia with olanzapine. *J Child Adolesc Psychopharmacol* 2000; **10**: 69–78.

Sikich L, Hamer RM, Bashford RA, et al. A pilot study of risperidone, olanzapine and haloperidol in psychotic youth: a double-blind, randomized, 8-week trial. *Neuropsychopharmacology* 2004; **29**: 13–145.

Spencer EK, Kafantaris V, Padron-Gayol MV, Rosenber CL, Campbell M. Haloperidol in schizophrenic children: early findings from a study in progress. *Psychopharmacol Bull* 1992; **28**: 183–6.

Spencer EK, Campbell M. Children with schizophrenia: diagnosis, phenomenology and pharmacotherapy. *Schizophr Bull* 1994; **20**: 713–25.

Sporn A, Gogtay N, Ortiz-Aguayo R, et al. Clozapine-induced neutropenia in children: management with lithium carbonate. *J Child Adolesc Psychopharmacol* 2003; **13**: 401–4.

Sporn AL, Addington AM, Gogtay N, et al. Pervasive developmental disorder and childhood-onset schizophrenia; comorbid disorder or a phenotypic variant of a very early onset illness? *Biol Psychiatry* 2004; **55**: 989–94.

Stahl SM. *Essential psychopharmacology*, 2nd edn. Cambridge: Cambridge University Press; 2000.

Staller JA. Intramuscular ziprasidone in youth: a retrospective chart review. *J Child Adolesc Psychopharmacol* 2004; **14**: 590–2.

Stayer C, Sporn A, Gogtay N, et al. Multidimensionally impaired: the good news. *J Child Adolesc Psychopharmacol* 2005; **15**: 510–19.

Strauss ME, Reynolds KS, Jayaram G, et al. Efects of anticholinergic medication on memory in schizophrenia. *Schizophr Res* 1990; **3**: 127–9.

Szighety E, Wiznitzer M, Branky LA, et al. Risperidone-induced hepatotoxicity in children and adolescents?: a chart review. *J Child Adolesc Psychopharmacol* 1999; **9**: 93–8.

Tandon R, Greden JF. Cholinergic hyperactivity and negative schizophrenic symptoms. A model of cholinergic/dopaminergic interactions in schizophrenia. *Arch Gen Psychiatry* 1989; **46**: 745–53.

Theisen FM, Linden A, Geller F, et al. Prevalence of obesity in adolescent and young adult patients with and without schizophrenia and in relationship to antipsychotic medication. *J Psychiatr Res* 2001; **35**: 339–45.

Toren P, Laor N, Weizman A. Use of atypical neuroleptics in child and adolescent psychiatry. *J Clin Psychiatry* 1998; **59**: 644–56.

Towbin KE, Dykens EM, Pearson GS, Cohen DJ. Conceptualizing "borderline syndrome of childhood" and "childhood schizophrenia" as a developmental disorder. *J Am Acad Child Adolesc Psychiatry* 1993; **32**: 775–82.

Tsai GE, Yang P, Chung LC, et al. D-Serine added to clozapine for the treatment of schizophrenia. *Am J Psychiatry* 1999; **156**: 1822–5.

Tsuang MT, Stone WS, Seidman LJ, et al. Treatment of non-psychotic relatives of patients with schizophrenia: four cases studies. *Biol Psychiatry* 1999; **45**: 1412–18.

Tsuang MT, Stone WS, Faraone SV. Towards the prevention of schizophrenia. *Biol Psychiatry* 2000; **48**: 349–56.

Turetz M, Mozes T, Toren P, et al. An open trial of clozapine in neuroleptic-resistant childhood-onset schizophrenia. *Br J Psychiatry* 1997; **170**: 507–10.

Ty EB, Rothner AD. Neuroleptic malignant syndrome in children and adolescents. *J Child Neurol* 2001; **16**: 157–630.

Ulloa RE, Birmaher B, Axelson D, et al. Psychosis in a pediatric mood and anxiety disorders clinic: phenomenology and clinical correlates. *J Am Acad Child Adolesc Psychiatry* 2000; **39**: 337–45.

Van der Gaag RJ, Buitelaar J, Van den Ban E, et al. A controlled multivariate chart review of multiple complex developmental disorder. *J Am Acad Child Adolesc Psychiatry* 1995; **34**: 1096–106.

Volkmar FR, Cohen DJ. Comorbid association of autism and schizophrenia. *Am J Psychiatry* 1991; **148**: 1705–7.

Werry JS, Taylor E. Schizophrenia and allied disorders. In: Rutter M, ed. *Child and adolescent psychiatry*. London: Blackwell Publishing; 1994.

Werry JS, McClellan J, Chard L. Early-onset schizophrenia, bipolar and schizoaffective disorders: a clinical follow-up study. *J Am Acad Child Adolesc Psychiatry* 1991; **30**: 457–65.

Wolff S. Schizoid personality in childhood and adult life. III. The childhood picture. *Br J Psychiatry* 1991; **159**: 629–35.

Woods SW, Martin A, Spector SG, McGlashan TH. Effects of development on olanzapine-associated adverse events. *J Am Acad Child Adolesc Psychiatry* 2002; **41**: 1409–11.

Woods SW, Breier A, Zipursky RB, et al. Randomized trial of olanzapine versus placebo in the symptomatic acute treatment of the schizophrenic prodrome. *Biol Psychiatry* 2003; **54**: 453–64.

Wudarski M, Nicolson R, Hamburger SD, et al. Elevated prolactin in pediatric patients on typical and atypical antipsychotics. *J Child Adolesc Psychopharmacol* 1999; **9**: 239–45.

Yildiz A, Sachs GS, Turgay A. Pharmacological management of agitation in emergency settings. *Emerg Med J* 2003; **20**: 339–46.

Zuddas A, Pintor M, Cianchetti C. Risperidone for negative symptoms. *J Am Acad Child Adolesc Psychiatry* 1996; **35**: 838–9.

chapter 9

Pharmacologic treatment of children and adolescents with attention deficit hyperactivity disorder

Benedetto Vitiello, Alessandro Zuddas, and Gabriele Masi

Attention deficit hyperactivity disorder (ADHD) is a syndrome characterized by levels of hyperactivity, inattention, and impulsivity that are:

1. developmentally abnormal
2. persistent in time
3. not better explained by psychosocial circumstances or other medical or mental illnesses, and
4. causing substantial functional impairment in more than one setting, most typically home and school.

This definition is based on the DSM-IV classification system (American Psychiatric Association, 1994). The hyperkinetic disorder of the ICD-10 classification is a particularly severe and pervasive form of ADHD and is thus subsumed within the broader DSM-IV definition. ADHD is further divided into an inattentive, hyperactive, or combined type.

ADHD is a condition of still unclear etiology, which tends to run in families and has been associated with specific genetic polymorphisms related to the expression of the dopamine transporter and of the D4 dopamine receptor gene. In general terms, it can be conceptualized as being the result of an interaction between a genetic predisposition and environmental factors. For a minority of subjects, ADHD can be linked to a specific brain insult such as encephalitis, pre- or perinatal trauma, or heavy metal poisoning. Dietary etiologic hypotheses have been raised at different times, but never proven.

Although ADHD subjects as a group have been found to present differences in brain volumetric measurements (smaller brain, prefrontal areas, and basal ganglia) and are more likely to have certain genetic polymorphisms than normal controls, these differences do not have adequate specificity, sensitivity, or predictive value to serve as diagnostic markers. Likewise, cognitive performance testing, such as the continuous performance tests, can help document deficits, but are not diagnostic. Thus, ADHD is currently still an entirely descriptive diagnosis based on careful history collection and comprehensive medical and psychiatric examination (American Academy of Pediatrics, 2000). It is estimated that from 3 to 8% of school-age children meet criteria of ADHD. ADHD is from 2 to 3 times more common in boys than in girls in the population, and it also tends to be more commonly diagnosed in boys than in girls.

ADHD symptoms become evident before 7 years, and often as early as 3 years of age. Most children are diagnosed in elementary school when behavioral problems and academic difficulties emerge. Once thought to subside at puberty, ADHD has been found to persist into adolescence in 60–80% of the cases, and to continue into adulthood in at least one third of the cases. ADHD increases the risk for school failure, accidents, nicotine dependence, and, when associated with conduct disorder, substance abuse. In about two thirds of cases, ADHD is accompanied by other conditions, such as oppositional and defiant disorder, conduct disorder, anxiety disorders, and learning disabilities in children. In adolescence, ADHD can be associated with delinquent behavior and use of alcohol, nicotine, marijuana, and other substances of abuse.

Approach to treatment

Any treatment plan must be based on a comprehensive diagnostic evaluation, whose importance cannot be overemphasized (American Academy of Pediatrics, 2001). In approaching treatment, the clinician must have documentation that the child meets the criteria for a diagnosis of ADHD, and must also be aware of the presence of any possible concomitant medical or psychiatric condition or learning disability. As always in medicine, who is being treated is the child as an individual in her/his particular social context, and not the disorder.

Before starting treatment, it is important to identify the target outcomes for each individual patient. For example, a possible treatment target can be a decrease in certain inappropriate behaviors, improvement in social interactions, or the degree of accuracy, completion, and/or timeliness of academic work. Specifying and quantifying the target outcomes upfront help guide the clinical management of the child with ADHD.

To this end, it is essential to document the severity of ADHD symptoms before and during treatment. ADHD severity can be measured using one of the several symptom rating scales that have been developed for children and adolescents with ADHD, such as the Conners Parent Rating Scale – Revised, the Conners Teacher Rating Scale – Revised, the IOWA Conners Teacher Rating Scale, or the Swanson, Nolan, and Pelham (SNAP-IV). Some of these scales can be found at the Internet site www.adhd.net, others are available in the scientific literature or commercially (Swanson, 1992; Conners et al, 1998).

Either behavior modification ("behavior therapy") or pharmacotherapy with stimulants can be considered as first-step treatment for children with ADHD (American Academy of Pediatrics, 2001). Treatment with stimulant medication, however, has been generally found to be more effective than psychotherapy in ADHD (Jadad et al, 1999; MTA Cooperative Group, 1999). Intensive pharmacotherapy is superior to intensive behavior therapy for decreasing ADHD symptoms in school-age children (MTA Cooperative Group, 1999). No study, however, has yet systematically examined the advantages and disadvantages of starting treatment with either modality. In usual practice, the treatment choice may be influenced by several factors, such as age of the child, severity of ADHD, comorbidity, presence of inconsistent parenting, availability of therapists in the community, cost considerations, and parents' preference (Table 9.1).

Thus, for children under age 6, it is preferable to start with behavior therapy before considering pharmacotherapy in order to minimize exposure to medication at such a young age. When parents are inconsistent in their discipline and limit settings, treatment may first aim at correcting these deficiencies with behavior therapy and parent training. For severe ADHD with high levels of hyperactivity and impulsiveness, behavior therapy alone is less likely to be sufficient, and pharmacotherapy may be preferable. When ADHD is comorbid with anxiety or conduct disorder, behavior therapy may be

Table 9.1 Pharmacotherapy or behavior therapy as the first-step treatment?

To consider	Approach
Age of the child	Under 6 years, it is preferable to start with behavior therapy
Comorbidity	If comorbid with anxiety, behavior therapy may be the first choice
	If comorbid with substance abuse, behavior therapy may be the first choice
Poor parenting	Behavior therapy with parent training
Severity of ADHD	For severe ADHD, medication, alone or in combination, may be the first choice
Cost	Pharmacotherapy is usually less expensive than intensive behavior therapy
Parental preference	Parents tend to prefer non-pharmacologic interventions before considering medication

preferable as the first step. Pharmacotherapy is usually less expensive than intensive behavior therapy, and this can be a practical consideration for families. Parents, however, tend to prefer non-pharmacologic interventions before trying medications, and parental preference is obviously an important variable in choosing treatment.

The combination of behavior therapy and pharmacologic treatment does not, in general, lead to substantially better control of ADHD symptoms than pharmacologic treatment alone, although the combined use may help with comorbidities (MTA Cooperative Group, 1999). There are also suggestions that children receiving combined treatment can be improved on lower doses of medication than similar children receiving pharmacotherapy alone (Vitiello et al, 2001). If pharmacotherapy as first step is effective, there is little advantage in adding behavior therapy, at least for children without learning disabilities or other major comorbidities (Abikoff et al, 2004).

Once the decision to use pharmacotherapy is made and a particular medication is selected, the clinician's first task it to identify the best dose for the individual patient. As in other areas of pharmacology, there is substantial intersubject variability in response treatment with respect to both therapeutic benefit and sensitivity to adverse effects. The best dose can be defined as the lowest dose that results in the desired outcome, is well tolerated, and does not increase the risk for future toxicities. During treatment, clinical monitoring focuses on the individual target outcomes and on possible adverse effects of treatment. There is evidence that closer monitoring with more frequent office visits, review of progress, and dose adjustments results in much better improvement than is achieved with less intensive management (MTA Cooperative Group, 1999).

In general, the concomitant administration of more than one medication for ADHD should always be approached with caution and, if possible, avoided. Very little research has been conducted on the efficacy and safety of combined pharmacologic treatment. If the response to a single agent at adequate doses is insufficient, it is usually preferable to discontinue that medication and try another one.

Stimulant medications

The central nervous system stimulants methylphenidate and amphetamines are the first-line medication treatments for ADHD (Table 9.2). Stimulants are agents that increase the activity of the brainstem arousal system and enhance alertness, attention, and ability to concentrate on and perform physical and mental tasks. Ability to tolerate fatigue and boredom is enhanced, while appetite and sleep are reduced in a dose-dependent manner. Their onset of action is rapid, with effects evident within an hour. From this profile, it is evident that stimulants are "action promoting" agents, which help performance while suppressing physiologic and mental stimuli that can interfere with goal-oriented activity.

Table 9.2 Pharmacotherapy for school-age children with ADHD

First-line	Methylphenidate or an amphetamine preparation
Second-line	The other stimulant (methylphenidate or amphetamine) not used as initial treatment
Third-line	Atomoxetine
Fourth-line	Clonidine or bupropion
Fifth-line	Imipramine or nortriptyline

Stimulants have been used for more than 60 years to reduce hyperactivity and improve attention in children, and currently constitute the recommended first-choice treatment for the pharmacologic management of ADHD (American Academy of Pediatrics, 2001; Greenhill et al, 2002; Kutcher et al, 2004).

Stimulants are sympathomimetic amines that act by releasing norepinephrine and dopamine from their storage sites in presynaptic terminals (in the case of amphetamines) or by increasing the availability of these neurotransmitters in the synaptic cleft through inhibition of their neuronal reuptake (in the case of methylphenidate).

Stimulants are drugs of potential abuse and, as such, are subject to the prescribing procedures and restrictions reserved for this type of drugs. Most notably, they can be dispensed only upon presentation of a written, non-refillable prescription. Both methylphenidate and cocaine block the presynaptic transporter of dopamine, but the addictive effects leading to abuse and dependence are dependent on the speed with which the blockage occurs, which is rapid in the case of cocaine and slow for oral methylphenidate (Volkow and Swanson, 2003). Thus, the therapeutic administration of oral doses of stimulants for the treatment of ADHD does not lead per se to abuse or dependence. To minimize the risk that stimulants prescribed for the treatment of ADHD may be diverted to non-therapeutic uses, it is important to ensure that a responsible adult be in charge of the prescription and the dispensed medication.

Stimulants are the most commonly prescribed psychotropic medications in the US, with an estimated 2.7 million children and adolescents receiving this treatment in 2002 (Zuvekas et al, 2006). There are suggestions that these drugs may be both over- and underutilized. Epidemiologic surveys have indicated that, while many children with ADHD are untreated, others are prescribed stimulants without meeting the diagnostic criteria for ADHD. Because stimulants are cognitive enhancers and can improve behavior and academic performance even among non-ADHD individuals, misuse is a concrete possibility. Use of these medications for purposes other than the treatment of ADHD has to be considered an inappropriate practice of unproven benefit and questionable safety.

The clinician prescribing stimulants for ADHD should be aware of the benefits, risks, and limitations of these medications, and commit to a careful diagnostic evaluation and ongoing monitoring (Tables 9.3–9.5)

Efficacy

The effects of stimulants in school-age children with ADHD have been extensively studied. Their effectiveness in decreasing hyperactivity, distractibility, impulsivity, and other manifestations of disruptive behavior, such as aggression and argumentativeness, is well documented (Table 9.3). The response rate to one stimulant trial is at least 70% and, if non-responders are treated with another stimulant, the cumulative response rate is at least 80% (Elia et al, 1991; Greenhill et al, 2001). Academic performance is also improved: children with

Table 9.3   Stimulant effects: what is known and what remains unknown

Outcome	Level of evidence for effect on the target outcome at the recommended dosage[a]
Reduction of ADHD symptoms	Strong
Reduction of oppositional behavior, aggression	Strong
Completion of school work	Strong
Improvement in social skills	Strong
Improvement in peer interactions	Strong
Improvement in family interactions	Strong
Improvement in academic achievement (better grades, higher educational level)	Insufficient data
Reduced risk of accidents	Insufficient data
Decrease in physical growth	Moderate, dose-dependent
Induction of hypertension	None
Induction of arrhythmias	None
Induction of seizures	None in children who do not have epilepsy
Decreased risk for substance abuse	Weak
Increased risk for substance abuse	Little and inconsistent
Induction of mania	Insufficient data
Induction or worsening of tics	Some, but inconsistent (improvement can also occur with stimulant treatment)

[a]Evidence refers to children aged 6 years and above

ADHD taking stimulant treatment can complete more reading and mathematics assignments, and with fewer errors (Elia et al, 1993; Swanson et al, 2004a). The therapeutic benefits also include improvement in the child's interpersonal relationship with family and peers, and decreased anxiety (MTA Cooperative Group, 1999). The long-term and distal effects of stimulants have been less well investigated, primarily because it is extremely difficult to run controlled studies for years. The benefits of optimally titrated and intensively monitored stimulant treatment have been documented for up to about 2 years of treatment (MTA Cooperative Group, 2004a), but it remains unclear whether successful control of ADHD symptoms during childhood results in better prognosis in adult years.

Safety

Granted that all medications can have unwanted effects and that "safety" is a relative concept, stimulants can claim a highly favorable balance between benefits and risks when used at the recommended doses for the treatment of ADHD. The most common side-effects of stimulants are decreased appetite, stomach ache, nausea, headache, insomnia, and nervousness (Efron et al, 1997; Greenhill et al, 2001). When the dose is too high or the child very sensitive to drug effects, the affect can become blunted and the child appears flat, without her/his normal range of emotional expressions. This listless appearance is usually noticed by both parents and peers, and the child may be described as "sad" or "too serious." Occasionally, changes in mood with tearfulness and high emotionality emerge at the end of day, when the medication wears off. In some cases, adjustments in dosage and/or redistribution of the dose during the day help, but in others the drug needs to be discontinued and replaced by an alternative treatment (Table 9.6). It is estimated that less than 5% of school-age children are unable to tolerate the side-effects of stimulants (Greenhill et al, 2001).

Long-term treatment with stimulants has a dose-related effect on growth. When methylphenidate is given at doses of about 3–40 mg/day continuously for 7 days a week, growth is delayed by an average of about 3 kg for weight and 1.5 cm for height (MTA Cooperative Group, 2004b). The effect on weight is due to the well-known stimulant-induced decrease in appetite and food intake. The effect on height is less well understood and it is unclear whether

Table 9.4 Checklist of what to know prior to prescribing a stimulant medication

Valid diagnosis of ADHD?	If no, stimulants are not indicated
Presence of comorbidities?	To be taken into account during treatment
History of simple tics or Tourette's disorder?	If so, carefully weigh possible advantages and risks of medication, and discuss with parents; plan for close monitoring of tics during treatment
History of cardiovascular symptoms (e.g. fainting) or heart abnormalities?	Obtain ECG and cardiologic consultation
Family history of malignant hypertension, stroke under age 40, or sudden unexplained death?	Obtain ECG and cardiologic consultation
Family history of mania, psychosis?	If so, carefully weigh possible advantages and risks of medication and discuss with parents; plan for close monitoring of mood during treatment
History of substance abuse at home?	Stimulant may not be appropriate; consider an alternative medication
Previous treatment with stimulants?	Inquire on dosage used and consequent benefit and adverse events
What are the specific target outcomes?	Specify which are the desirable improvement areas that treatment is expected to produce in the individual child
Quantify ADHD symptom severity	Necessary to document medication effects
Measure and record weight and height with relative normed percentiles	Necessary to document medication effects
Measure and record blood pressure and pulse	Necessary to document medication effects
Document presence or absence of tics	Necessary to infer medication effects
Document presence or absence of sleep difficulties	Necessary to infer medication effects

it is mediated by decreased caloric intake. Measurement of weight and height before starting treatment and then periodically, every 3–6 months for weight and 6–12 months for height, is recommended.

Stimulants have cardiovascular effects that are statistically, but not clinically significant. After one year of methylphenidate treatment, increases in systolic (average 3.3 mmHg) and diastolic (1.1 mmHg) blood pressure and in heart rate (3.9 beats/min) have been reported. These are minor, not clinically significant changes for children who do not have cardiovascular disease (Wilens et al, 2004). Likewise, no clinically significant cardiologic or electrocardiographic changes have been observed with amphetamine use at least at doses up to 15 mg/day (Findling et al, 2001). In any case, a physical examination, with recording of blood pressure and heart rate, is recommended before stimulant treatment is started. The presence of abnormal heart murmurs should be further investigated. Unless there is a personal history of hypertension, fainting, heart disease, structural cardiac, or arrhythmias, or a family history of congenital heart disorders or of sudden unexplained death, it is not necessary to obtain an ECG before or during treatment.

Hematologic and plasma tests are not required for stimulant use in ADHD. There is no evidence that stimulants increase the risk for hypertension, cardiovascular illness in general, cancer, or liver failure.

Stimulants decrease the seizure threshold, but only at much higher doses than used therapeutically in ADHD; this effect is clinically significant and translates into an increased risk for seizures. For children with epilepsy and ADHD, stimulants can be safely used in combination with anticonvulsant medications, but little research has been thus far conducted on this approach.

Acute intoxication by stimulants can occur after intake that is at least twice the maximum recommended dose. Symptoms of intoxication can include restlessness, tremor, confusion, hallucinations, sweating, rapid respiration, tachycardia, hypertension or hypotension, nausea, vomiting, seizures, and coma. The extent and severity of these symptoms tend to be proportional to the dose ingested.

Carcinogenesis and mutagenesis studies

Amphetamines and methylphenidate have been extensively used in clinical practice for more than 40 years, and no link has been established between their use and increased risk of cancer.

Methylphenidate was tested in a number of in vitro and animal studies. In vitro, it was not mutagenic in the Ames mutation test or in the mouse lymphoma cell forward mutation assay, while chromosome aberrations were increased in cultured hamster ovary cells (Physician's Desk Reference 2005). Other studies, also included in the FDA-approved labeling information for methylphenidate, looked at the incidence of cancer in animals treated with this drug. In a particular brand of mice (B6C3F1), methylphenidate, given at weight-corrected doses 30 times higher than the maximum recommended human dose, caused an increase in hepatocellular adenomas (a benign, non-invasive tumor of the liver) and, in male mice only, in hepatoblastoma (a malignant tumor). No increase in tumors was found in rats, and actually a decreased incidence of breast cancer was found in female rats treated with methylphenidate.

More recently, in what was apparently the first in vivo study in humans, an increase in chromosomal and other cytogenetic aberrations was reported in the blood cells of a small group of children treated with methylphenidate for 3 months (El-Zein et al, 2005). This report is to be considered preliminary and not indicative per se of carcinogenesis (Preston et al, 2005). No similar studies have been conducted on amphetamines.

Stimulants and substance abuse

Stimulants are drugs of potential abuse. In animal models, both methylphenidate and amphetamine display the typical features of substances of abuse, such as compulsive self-administration, with neglect of other activities, including food intake, in order to satisfy the addiction. There are, however, important differences between therapeutic use and non-therapeutic abuse of stimulants that involve the dose, route of administration, and social context. When abused, stimulants are typically injected or snorted at doses that are much higher than therapeutic doses, in the search for euphoria. In ADHD, stimulants are used orally, at lower doses, and in an attempt to improve deportment and academic work. Euphoria is practically unknown among medicated children.

Concern has been raised that therapeutic use of stimulants may sensitize the brain of the child and possibly increase the risk for substance abuse later in life. The issue is complicated by the fact that ADHD itself, because of the impulsivity, impaired social judgment, and conduct disturbances with which it is often accompanied, can be a risk factor for substance abuse. It is practically impossible to run randomized clinical experiments for the many years required to test the hypothesis of whether treatment of ADHD with stimulants results in any changes, either a decrease or an increase, in substance abuse in early adulthood. Thus, only naturalistic follow-up of clinical samples is available. For the most part, these studies do not support the contention that stimulant treatment increases risk for substance abuse, and actually indicate that the risk is decreased (Barkley et al, 2003; Wilens et al, 2003).

The possibility remains that stimulant medication prescribed for the treatment of ADHD may be diverted by patients or families toward abuse. The presence of current substance abuse in the family is a contraindication for stimulant prescription. A history of substance abuse, without current abuse, is a relative contraindication, but each case must be carefully considered on an individual basis. The most recent extended-release formulations of stimulants are less prone to diversion because these preparations cannot be easily crushed into powder for injection or snorting, and also because the once-a-day administration makes parental supervision easier to enforce.

Contraindications to stimulant treatment

The presence of florid psychosis or mania is a contraindication to the use of stimulants, which can worsen these conditions by stimulating the dopaminergic transmission. In cases of well-controlled psychosis or mania, use of stimulants for comorbid ADHD can be considered on an individual basis in combination with appropriate antipsychotic or antimanic treatment.

Comorbid ADHD and substance abuse can occur in adolescence and is generally a reason for avoiding stimulants and considering non-stimulant treatment. Likewise, current substance abuse in the child's household is a contraindication for the use of stimulants unless the medication can be completely handled by another responsible adult. History of past substance abuse in the family is a relative contraindication.

Tourette's disorder, which is comorbid with ADHD in about half of the cases, was once considered an absolute contraindication to stimulants for fear that tics would worsen with treatment. A number of studies have, however, shown that stimulants are quite effective in controlling ADHD in the context of Tourette's disorder and do not generally worsen motor or vocal tics (Castellanos et al, 1997;

Tourette Syndrome Study Group, 2002). Methylphenidate tends to be better tolerated than amphetamines (Castellanos et al, 1997). Thus, stimulants, and methylphenidate in particular, should be considered an appropriate treatment option for children with ADHD and tic disorders, but careful monitoring during treatment is required. If the tics worsen, the stimulant should be suspended and other treatments considered. It is critical to document the type and severity of tics before starting treatment in order to establish a baseline against which to assess treatment-associated changes.

Eating disorders, especially severe anorexia and bulimia, are reasons to avoid stimulants, which can further disrupt appetite regulation. Other contraindications are hypertension, tachycardia, or arrhythmias. Individual exceptions can be made after cardiologic tests and consultation.

Clinical monitoring during stimulant treatment

During stimulant treatment, regular clinical monitoring, with monthly visits and dose adjustments based on residual symptoms and tolerability, results in substantially greater improvement than with less intense management (MTA Collaborative Group, 1999). Even when the initial dose is carefully chosen and tailored to the needs of the individual child, there is evidence that, for most patients, the dosage needs to be adjusted, at least during the first year of treatment (Vitiello et al, 2001). Growth, vital signs, and the presence of possible adverse events need to be periodically monitored, and the severity of ADHD measured (Table 9.5).

It is matter of debate whether continuous stimulant treatment 7 days a week and throughout the year is a more effective strategy than a less intense approach, without treatment on weekends or summer vacations. There is probably a large individual variability in the need for continuous treatment. For children with more severe and pervasive hyperactivity and impulsivity, the benefit of the medication is likely to extend to non-school situations and, in these cases, continuous treatment may be more appropriate.

Because ADHD is a chronic condition, treatment is usually administered for extended periods, usually years. It is, however, good practise to verify the need of continuous treatment about once a year. This can be easily accomplished in the case of stimulants by discontinuing

Table 9.5 Monitoring during treatment with methylphenidate or amphetamines

ADHD symptom severity	After the 1st week of treatment, then at least monthly until a stable and effective dose is found; at least quarterly afterwards
Comprehensive adverse events check	After the 1st week of treatment, then at least monthly until a stable, well-tolerated dose is found; at least quarterly afterwards
Presence and severity of comorbidities	At least monthly initially, at least quarterly afterwards
Heart rate and blood pressure	At least quarterly initially, then every 6 months
Weight	At least monthly initially, then every 6 months
Height	At least yearly

the medication for a few days while monitoring the child's behavior at home and in school (ideally, without informing the teacher that the child is off treatment in order to avoid biases in the feedback).

Methylphenidate

Methylphenidate is the most commonly used and most extensively studied medication for ADHD treatment. Different formulations exist, which primarily differ as to the timing with which the medication is released in the stomach for systemic absorption (Table 9.7). Racemic methylphenidate is made of both *d*- and *l*-threo-enantiomers in a 50/50 ratio. The *d*-threo-enantiomer is more pharmacologically active than the *l*-threo-enantiomer. All the currently marketed preparations are racemic, except for the more recently introduced dexmethylphenidate, which contains only the *d*-threo-enantiomer. The *d*-threo-enantiomer is responsible for the clinical efficacy of methylphenidate (Quinn et al, 2004). The advantages of using the *d*-threo-enantiomer over the racemic are, however, unclear.

Pharmacokinetics

Methylphenidate is rapidly absorbed from the gastrointestinal tract, with a peak plasma concentration reached at about 1.5–3 hours

Table 9.6   Approach to adverse events during stimulant treatment

Adverse event	*Possible approach*
Loss of appetite (e.g. no food intake at lunch)	Decrease dose, if clinically possible
	Increase caloric intake at breakfast and dinner
	If early in treatment, look for possible tolerance to this side-effect over time
	Monitor weight
Loss of weight	Decrease dose (unless child is overweight)
	Increase caloric intake at breakfast and dinner; add caloric snacks in between
	Consider lower dose or no medication during weekend or part of it
	Keep monitoring weight. Tolerance to anorexigenic effect often develops
Early insomnia (difficulty falling asleep)	If using immediate-release preparations, allow no dosing after 3 pm
	If using extended-release preparations, reduce dosing or start treatment early in the morning and give medication before breakfast to allow more rapid absorption
	Be sure that there is an appropriate bedtime routine (e.g. reading)
	If it occurs while on amphetamine, try methylphenidate as it has a shorter duration of action
Blunted affect ("zombie"-like appearance)	Decrease dose, if possible. Otherwise, try different preparation or medication
Tics (new onset)	Discontinue treatment and see if tics go away. Restart treatment and see if tics come back. If so, use different medication
Stereotypic movements (e.g. skin picking)	Decrease dose, if clinically possible
Growth delay (e.g. from 10th to 5th percentile)	Decrease dose
	Allow "drug holidays" during weekends and school vacations, if clinically possible
	Obtain bone age reading (radiograph of left hand) to document extent of delay and potential for growth

Table 9.7 Most commonly used stimulant preparations

Medication	Marketed as	Release type	Duration of action (hours)	Usual dose mg/day	mg/kg/day	Dosing
Methylphenidate (*dl*-threo-enantiomers)	Methylphenidate HCl tablets	Immediate	3–4	10–60	0.3–1.5	bid/tid
	Ritalin tablets	Immediate	3–4	10–60	0.3–1.5	bid/tid
	Methylin tablets	Immediate	3–4	10–60	0.3–1.5	bid/tid
	Methylphenidate HCl ER tablets	Extended, sustained	8–9	10–60	0.3–1.5	Once a day
	Methylin ER tablets	Extended, sustained	8–9	10–60	0.3–1.5	Once a day
	Ritalin SR tablets	Extended, sustained	8–9	10–60	0.3–1.5	Once a day
	Metadate ER tablets	Extended, sustained	8–9	10–60	0.3–1.5	Once a day
	Ritalin LA capsules	Extended, biphasic	8–9	10–60	0.3–1.5	Once a day
	Metadate CD capsules	Extended, biphasic	8–9	10–60	0.3–1.5	Once a day
	Concerta tablets	Extended, biphasic	12	18–54	0.3–1.5	Once a day
Dexmethylphenidate (*d*-threo-enantiomer)	Focalin tablets	Immediate	3–4	5–20	0.2–0.7	bid
Amphetamine (*dl*-enantiomers)	Amphetamine racemic	Immediate	4–5	10–14	0.3–1.0	bid
Dextroamphetamine (*d*-amphetamine)	Dextroamphetamine tablets	Immediate	4–5	5–30	0.2–0.7	bid
	Dexedrine tablets	Immediate	4–5	5–30	0.2–0.7	bid
	Dextrostat tablets	Immediate	4–5	5–30	0.2–0.7	bid
	Dextroamphetamine ER capsules	Extended	8–9	5–30	0.2–0.7	Once a day
	Dexedrine spansules	Extended	8–9	5–30	0.2–0.7	Once a day
Amphetamine + *d*-amphetamine	Adderall tablets	Immediate	4–5	10–40	0.3–1.0	bid
	Adderall XR capsules	Extended	8–9	10–40	0.3–1.0	bid

after administration. Food delays the time to maximum plasma concentration by about 1 hour: mean peak concentration is 1.5 hours when fasting as compared with 2.5 hours after a heavy breakfast. For this reason, it is usually recommended to give the medication just before breakfast.

Methylphenidate is metabolized primarily through de-esterification to ritalinic acid, which has no clinically significant pharmacologic activity and is excreted in the urine. The elimination plasma half-life is about 4.5 hours, with a 95% confidence interval of 3.1–8.1 hours (Shader et al, 1999). Because of this short half-life, the steady state is never achieved during treatment and there is no carry-over of medication from one day into the next. The metabolism and pharmacokinetics of methylphenidate are similar in school-age children and in adults.

Interaction with other drugs

Methylphenidate has little interference with the metabolism and pharmacokinetics of other drugs. It can, however, inhibit the metabolism of some anticonvulsants, such as phenobarbital, phenytoin, and primidone, and some antidepressants, such as tricyclics and selective serotonin re-uptake inhibitors (SSRIs). In addition, methylphenidate can interact pharmacodynamically with other drugs that also have sympathomimetic effects. Thus, the concurrent use of methylphenidate and theophylline is more likely to cause tachycardia, tremor, and nervousness than either drug given in isolation.

Because ADHD is often accompanied by other psychiatric conditions, such as mood or anxiety disorders, the combined use of methylphenidate with another psychotropic medication, such as an SSRI, is not uncommon and is usually considered safe.

Concerns were raised in the early 1990s about the safety of the concurrent administration of methylphenidate and clonidine to children with ADHD. Four cases of sudden death were reported in children taking this combination (Cantwell et al, 1997). However, no cause–effect link between these drugs and cardiovascular adverse events has been established. Recently conducted studies have not revealed particular clinical or ECG abnormalities during treatment with these drugs (Tourette Syndrome Study Group, 2002). Caution is, however, recommended when prescribing concomitant treatment with medications that can affect the cardiovascular system through different mechanisms.

Duration of action: immediate- versus extended-release formulations

The onset of action of methylphenidate is rapid, within an hour after oral administration of the immediate-release or the more recent extended-release biphasic preparations. The duration of action of the absorbed drug is short: about 3–4 hours. For adequate control of ADHD, immediate-release methylphenidate must be administered at least twice a day, at breakfast and lunch-time (bid) and usually also in mid-afternoon at about 3.30 pm (tid). To obviate the inconvenience of repeated doses, which typically requires the involvement of school personnel for the midday dosing, formulations with different rates of absorption have been developed to ensure an extended duration of action with a once-a-day administration.

The extended-release formulations of methylphenidate can be differentiated into a first generation of sustained-release preparations and a second generation of biphasic extended-release. The former are tablets with different coatings of immediate- and slower-release medication. There is, however, substantial variability in absorption among children. The onset of action, in particular, can be delayed and may require the concomitant administration with a low dose of immediate-release preparation. In addition, the therapeutic effect may attenuate in the afternoon.

The observation that optimal clinical effect seems to be associated with increasing plasma levels of methylphenidate led to the development of a second generation of preparations with bimodal-release systems that ensure an initial sharp plasma peak occurring about 1.5 hours after dosing, followed by a second peak about 3 hours later, and a gradual decline. These biphasic extended-release preparations are usually capsules containing beads of medication with different release timing (30% of the beads are immediate-release and 70% are slower-release). One particular preparation (OROS methylphenidate) uses a capsule with an osmotic pump to produce continuously ascending plasma levels of methylphenidate, with a peak at 6–8 hours after dosing. Using these extended-release preparations, ADHD symptoms can be adequately controlled for 8 to 10 hours following a single morning dose (Stein et al, 2003; Swanson et al, 2003).

Dosage

The target dose for each individual child is the lowest possible dose that produces the desired outcome without unwanted effects. With immediate-release methylphenidate, the starting dose is usually 5 mg bid, then raised to tid, and further increased gradually by 5 mg/day as often as every 3–4 days, based on observed improvement and side-effects. The effective daily dose can be expected to be in the range between 0.3 and 1.5 mg/kg (Table 9.7). The maximum recommended dose is 60 mg/day. Individual children may require higher doses, but more intense monitoring of adverse events is needed in these cases.

For extended-release methylphenidate, the once-a-day dose is equivalent to immediate-release methylphenidate given three times a day (Wolraich et al, 2001). In the initial dose-finding phase of treatment, the clinician can either titrate an immediate-release formulation to determine the optimal daily dosage, and then administer it in the morning as an extended-release preparation, or start with the lowest possible dose of the extended-release in the morning, and gradually adjust the dose based on response.

These considerations apply to the treatment of children aged 6 years and older. For younger children, methylphenidate is not an officially approved medication, although some studies have been conducted that show its efficacy and tolerability profile, as addressed in the section on special populations.

Amphetamines

Racemic amphetamine contains equal amounts of *d*- and *l*-amphetamine. Most of the stimulant pharmacologic activity is due to *d*-amphetamine, while *l*-amphetamine is only weakly active. Racemic amphetamine is the oldest stimulant preparation used therapeutically to treat ADHD since the seminal observations of Bradley in 1937. It is, however, seldom used any more and is not commercially available in most countries. Amphetamine preparations used in ADHD are either *d*-amphetamine or a mixture of *d*-amphetamine and *dl*-amphetamine (Adderall).

Pharmacokinetics

Absorption is fast, with peak plasma levels at about 3 hours after oral administration. Food does not affect total absorption, but delays it. Metabolism is through the liver enzymes. Children eliminate amphetamine faster than adults, the elimination plasma life of *d*-amphetamine being about 7.5 hours in 7–12-year-old children as compared with about 10 hours in adults (Greenhill et al, 2003).

Acidification of the urine increases urinary excretion of amphetamines. Ingestion of acidic substances such as ascorbic acid or fruit juice lowers absorption, and gastrointestinal alkalinizing agents, such as sodium bicarbonate, increase absorption.

Interaction with other drugs

As for methylphenidate, most of the clinically significant drug–drug interactions are pharmacodynamically determined, due to the potentiation of stimulating effects of other drugs on the cardiovascular or central nervous system.

Onset and duration of action

Consistent with the pharmacokinetics profile, the onset of action of amphetamines is rapid, within 1 hour after administration. For immediate-release preparations, the duration of action is around 4–5 hours, which is longer than for methylphenidate, but still requires a bid administration to ensure adequate coverage. Extended-release formulations exist for both *d*-amphetamine and Adderall (Table 9.7). Adderall XR 20mg provides comparable plasma concentrations to Adderall immediate-release 10mg bid administered 4 hours apart. Its administration produces ascending plasma levels of amphetamine up to a peak at about 7 hours after dosing, followed by a gradual decline that leaves, however, detectable plasma levels 24 hours after dosing.

Dosage

Most considerations already made for methylphenidate apply also to amphetamine preparations, with two important differences. First, the per mg potency of *d*-amphetamine is about twice that of methylphenidate. Thus, 5 mg of *d*-amphetamine are roughly equivalent to 10 mg of methylphenidate in pharmacologic efficacy. Second, the duration of action of amphetamines is somewhat longer than that of methylphenidate so that a tid administration is usually not necessary.

For immediate-release preparations, the starting dose varies from 2.5 to 5 mg bid, and for extended-release preparations from 5 to 10 mg once a day at breakfast, with gradual increases at 4–5-day intervals based on therapeutic response and side-effects.

Methylphenidate or amphetamine?

Methylphenidate and amphetamine have comparable efficacy. Response rate of about 70% and, if non-responders to one are give a trial of the other, the cumulative response rate to the two is at least 80%. Amphetamine has a slightly longer duration of action (4–5 hours) than methylphenidate (3–4 hours) after oral administration of immediate-release preparations. However, this difference has become less clinically important after the introduction of extended-release methylphenidate preparations. The shorter duration of action of methylphenidate can actually be advantageous as it is less likely to suppress appetite at dinner or interfere with sleep.

The side-effect profiles of methylphenidate and amphetamine are also similar. Amphetamines may have more of an effect on the cardio-vascular system. Recent concerns were raised about cases of sudden unexplained death occurring during treatment with mixed salts of amphetamines (Adderall), but a causal link has not been established. Some clinicians prefer to obtain an ECG before starting treatment with amphetamine, but the actual clinical value of this practise is unproven.

The main difference of practical importance between the two medications seems to be that *d*-amphetamine is twice as potent as methylphenidate on a per mg basis. This makes methylphenidate somewhat easier to titrate at lower doses. It is important to appreciate that, although the efficacies of methylphenidate and amphetamine are basically equivalent, there is considerable individual variability. For reasons that are not clear yet, but may relate to the genetically determined expression of dopamine receptors and/or transporter, some children improve and tolerate one drug better than the other. Because no predictors of differential response are available at this time, it is recommended that non-responders to methylphenidate be tried on an amphetamine preparation, and vice versa.

Other stimulants

Pemoline is a long-acting stimulant whose range of doses is between 37.5 and 112.5 mg (1–3 mg/kg) once a day in the morning. Its efficacy in ADHD is well documented, but because of its potential for liver toxicity it is now seldom used. The degree of liver injury can be variable, ranging from a mild transient increase in serum transaminases to liver failure and consequent death. Periodic monitoring of liver enzymes can help detect some but not all cases, and may not completely avert the risk for liver failure. Hepatotoxicity can emerge at any time during treatment, at times after many months of use.

Methamphetamine is also marketed for the treatment of ADHD in the US, but it is seldom used because of its high potential for abuse and less favorable safety profile.

Non-stimulant medications

There are a number of non-stimulant compounds that have been proven to be effective in decreasing the symptoms of ADHD in school-age children (Spencer et al, 2004) (Tables 9.8 and 9.9). Currently, only atomoxetine is approved by the Food and Drug Administration for the treatment of school-age children with ADHD (Michelson et al, 2001). In general, the magnitude of the effect of non-stimulant medications in ADHD is smaller than for stimulants. In addition, the onset of the therapeutic action is less immediate than in the case of stimulants, and may require a week or two to become fully evident. None of these non-stimulant medications is a drug of potential abuse, and this is a clear advantage in treating ADHD in the context of substance abuse.

Table 9.8 Possible reasons for using a non-stimulant medication

Inadequate response to adequate doses of methylphenidate and of an amphetamine

Poor tolerability to methylphenidate and an amphetamine

Major intolerance to methylphenidate or amphetamine administration (e.g. psychotic reaction, mania, severe tic movements)

Presence of hypertension, tachycardia, or arrhythmias

Comorbid eating disorder

Comorbid substance abuse

Substance abuse in the family

Table 9.9   Non-stimulant medications in the treatment of ADHD

| Medication | Usual dose | | | Evidence for efficacy in ADHD[a] |
	mg/day	mg/kg/day	Dosing	
Atomoxetine				Good
for body weight up to 70 kg	10–80	0.5–1.2	bid or once in am	
for body weight above 70 kg	40–100		bid or once in am	
Clonidine	0.1–0.4	0.05–0.3	bid/tid	Fair in ADHD comorbid with Tourette's disorder
Guanfacine	0.5–4	0.02–0.06	bid	Tentative, less studied than clonidine
Bupropion	100–300	3–6	bid	Fair
Imipramine	20–150	0.7–3.5	bid	Good[b]
Desipramine	20–100	0.7–3.5	bid	Good[b]
Nortriptyline	10–150	0.4–2	bid	Fair[b]

[a]Level of evidence: good (A): efficacy proven by two or more randomized controlled clinical trials; fair (B): efficacy supported by only one randomized controlled clinical trial; and tentative (C): efficacy suggested by uncontrolled studies or case reports.

[b]The evidence for efficacy of the tricyclic medications imipramine, desipramine, and nortriptyline must be weighed against their side-effects and potentially lethal cardiotoxicity in overdose.

Atomoxetine

Atomoxetine is the only non-stimulant medication that is officially approved for the treatment of ADHD in patients aged 6 and older. It is a selective inhibitor of the synaptic re-uptake of norepinephrine. It enhances adrenergic transmission in a similar way to the older tricyclic antidepressants, with the advantage, however, of superior tolerability and safety. In fact, atomoxetine does not have any significant cardiotoxicity or anticholinergic effects. It is generally considered less effective than stimulant medications and, therefore, generally a drug of third choice, after trying sequentially methylphenidate and amphetamine preparations. In those countries where amphetamines are not available on the market, atomoxetine is the logical second-choice pharmacotherapy for ADHD.

Efficacy

Atomoxetine has been shown to be effective in decreasing hyperactivity, impulsivity, and inattention in school-age children with ADHD as compared with placebo (Michelson et al, 2001). The effect can be clinically evident at the end of the first week of treatment, but full therapeutic activity may not emerge until after 2–4 weeks of treatment. The therapeutic benefit persists in time and is not subject to attenuation or tolerance (Buitelaar et al, 2004). This long-term efficacy was demonstrated experimentally with a double-blind, placebo-controlled study for one year followed by a blinded discontinuation that showed symptom relapse when placebo was substituted for atomoxetine (Michelson et al, 2004).

Safety

Atomoxetine is in general a well-tolerated medication and its side-effects are usually mild and seldom lead to discontinuation of the drug (Werricke and Kratochvil, 2002). The most common side-effects are gastric upset, nausea, vomiting, dizziness, tiredness, decreased appetite, and insomnia. Because it is pharmacologically related to the antidepressants, atomoxetine was included by the European Medicines Agency among the drugs that can increase the risk for agitation and suicidal behavior, and should not therefore be prescribed to depressed children or adolescents (European Medicines Agency, 2005). A recent review of safety data from 12 controlled clinical trials of atomoxetine (11 in ADHD and 1 in enuresis), involving a total of about 2,200 patients, found an increased risk of suicidal thinking on atomoxetine (0.4%) as compared with placebo (0.0%). Consequently, a warning was issued by the U.S. FDA about this risk and the need for clinical monitoring (U.S. FDA, 2005).

Atomoxetine can increase blood pressure and heart rate. At a group level, these changes do not seem to have clinical significance, but there is individual variability and the clinician should measure vital signs before starting treatment and then periodically (at least monthly first, then at least quarterly) afterwards.

Treatment with atomoxetine can be associated with decreased appetite and weight loss. In a 9-week study, the atomoxetine-treated group lost an average of 0.4kg, while the placebo group gained on average 1.5kg. As for stimulant medications, there can be an effect on height, with slower growth on atomoxetine, but the clinical significance of these changes is unclear. Thus, after 18 months of treatment, the average height percentile moved from 54 to 50 and the weight percentile from 68 to 60.

By December 2004, after an estimated 2 million patients had been treated with atomoxetine, two cases of severe liver toxicity had been reported. Both cases fully recovered after drug discontinuation. Because of this rare, but potentially life-threatening reaction, it is recommended that parents be informed of the potential risk and requested to report the emergence of pruritus, jaundice, dark urine, upper right-sided abdominal tenderness, or unexplained flu-like symptoms to the prescribing clinician. If liver toxicity is suspected, the drug should be immediately discontinued and the liver function monitored.

Pharmacokinetics

Atomoxetine is metabolized mainly through the hepatic cytochrome P450 2D6 enzymatic system (CYP 2D6), with the production of metabolites devoid of clinically significant activity. About 8% of Caucasians and 2% of African Americans have genetically determined low CYP 2D6 activity ("poor metabolizers"). Poor metabolizers metabolize atomoxetine, like any other drugs whose metabolism is CYP 2D6-dependent, much more slowly. The consequence is that plasma levels of atomoxetine can be 10-fold higher in these subjects than in subjects with normal CYP 2D6 activity ("extensive metabolizers"). Thus, the mean elimination half-life of atomoxetine is about 5 hours in children or adults who are extensive metabolizers, but 22 hours in poor metabolizers.

Interaction with other drugs

Concomitant administration of fluoxetine, a drug that inhibits the CYP 2D6 activity, results in higher plasma levels of atomoxetine. Likewise, one should expect slower metabolism of atomoxetine and higher plasma levels during concomitant use of other drugs that inhibit the CYP 2D6 system.

No rationale or supporting data currently exist for combining atomoxetine with stimulants or any other drug for the treatment of ADHD. Possible interactions between atomoxetine and other drugs for ADHD treatment have not been systematically studied.

Dosage

The general approach to dosing is to start treatment with a low dose of medication, increase it gradually, no faster than once every 3 days, and monitor clinically for efficacy and possible adverse events. Dosing can be either bid or once-a-day in the morning. The dosage is guided by body weight.

For body weight no greater than 70 kg, the starting dose is 0.5 mg/kg per day, then it is gradually increased at intervals no shorter than 3 days up to a target dose of 1.2 mg/kg per day, with a maximum daily dose of about 80 mg.

For body weight above 70 kg, the starting dose is 40 mg/day, then gradually increased up to a target dose of 80 mg/day. In some cases, the dose can be slowly raised up to 100 mg/day. In general, there is no evidence that using doses greater than 1.2 mg/kg per day or 100 mg/day will lead to better efficacy than lower doses for ADHD. But for comorbid conduct problems, such as oppositional and defiant behaviors, doses of about 1.8 mg/kg per day have been found to be more effective (Newcorn et al, 2005).

Clonidine

Clonidine is an alpha-2 receptor agonist that downregulates adrenergic transmission, thus causing hypotension and other effects of decreased autonomic sympathetic activity. Clonidine acts on the brain with sedative and anti-anxiety effects. It is marketed for the treatment of hypertension, but also used off label for the treatment of ADHD and, in adults, for the management of symptoms of withdrawal from drugs of abuse.

Efficacy

The evidence for the efficacy of clonidine in ADHD is much weaker than for stimulants and atomoxetine. The results of the few high-quality studies that have been thus far reported do not unequivocally support its efficacy.

The better evidence for efficacy currently exists in children with ADHD and tic movement disorder, such as Tourette's disorder. A multi-site trial found that clonidine was better than placebo, especially for impulsivity and hyperactivity, and the combination of clonidine with methylphenidate was more effective than each drug in isolation (Tourette Syndrome Study Group, 2002). A previous controlled study, however, had not found it to be effective for either tics or ADHD control (Singer et al, 1995).

It can be inferred that clonidine can indeed help for the hyperactive, impulsive, and disruptive behavior components of ADHD, but this effect is not of the same magnitude and consistency of that of stimulant medication. Furthermore, while stimulants are cognitive enhancers and improve performance on academic tasks, clonidine is a sedative agent and its effect on cognition is uncertain and potentially negative.

It has become common practice for some clinicians to add clonidine to methylphenidate for children with ADHD with comorbid oppositional defiant or conduct disorder in an effort to obtain more complete control of symptoms. This practice is indeed supported by some controlled investigations (Hazell and Stuart, 2003).

The sedative effect of clonidine has been used to induce sleep in children with early insomnia, either idiopathic or consequent to use of stimulant medication. While this practice is apparently not uncommon in some communities, no adequate testing of its potential benefit and harms has been conducted.

Safety

Clonidine has prominent cardiovascular and central nervous system effects that lead to decreased blood pressure and can result in symptoms of orthostatic hypotension, such as dizziness, palpitations, and rapid heart beat, upon standing. Bradycardia is also a possible side-effect. Other common side-effects are dry mouth and sedation. Sedation can be of moderate or severe degree in more than a quarter of the subjects (Tourette Syndrome Study Group, 2002).

Blood pressure and heart rate must be measured before and during treatment. ECG monitoring is not usually required, unless there is a personal or family history of arrhythmias, cardiac malformations, or sudden unexpected death.

There is usually tolerance to the hypotensive effect of clonidine and this has important implications for drug discontinuation. If clonidine is abruptly discontinued, rebound hypertension can ensue. Gradual tapering off, by decreasing the daily dose by 0.05 mg every 3–4 days, and blood pressure monitoring are recommended.

In the 1990s, concern was raised about the safety of combining clonidine with methylphenidate, following the report of four children who suffered sudden and unexpected death while receiving this combination. While alternative explanations were advanced for some of these cases (two had underlying heart abnormalities) and no causal link between treatment and death was established, a high level of caution is recommended when using this combination. Children with known heart disturbances or family history of sudden death should not receive this treatment. For the others, in addition to checking blood pressure and pulse, an ECG is also recommended before combining clonidine with stimulant medication, and then periodically during treatment.

Use in children under 6 years is in any case not recommended.

Pharmacokinetics

From studies in adults, clonidine is known to be rapidly absorbed after oral ingestion and to have an elimination half-life of about 13 hours after multiple dosing. It is metabolized by liver enzymes. It can interact with other concomitantly administered medications through pharmacokinetic or pharmacodynamic mechanisms. Clinicians considering using clonidine in combination with other drugs are referred to the relevant prescribing label information.

Dosage

The starting dose is between 0.025 and 0.05 mg/day, gradually increased every 3–4 days to maintenance doses between 0.1 and 0.4 mg/day. To avoid sedation, the daily dose is usually divided into three doses. Transdermal delivery systems ("skin patch") exist that deliver 0.1, 0.2, or 0.3 mg/day for a week. Anecdotal reports, but no systematic investigation of the efficacy and safety of the skin patch in ADHD are available; the data are too limited to support skin delivery systems in children at this time.

Guanfacine

Guanfacine is pharmacologically similar to clonidine. It is a more recently introduced alpha-2 adrenergic receptor agonist, with longer duration of action and less sedating activity than clonidine. Its elimination plasma half-life is 10–30 hours (mean 17 hours) in adults. A double-blind, placebo-controlled trial supports the efficacy of guanfacine for children with ADHD and tics (Scahill et al, 2001). The starting dose is 0.5 mg at bedtime, gradually increased every 4–5 days by adding 0.5 mg in the morning up to 1.5 mg/day. In the absence of more informative experimental data in ADHD, the same considerations about cardiovascular effects that were made for clonidine apply also to guanfacine.

Bupropion

Bupropion is an antidepressant that was shown to be better than placebo in decreasing ADHD symptoms in children (Conners et al, 1996). Its efficacy is, however, lower than that of stimulants. Preliminary studies suggest that it may be an appropriate treatment for adolescents with comorbid ADHD and depression (Daviss et al, 2001).

The mechanism of action of bupropion remains unclear. It is a weak inhibitor of the presynaptic re-uptake of norepinephrine, dopamine, and serotonin. It is rapidly absorbed after oral administration and has mean elimination half-life at steady state of about 12 hours in youths, which is shorter than in adults (21 hours) (Davis et al. 2005). It is metabolized primarily though the CYP2B6 system into hydroxy-bupropion, which is active but less potent.

The starting dose is 100 mg/day and maintenance doses range from 100 to 300 mg/day. Given the shorter half-life, a bid administration is recommended in children and adolescents. Clinical benefit may start becoming evident after about 3 days of treatment, but it can take longer for the full effects to emerge.

Bupropion can cause nausea, insomnia, and palpitations, but these side-effects are not frequent and seldom intolerable. Bupropion can also trigger tics and cause dermatologic reactions, such as rash and urticaria, at times severe enough to lead to discontinuing the drug. Bupropion increases the overall risk for seizures, but this effect is minimal if the dose is maintained within 300 mg/day. However, the possible effect of age on the risk for seizures has not been investigated.

Tricyclics

Tricyclics constitute the first generation of antidepressants, which were introduced in the 1960s and remained the usual treatment of mood and anxiety disorders in adults until the introduction of the SSRIs in the late 1980s. Some of them have also been tested in the treatment of ADHD in both children and adults. Imipramine, desipramine, nortriptyline, amitriptyline, and clomipramine have been found to be more effective than placebo for the control of ADHD symptoms, but in general less effective than stimulants (Biederman et al, 1989). None of them has been approved by the Food and Drug Administration for the treatment of ADHD. Not uncommonly prescribed off label for children with ADHD, tricyclics have become, however, less used because of concerns about their unwanted cardiovascular effects and potential toxicity.

Tricyclics enhance adrenergic activity by inhibiting the re-uptake of norepinephrine into presynpatic neurons. They also have anticholinergic activity, which is responsible for some of their side-effects such as dry mouth, constipation, tachycardia, and sedation, and quinidine-like effects, which are responsible for delayed electrical conduction in the heart and related potential cardiotoxicity. Blood pressure is sometimes increased due to adrenergic stimulation.

Pharmacokinetics

Tricyclics are metabolized by hepatic microsomal enzymes, primarily the CYP 2D6. Between 5 and 10% of Caucasians and about 2% of African Americans have a genetic polymorphism that causes slow metabolization through the CYP 2D6 system and consequently plasma levels of tricyclic medication that are up to 10-fold higher than in normal metabolizers. The half-life of tricyclics is therefore subject to extremely large intersubject variability. On average, metabolism tends to be faster in children than in adults because of their greater hepatic parenchyma relative to body mass during development. The elimination plasma half-life of imipramine can range from 6 to 24 hours and that of desipramine from 12 to 76 hours in adults. Nortriptyline pharmacokinetics was studied in children and its elimination plasma half-life was found to range from 11 to 42 hours in 5–12-year-olds and from 14 to 89 hours in 13–16-year-olds (Geller et al, 1987).

The concomitant administration of other drugs that are metabolized by the CYP 2D6 system prolongs the metabolism of tricyclics and increases plasma levels.

Risk/benefit analysis

Safety considerations are prominent when considering a tricyclic medication as a treatment for children with ADHD. The evidence for efficacy is generally good, although tricyclics are less effective than stimulants. However, the concerns about possible cardiotoxicity, especially in accidental or intentional overdose, detract from their use. In fact, the possibility that the child, siblings, or other family members overdose on a prescribed medication must always be taken into account by the treating clinician. Tricyclics delay electrical conduction in the heart in a dose-related way and doses 5–10 times higher than those used therapeutically can lead to complete heart block and death.

Also worrisome is the fact that instances of sudden and unexplained deaths have been reported in children receiving therapeutic doses of tricyclics, most often desipramine. Some of these events occurred during, or soon after strenuous physical exercise. While a cause–effect relationship between therapeutic doses of tricyclics and sudden unexplained death has not been proven, the use of tricyclics has much declined after these reports.

Tricyclics may be a treatment to consider for children with ADHD and tic disorders after both stimulant and atomoxetine have proven either poorly tolerated or ineffective. A placebo-controlled trial in these patients found desipramine to be quite effective and, overall, well tolerated (Spencer et al, 2002).

If treatment with a tricyclic is undertaken, careful pretreatment assessment and monitoring during treatment are necessary. In addition, parents should be informed of the potential risks and advised to keep the prescribed medication in a safe place away from the child's reach.

Approach to treatment with tricyclics

Before starting treatment, the child should receive a complete physical examination, with an ECG recording. Treatment should be considered only if the following limits are not exceeded on the ECG: 200 ms for the PR, 120 ms for the QRS, and 450 ms for the QTc, and the heart rate should be regular and not higher than 100 bpm. If there is a personal history of arrhythmias, dizziness, fainting, palpitations, or heart abnormalities, a more thorough evaluation by a cardiologist is a appropriate. A family history of sudden unexpected death or life-threatening arrhythmias should be a reason for avoiding the use of tricyclic medication.

The tricyclic whose efficacy in ADHD has been best documented is desipramine. It is, however, unfortunate that most of the sudden deaths were associated with therapeutic doses of desipramine (in spite of the wider use of imipramine). It should be noted that desipramine is an active metabolite of imipramine, and that administration of imipramine results in plasma levels of desipramine. Despite the numerous unknowns about tricyclics and cardiotoxicity, it may be prudent, if a tricyclic is to be used at all, to consider imipramine or nortriptyline ahead of desipramine.

The starting dose is usually about 10–25 mg once a day, then gradually raised in a few days to bid and further adjusted on the basis of clinical effects and side-effects. Clinical effects can become evident in a few days, but the full response may take weeks and the dose usually needs multiple adjustments. The usual therapeutic dose is between 0.7 and 3.5 mg/kg per day. In some cases, especially when the patient is a fast metabolizer, the dose can be gradually increased above 3 mg/kg per day, without exceeding in any case 5 mg/kg per day. It is recommended to check the plasma levels at the steady state to make sure that the subject is not a slow metabolizer. Plasma levels of imipramine and desipramine combined are usually around 80–225 ng/ml, and should not exceed 300 ng/ml.

An ECG should be obtained before starting treatment and then after reaching the steady state (usually after 4 days on a stable dose), and then repeated if the dose is increased above 3 mg/kg per day. During long-term maintenance treatment on a stable dose, the ECG should be repeated at least annually. If the PR exceeds 200 ms, QRS 120 ms, or QTc 450 ms, the medication should not be started. If these limits are exceeded during treatment, the dose should be reduced and cardiologic consultation sought about the wisdom of continuing treatment.

Abrupt discontinuation of tricyclic treatment can trigger withdrawal symptoms, such as nausea, vomiting, headache, lethargy, and flu-like symptoms. To prevent withdrawal symptoms, the medication must be tapered off gradually, decreasing the dose by 10–25 mg every 2–3 days until complete discontinuation.

Other drugs

Modafinil is a "wakefulness-promoting agent," of unknown mechanism and unrelated to the sympathomimetic stimulants. It is marketed for the treatment of narcolepsy and has been occasionally used for the management of inattention in adults. Clinical trials in children with ADHD are in progress. There are currently not enough data to consider modafinil an effective and safe medication for ADHD.

Special populations

Preschoolers

Most treatment research in ADHD has been conducted in children of 6–10 years of age. The official label of methylphenidate warns that this drug is not approved for use under age 6. Amphetamine is approved for use down to age 3 years, but not because it has been better investigated, rather because it is an older drug and the label information simply reflects the lower regulatory standards of 50 years ago.

A few controlled studies have actually been reported on the use of methylphenidate in children aged 3–5 years of age. They are all rather small, except for the recently completed Preschoolers with ADHD Treatment Study (PATS), a publicly funded, multi-site trial that randomized about 160 children to placebo or methylphenidate 1.25, 2.5, 5, or 7.5 mg tid (Greenhill et al, 2005).

In PATS, while 1.25 mg was not significantly different from placebo, there was a proportional improvement in ADHD symptoms across the 2.5–7.5 mg dose range. The magnitude of the effect compared with placebo was somewhat lower than typically observed in school-age children. Methylphenidate presented the typical profile of side-effects of stimulant medication in older children, but the frequency and severity of adverse events were greater and led to treatment discontinuation in about 9% of cases. In particular, mood lability seems to be more common among children below 6 years of age. Continuous treatment for about 9–10 months was associated with a slight but detectable decrease in height and weight (Swanson et al, 2004b). PATS utilized immediate-release methylphenidate. No studies of extended-release formulations have been reported in preschoolers.

Based on current data, it seems reasonable to treat children aged 3–5 years with behavior therapy first and, in case of inadequate response, to use methylphenidate starting with 5 mg/day and increasing up to 15–20 mg/day. Growth needs to be closely monitored.

Children with Tourette's disorder

About half of the children with Tourette's disorder also have ADHD. For many of these children, the ADHD symptoms are a major source of impairment, often greater than the tics themselves. Contrary to what was held until the late 1990s, there is now evidence from controlled studies that stimulants usually do not worsen tics, even though this may in fact occur in a minority of Tourette's patients.

In children with both ADHD and Tourette's disorder, the combination of methylphenidate and clonidine is the most effective treatment (Tourette Syndrome Study Group, 2002). Combined pharmacologic treatment, however, should be in general considered only if monotherapy has proven insufficient. It seems therefore reasonable to use clonidine first if the tics are prominent and severe, and to consider adding methylphenidate for residual ADHD symptoms. If, on the other hand, it is ADHD that causes more impairment to the child than the tics, it may be appropriate to start with methylphenidate first, and consider adding clonidine in the case of incomplete response.

As already addressed among the safety considerations for stimulants, the combined use of methylphenidate and clonidine requires attention to potential cardiovascular adverse effects, which include pretreatment screening and then monitoring during treatment.

Children with autism or other pervasive developmental disorders (PDDs)

According to the current nosologic system, a formal diagnosis of ADHD is not possible in the context of autism or other PDDs (American Psychiatric Association, 1994). However, children with these severe developmental disorders do often suffer from hyperactivity, inattention, and impulsiveness that cause substantial impairment in their ability to learn and interact with others.

A multi-site trial of methylphenidate immediate-release, 7.5–25 mg/day, given with tid dosing to children with autism or other PDDs, and significant ADHD symptoms was recently completed (RUPP Autism Network, 2005). The data indicate that this medication is effective in reducing ADHD symptom severity, but only in about 50% of the cases, a rate that is substantially lower than that observed in non-PDD children with ADHD. The rate of children unable to tolerate the side-effects of methylphenidate was higher (18%) compared with normal children (less than 5%).

Thus, methylphenidate can be considered for children with prominent ADHD symptoms in the context of autism or other PDDs, but its relatively low efficacy and tolerability must be taken into account.

Patients with bipolar disorder

Bipolar disorder has recently been found to be more common among children than once thought. Although bipolar disorder and ADHD share some common symptoms, such as increased motor activity and distractibility, the two disorders can be distinguished based on other more specific manic symptoms such as elation, grandiosity, flight of ideas/racing thoughts, decreased need for sleep, and hypersexuality (Geller et al, 2002). ADHD can be comorbid with bipolar disorder, and children successfully treated with mood stabilizers can still suffer from ADHD symptoms. The use of stimulants in bipolar disorder untreated with mood stabilizer is to be avoided because of potential worsening of mania. However, stimulant medication can be successfully added after the bipolar disorder has been treated with a mood stabilizer, as recently shown by a randomized, placebo-controlled trial of amphetamine added to divalproex in 6–17-year-old patients (Scheffer et al, 2005).

Adolescents with substance abuse

As already addressed in the stimulant section of this chapter, presence of concomitant substance abuse is generally a cause for avoiding stimulants in the treatment of ADHD. Behavior therapy and/or a non-stimulant medication, such as atomoxetine, are reasonable alternatives in these cases.

Alternatives to medication treatment

Behavioral therapy is an effective, though less potent, treatment for children with ADHD. As previously discussed, it can be an obvious alternative to medication (Table 9.1). No other intervention has been proven to be effective in ADHD. In spite of the considerable interest in non-pharmacologic treatment of ADHD among the public, there is currently no evidence that dietary manipulation, including also micronutrient and vitamin supplementation, is generally useful in ADHD. Likewise, there is no convincing evidence that relaxation techniques, meditation, biofeedback, or sports involvement have specific efficacy for clinically significant hyperactivity.

Tutoring, organizational skill remediation, and computerized training of working memory to correct executive functioning can certainly add to the benefit of pharmacotherapy or behavioral therapy, but are seldom sufficient for clinical ADHD.

Frequently asked questions

1. Q: For treating a child who has never been medicated, should methylphenidate or an amphetamine be the first choice?

    A: Either methylphenidate or amphetamine can be considered as first-step treatment. The response rate to each medication is comparable. If the child does not improve on one stimulant, the other one should be tried because there is at least a 50% chance that he/she will respond to the second.

2. Q: What to do for a child who has received adequate doses of methylphenidate, but, even though improved, still has clinically significant symptoms?

    A: If the residual symptoms are limited to a particular part of the day (e.g. early morning, afternoon, evening), it may be possible to redistribute the daily dose in a way to cover better the entire day. If the need for improvement is pervasive and the dose cannot be further increased, an amphetamine preparation should be substituted for methylphenidate.

3. Q: A child is much improved on a stimulant medication but has been making repeated throat-clearing noises. What could be the best approach to treatment?

    A: Check if the throat-clearing noise is explained by sinusitis, allergies, or other upper respiratory conditions. If a vocal tic is suspected, it may be appropriate to discontinue the stimulant; verify whether the noise subsides, and, if it does, re-introduce the stimulant to see if the noise re-appears. If it does, an alternative non-stimulant treatment is usually preferable. Individual exceptions apply.

4. Q: What would be a reasonable treatment plan for a 4-year-old child with high levels of impulsivity and hyperactivity that make it difficult for him to attend preschool?

A: An intensive course of behavior therapy for 2–3 months should be tried. If it is not sufficient in controling ADHD, methylphenidate 5 mg/day can be started and adjusted up to about 20 mg/day.

5. Q: A 10-year-old has been on stimulant medication since age 6. He is functioning well in school when on medication, but, upon discontinuation, ADHD symptoms come back. At a recent visit, it was noted that his growth has been delayed. Compared with age 6, he has moved from the 50th to 25th percentile for weight and from the 25th to the 10th percentile for height. What to do?

   A: Consider reducing the dose, if clinically possible, and interrupting treatment on weekends and summer vacations. Also, check bone age with a radiograph of the left hand to document the degree of delay and potential for future growth.

6. Q: A 6-year-old girl cannot swallow the stimulant medication capsule.

   A: Unless this is an osmotic capsule, it can be opened and the content poured on apple sauce and immediately ingested.

7. Q: A 15-year-old boy is falling behind in school as academic tasks become more complex and challenging. Since early elementary, he had been noted to have a short attention span and some hyperactivity, but he had been able to do his work and get As and Bs. However, now his grades are failing, despite intensive tutoring. A diagnostic evaluation shows that he meets criteria for ADHD inattentive type. What to do?

   A: Stimulant treatment is an effective treatment of ADHD inattentive type and could be tried in this case.

8. Q: Should the dosage of stimulant medication be different for treating ADHD inattentive type from that used for the hyperactive or combined?

   A: Based on current, limited evidence, the dosage is similar for all the three types of ADHD.

9. Q: Does treatment with stimulant medication predispose to substance abuse later in life?

A: The current evidence does not support this concern and actually suggests that therapeutic use of stimulants to control ADHD may decrease the risk for substance abuse.

10. Q: A 7-year-old boy treated with stimulant medication is much improved as to ADHD symptoms, but looks blunted in his affect, does not smile, or show his emotions as before. He looks sad and unable to enjoy play as usual.

A: It is certainly possible that the stimulant is causing the restricted range of emotional expression. The dose should be lowered, if clinically possible. If not, an alternative stimulant should be tried. If the affect is still blunted, a non-stimulant should be instituted.

References

Abikoff H, Hechtman L, Klein RG, et al. Symptomatic improvement in children with ADHD treated with long-term methylphenidate and multimodal psychosocial treatment. *J Am Acad Child Adolesc Psychiatry* 2004; **43**: 802–11.

Agency of Health Care Policy and Research. *Treatment of attention deficit/hyperactivity disorder.* AHCPR Publication No 99-E017, December 1999. Rockville, MD. http://www.ahrq.gov/clinic/adhdsum.htm.

American Academy of Pediatrics. Diagnosis and evaluation of the child with attention-deficit/hyperactivity disorder. *Pediatrics* 2000; **105**: 1158–70.

American Academy of Pediatrics. Clinical practice guideline: treatment of the school-aged child with attention-deficit/hyperactivity disorder. *Pediatrics* 2001; **108**: 1033–44.

American Psychiatric Association. *Diagnostic and statistical manual of mental disorders,* 4th edn. Washington, DC: American Psychiatric Association, 1994.

Barkley RA, Fischer M, Smallish L, Fletcher K. Does the treatment of attention-deficit/hyperactivity disorder with stimulants contribute to drug use/abuse? A 13-year prospective study. *Pediatrics* 2003; **111**: 97–109.

Biederman J, Baldessarini RJ, Wright V, Knee D, Harmatz JS. A double-blind placebo controlled study of desipramine in the treatment of ADD: I. Efficacy. *J Am Acad Child Adolesc Psychiatry* 1989; **28**: 777–84.

Bradley C. The behavior of children receiving Benzedrine. *Am J Psychiatry* 1937; **94**: 577–85.

Buitelaar JK, Danckaerts M, Gillberg C, et al. Atomoxetine International Study Group. A prospective, multicenter, open-label assessment of atomoxetine in non-North American children and adolescents with ADHD. *Eur Child Adolesc Psychiatry* 2004; **13**: 249–57.

Cantwell DP, Swanson J, Connor DF. Case study: adverse response to clonidine. *J Am Acad Child Adolesc Psychiatry* 1997; **36**: 539–44.

Castellanos FX, Giedd JN, Elia J, et al. Controlled stimulant treatment of ADHD and comorbid Tourette's syndrome: effects of stimulant and dose. *J Am Acad Child Adolesc Psychiatry* 1997; **36**: 589–96.

Conners CK, Casat CD, Gualtieri CT, et al. Bupropion hydrochloride in attention deficit disorder with hyperactivity. *J Am Acad Child Adolesc Psychiatry* 1996; **35**: 1314–21.

Conners CK, Sitarenios G, Parker JD, Epstein JN. The revised Conners' Parent Rating Scale (CPRS-R): factor structure, reliability, and criterion validity. *J Abnorm Child Psychol* 1998; **26**: 257–68.

Daviss WB, Bentivoglio P, Racusin R, et al. Bupropion sustained release in adolescents with comorbid attention-deficit/hyperactivity disorder and depression. *J Am Acad Child Adolesc Psychiatry* 2001; **40**: 307–14.

Daviss WB, Perel JM, Rudolph GR, et al. Steady-state pharmokinetics of bupropion SR in juvenile patients. *J Am Acad Child Adolesc Psychiatry* 2005; **44**: 349–57.

Efron D, Jarman F, Barker M. Side-effects of methylphenidate and dexamphetamine in children with attention deficit hyperactivity disorder: a double-blind, crossover trial. *Pediatrics* 1997; **100**: 662–6.

Elia J, Borcherding BG, Rapoport JL, Keysor CS. Methylphenidate and dextroamphetamine treatments of hyperactivity: are there true nonresponders? *Psychiatry Res* 1991; **36**: 141–55.

Elia J, Welsh PA, Gullotta CS, Rapoport JL. Classroom academic performance: improvement with both methylphenidate and dextroamphetamine in ADHD boys. *J Child Psychol Psychiatry* 1993; **34**: 785–804.

El-Zein RA, Abdel-Rahman SZ, Hay MJ, et al. Cytogenetic effects in children treated with methylphenidate. *Cancer Lett* 2005; **230**: 284–91.

European Medicines Agency. *European Medicines Agency finalises review of antidepressants in children and adolescents.* Doc. Ref. EMEA/CHMP/128918. London; 25 April 2005 (http://www.emea.eu.int).

Findling RL, Short EJ, Manos MJ. Short-term cardiovascular effects of methylphenidate and Adderall. *J Am Acad Child Adolesc Psychiatry* 2001; **40**: 525–9.

Geller B, Cooper TB, Schluchter MD, Warham JE, Carr LG. Child and adolescent nortriptyline single dose pharmacokinetic parameters: final report. *J Clin Psychopharmacol* 1987; **7**: 321–3.

Geller B, Zimerman B, Williams M, et al. DSM-IV mania symptoms in a prepubertal and early adolescent bipolar disorder phenotype compared to attention-deficit hyperactive and normal controls. *J Child Adolesc Psychopharmacol* 2002; **12**: 11–25.

Greenhill LL, Swanson JM, Vitiello B, et al. Impairment and deportment responses to different methylphenidate doses in children with ADHD: the MTA titration trial. *J Am Acad Child Adolesc Psychiatry* 2001; **40**: 180–7.

Greenhill LL, Pliszka S, Dulcan MK, and the Workgroup on Quality Issues. American Academy of Child and Adolescent Psychiatry – practice parameter for the use of stimulant medications in the treatment of children, adolescents, and adults. *J Am Acad Child Adolesc Psychiatry* 2002; **41**: 26S–49S.

Greenhill LL, Swanson JM, Steinhoff K, et al. A pharmacokinetic/pharmacodynamic study comparing a single morning dose of Adderall to twice-daily dosing in children with ADHD. *J Am Acad Child Adolesc Psychiatry* 2003; **42**: 1234–41.

Greenhill LL, Abikoff H, Chuangs S, et al. Efficacy and safety of Immediate-release methylphenidate treatment for preschoolers with ADHD. *J Am Acad Child Adolesc Psychiatry* 2006 (in press).

Hazell PL, Stuart JE. A randomized controlled trial of clonidine added to psychostimulant medication for hyperactive and aggressive children. *J Am Acad Child Adolesc Psychiatry* 2003; **42**: 886–94.

Jadad AR, Boyle M, Cunningham C, et al. *Treatment of attention-deficit/hyperactivity disorder.* Evidence Report/Technology Assessment No. 11. (Prepared by McMaster University under Contract No 290-97-0017.) AHRQ Publication No 00-E005. Rockville, MD:

Agency for Healthcare Research and Quality; November 1999. (Available at website: http://www.ncbi.nlm.nih.gov/books/bv.fcgi?rid=hstat1.section.14979.)

Kutcher S, Aman M, Brooks SJ, et al. International consensus statement on attention-deficit/hyperactivity disorder (ADHD) and disruptive behaviour disorders (DBDs): clinical implications and treatment practice suggestions. *Eur Neuropsychopharmacol* 2004; **14**: 11–28.

Mannuzza S, Klein RG, Moulton JL 3rd. Does stimulant treatment place children at risk for adult substance abuse? A controlled, prospective follow-up study. *J Child Adolesc Psychopharmacol* 2003; **13**: 273–82.

Michelson D, Faries D, Wernicke J, et al. Atomoxetine ADHD Study Group. Atomoxetine in the treatment of children and adolescents with attention-deficit/hyperactivity disorder: a randomized, placebo-controlled, dose-response study. *Pediatrics* 2001; **108**: E83.

Michelson D, Buitelaar JK, Danckaerts M, et al. Relapse prevention in pediatric patients with ADHD treated with atomoxetine: a randomized, double-blind, placebo-controlled study. *J Am Acad Child Adolesc Psychiatry* 2004; **43**: 896–904.

MTA Cooperative Group. A 14-month randomized clinical trial of treatment strategies for attention-deficit/hyperactivity disorder (ADHD). *Arch Gen Psychiatry* 1999; **56**: 1073–86.

MTA Cooperative Group. National Institute of Mental Health Multimodal Treatment Study of ADHD follow-up: 24-month outcomes of treatment strategies for attention-deficit/hyperactivity disorder. *Pediatrics* 2004a; **113**: 754–61.

MTA Cooperative Group. National Institute of Mental Health Multimodal Treatment Study of ADHD follow-up: changes in effectiveness and growth after the end of treatment. *Pediatrics* 2004b; **113**: 762–9.

Newcorn JH, Spencer TJ, Biederman J, Milton DR, Michelson D. Atomoxetine treatment in children and adolescents with attention-deficit/hyperactivity disorder and comorbid oppositional defiant disorder. *J Am Acad Child Adolesc Psychiatry* 2005; **44**: 240–8.

Physician's Desk Reference. 58th edn. Montvale, NJ: Thomson PDR; 2005.

Preston RJ, Kollins SH, Swanson JM, Greenhill LL, Vitiello B. Comments on Cytogenetics effects in children treated with methylphenidate by EL-Zein et al. *Cancer Lett* 2005; **230**: 292–4.

Quinn D, Wigal S, Swanson J, et al. Comparative pharmacodynamics and plasma concentrations of *d*-threo-methylphenidate hydrochloride after single doses of *d*-threo-methylphenidate hydrochloride and *d,l*-threo-methylphenidate hydrochloride in a double-blind, placebo-controlled, crossover laboratory school study in children with attention-deficit/hyperactivity disorder. *J Am Acad Child Adolesc Psychiatry* 2004; **43**: 1422–9.

Research Units on Pediatric Psychopharmacology (RUPP) Autism Network. A randomized controlled crossover trial of methylphendiate in pervasive developmental disorders and hyperactivity. *Arch Gen Psychiatry* 2005; **62**: 1266–74.

Scahill L, Chappell PB, Kim YS, et al. A placebo-controlled study of guanfacine in the treatment of children with tic disorders and attention deficit hyperactivity disorder. *Am J Psychiatry* 2001; **158**: 1067–74.

Scheffer RE, Kowatch RA, Carmody T, Rush AJ. Randomized, placebo-controlled trial of mixed amphetamine salts for symptoms of comorbid ADHD in pediatric bipolar disorder after mood stabilization with divalproex sodium. *Am J Psychiatry* 2005; **162**: 58–64.

Shader RI, Harmatz JS, Oesterheld JR, et al. Population pharmacokinetics of methylphenidate in children with attention-deficit hyperactivity disorder. *J Clin Pharmacol* 1999; **39**: 775–85.

Singer HS, Brown J, Quaskey S, et al. The treatment of attention-deficit hyperactivity disorder in Tourette's syndrome: a double-blind placebo-controlled study with clonidine and desipramine. *Pediatrics* 1995; **95**: 74–81.

Spencer T, Biederman J, Coffey B, et al. A double-blind comparison of desipramine and placebo in children and adolescents with chronic tic disorder and comorbid attention-deficit/hyperactivity disorder. *Arch Gen Psychiatry* 2002; **59**: 649–56.

Spencer T, Biederman J, Wilens T. Nonstimulant treatment of adult attention-deficit/hyperactivity disorder. *Psychiatr Clin North Am* 2004; **27**: 373–83.

Stein MA, Sarampote CS, Waldman ID, et al. A dose-response study of OROS methylphenidate in children with attention-deficit/hyperactivity disorder. *Pediatrics* 2003; **112**: e404.

Swanson JM. *School-based assessments and interventions for ADD students.* Irvine, CA: KC Publishing; 1992.

Swanson JM, Gupta S, Lam A, et al. Development of a new once-a-day formulation of methylphenidate for the treatment of attention-deficit/hyperactivity disorder: proof-of-concept and proof-of-product studies. *Arch Gen Psychiatry* 2003; **60**: 204–11.

Swanson JM, Wigal SB, Wigal T, et al. COMACS Study Group. A comparison of once-daily extended-release methylphenidate formulations in children with attention-deficit/hyperactivity disorder in the laboratory school (the COMACS Study). *Pediatrics* 2004a; **113**(3 Pt 1): e206–16.

Swanson JM and the PATS Cooperative Study Group: Adverse events and growth rates in PATS. Presentation at the 51st Anual Meeting of the American Academy of Child and Adolescent Psychiatry, Washington, DC, October 19–24, 2004b.

Tourette's Syndrome Study Group. Treatment of ADHD in children with tics: a randomized controlled trial. *Neurology* 2002; **58**: 527–36.

U.S. Food and Drug Administration. FDA Issues Public Health Advisory on Strattera (atomoxetine) for Attention Deficit Disorder. FDA News, September 29 2005, 5–65 (Available at Website: http://www.fda.gov/bbs/topics/NEWS/2005/NEW01237.html; access verified in October 31, 2005).

Vitiello B, Severe JB, Greenhill LL, et al. Methylphenidate dosage for children with ADHD over time under controlled conditions: lessons from the MTA. *J Am Acad Child Adolesc Psychiatry* 2001; **40**: 188–96.

Volkow ND, Swanson JM. Variables that affect the clinical use and abuse of methylphenidate in the treatment of ADHD. *Am J Psychiatry* 2003; **160**: 1909–18.

Wernicke JF, Kratochvil CJ. Safety profile of atomoxetine in the treatment of children and adolescents with ADHD. *J Clin Psychiatry* 2002; **63**: 50–5.

Wilens TE, Faraone SV, Biederman J, Gunawardene S. Does stimulant therapy of attention-deficit/hyperactivity disorder beget later substance abuse? A meta-analytic review of the literature. *Pediatrics* 2003; **111**: 179–85.

Wilens TE, Biederman J, Lerner M; Concerta Study Group. Effects of once-daily osmotic-release methylphenidate on blood pressure and heart rate in children with attention-deficit/hyperactivity disorder: results from a one-year follow-up study. *J Clin Psychopharmacol* 2004; **24**: 36–41.

Wolraich ML, Greenhill LL, Pelham W, et al. Randomized, controlled trial of OROS methylphenidate once a day in children with attention-deficit/hyperactivity disorder. *Pediatrics* 2001; **108**: 883–92.

Zuvekas S, Vitiello B, Norquist G. Recent national trends in the utilization of stimulant medications in the U.S. *Am J Psychiatry* (in press).

chapter 10

Pharmacologic treatment of children and adolescents with impulsive aggression and related behaviors

Benedetto Vitiello and Dario Calderoni

Aggressive behavior is one of the most common reasons for clinical referral in child psychiatry. Aggression does not constitute, however, a specific diagnostic category, and different types of aggression exist. Most notably, a distinction is made between a proactive, goal-oriented, planned, covert, predatory type characterized by low activation of the autonomic nervous system, and a reactive, impulsive, uncontrolled, overt, affective type characterized by high autonomic activation (Vitiello and Stoff, 1997). It is generally agreed that it is only the latter, "impulsive aggression," that constitutes a potential target for pharmacologic treatment (Jensen et al, 2005).

Impulsive aggression is characterized by recurrent outbursts of inappropriate, maladaptive behavior aimed at inflicting harm on others, self, or inanimate objects. The episodes occur suddenly, with little provocation, and are characterized by high affective activation, over which the subject has little control. Delinquency, which encompasses behaviors such as school truancy, vandalism, theft, and other violations of societal norms often committed by adolescents as a group ("gang activities"), is not per se an appropriate target for medication treatment. It is not uncommon, however, for a youth to have both types of aggression, with recurrent, uncontrolled episodes of impulsive aggression in addition to delinquency. In such cases, pharmacologic intervention can be beneficial for controlling impulsive aggression, but psychosocial interventions should be instituted to address the delinquent behavior.

Impulsive aggression is not a discrete psychiatric disorder, but rather a symptom that can appear in the context of a number of conditions, such as attention deficit/hyperactivity disorder (ADHD), conduct disorder, bipolar disorder, psychosis, depression, pervasive developmental disorders, mental retardation, post-traumatic stress disorder, Tourette's disorder, seizure disorder, or alcohol or substance abuse. Notably, even though aggression can be found in all these conditions, it is not a diagnostically defining symptom for any of them. Recurrent explosive disorder is the only diagnostic entity for which an aggressive episode is central, but this diagnosis is not commonly used in child psychiatry.

Approach to treatment

It is critical to conduct a comprehensive neuropsychiatric evaluation, including also an assessment of the social and environmental context in which aggression occurs (Figure 10.1). Pharmacologic treatment specifically targeted on aggression can be considered if the behavior is consistent with impulsive aggression, recurrent, pervasive, unresponsive to psychosocial intervention, and still present even after adequate treatment of the underlying psychiatric or medical condition (Table 10.1).

The decision to prescribe pharmacotherapy rather than attempt to control aggression exclusively with psychosocial intervention must be carefully made at the individual patient's level. Patients whose aggression is unpredictable and not likely to respond to behavioral interventions are candidates for pharmacotherapy (Schur et al, 2003). For children whose aggression occurs in the context of objectively stressful circumstances, addressing the environmental stressors is usually paramount and an extended period of observation of the child in a less stressful environment is recommended before initiating pharmacologic intervention. In fact, in a placebo-controlled study of children hospitalized for severe aggressive behavior, about half of the subjects showed substantial improvement, even without active medication (Malone et al, 1997). Behavioral therapy has been shown to be effective in reducing a number of disruptive behaviors, including

Comprehensive neuropsychiatric and psychosocial evaluation

Is aggression impulsive, uncontrolled, pervasive and recurrent?

Yes

No → Institute psychosocial interventions

Treat underlying disorder
(e.g. ADHD with stimulant,
bipolar with mood stabilizer,
psychosis with antipsychotic,
substance abuse with detoxification and
rehabilitation services)

Is aggression still present?

Yes

No → Continue treatment of underlying
condition

Try psychosocial treatment
targeted on aggression

Is aggression still present?

Yes

No → Continue psychosocial treatment

Start antiaggressive pharmacotherapy:[a]
antipsychotic
mood stabilizer
methylphenidate
alpha-2 adrenergic

Figure 10.1 *General approach to managing aggressive behavior*

[a]The choice of which medication to try first depends on the characteristics of the
individual patient and on current evidence for efficacy and adverse effects (see Table 10.2).

Table 10.1 Aggressive behavior for which pharmacotherapy may be appropriate

- Impulsive
- Uncontrolled
- Recurrent
- Pervasive and not limited to a particular setting or social context
- Causing substantial functional impairment
- Unresponsive to psychosocial interventions
- Still present after treatment of the underlying medical/psychiatric condition

aggressive behavior (Pelham et al, 2000). In any case, if pharmacologic treatment is prescribed, it should be part of a comprehensive and individualized clinical management plan including the appropriate psychosocial and educational interventions as needed by the child (Pappadopulos et al, 2003).

There are currently no specific laboratory markers or tests that can assist in ascertaining impulsive aggression. The assessment relies on clinical evaluation and interpretation. It is critically important to quantify the frequency and severity of aggression before and during treatment as a way of documenting possible treatment effects (Table 10.2). While no single instrument can be considered the standard tool, several rating scales have been used to measure aggression, such as the Overt Aggression Scale (Silver and Yudofsky, 1991; Kafantaris et al, 1996), the aggression subscale of the Child Behavior Checklist (Achenbach, 1991), the Children's Aggression Scale – Parent Version (Halperin et al, 2002), and individualized target symptom scoring (Arnold et al, 2003).

The primary aim of treatment is to reduce both the frequency and the severity of the aggressive episodes. At this time, no specific "antiaggressive" medication has been introduced into the pharmacopeia, but a variety of psychotropic agents that are marketed for other conditions are used also to treat aggression. Although aggression is a symptom that can be found in different conditions, there are suggestions that it may be equally responsive to treatment across conditions (Jensen et al, 2005). An antiaggressive effect, regardless

Table 10.2   Principles of medication management of impulsive aggression

1. Complete a complete diagnostic and psychosocial assessment

2. Attempt to treat first the underlying psychiatric syndrome

3. Use the most benign appropriate medication first (fewer side-effects and fewer potential adverse effects)

4. Use medication within a coordinated multimodal treatment plan (i.e. psychoeducational intervention)

5. Obtain exhaustive off-drug baseline data before drug treatment, using a validated, treatment-sensitive rating scale

6. Obtain data at regular intervals during drug treatment

7. Whenever possible avoid polypharmacy treatment

8. Explore the full range of a single medicine for an adequate length of time before augmentation or switching to another medication

9. Follow drug serum levels where appropriate (e.g. lithium)

10. Monitor for adverse effects with periodic clinical assessments and drug-specific laboratory tests (e.g. liver function tests during treatment with valproate)

of the underlying disorder, however, has been proven only for a few medications, such as the antipsychotics, and remains still hypothetical for other drugs used to control aggression.

Medications for the treatment of impulsive aggression

No medication currently carries a specific indication for impulsive aggression. Various and generally limited evidence supports the use of a few medications, which are reviewed here. These drugs have disparate pharmacologic activity, encompassing antidopaminergic, anticonvulsant, mood-stabilizing, alpha-2 adrenergic, and stimulant effects. A unified theory of how antiaggressive medication may operate is therefore lacking. The role of serotonin in aggressive behavior has been particularly investigated, but an attempt to design specific serotonergic agents that could function as "serenics" in the management of aggression has not been fruitful (Stoff and Cairns, 1997).

The decision of which drug to use for a particular child is based on the individual needs of the patient and a careful consideration of the benefit/risk profile of each medication. Almost no systematic research has been conducted in children under 5 years of age, so that the following considerations on the use of medications in aggression are relevant to children aged 5 and older. For younger children, the main approach includes treatment of the underlying condition and psychosocial interventions to control aggressive behavior.

Antipsychotics

Antipsychotics are the class of drugs for which there is currently the best evidence for antiaggressive properties across different conditions such as conduct disorder, autism, mental retardation, and psychotic disorders. Antipsychotics, however, are also associated with a number of adverse events and risk for toxicities. Typical antipsychotics commonly cause dystonias, tremor, muscle rigidity, sedation, hyperprolactinemia, and withdrawal dyskinesia. Chronic treatment can lead to tardive dyskinesia, which is related to the cumulative dose received. Less frequent, but potentially life-threatening, is the neuroleptic malignant syndrome, which is characterized by hyperpyrexia, muscle rigidity, and confusion, and can lead to coma and death.

Because of this problematic safety profile, typical antipsychotics have been practically replaced by atypical antipsychotics, whose use is associated with a much lower, although not absent, rate of the described adverse events. Atypical antipsychotics, however, can cause other types of adverse events, such as weight gain, obesity, impaired glucose tolerance, hyperlipidemia, and type II diabetes.

An issue that has not been fully investigated is the possible effect of antipsychotic treatment on cognition in children without psychosis. At this time, there is no evidence of a negative impact on the development of cognitive skills, and some data actually suggest that cognitive functioning can be improved (Campbell et al, 1982), but more data are clearly needed.

When considering antipsychotic treatment for patients with non-psychotic conditions, the potential for both benefit and harm must be carefully weighed for each patient in light of the severity of the aggression and the dysfunction that the condition causes. Placebo-controlled clinical trials support the efficacy of both typical (haloperidol) and atypical (risperidone) antipsychotics in decreasing aggression.

Atypical antipychotics

Risperidone   Risperidone is an atypical antipsychotic whose main pharmacologic activity occurs through the blockage of the dopamine-2 receptor and of the serotonin-2 receptor. It acts as an atypical antipsychotic, with few extrapyramidal adverse effects at low doses (up to about 4 mg/day in children), but it displays features of a typical antipsychotic, with common adverse effects, at higher doses. Risperidone is marketed for the treatment of schizophrenia and bipolar disorder in adults, and is also used in children and adolescents for the treatment of aggressive behavior.

Its efficacy has been shown in four separate placebo-controlled studies ranging from 4 to 12 weeks in 5–17-year-old subjects with aggression in the context of conduct disorder, mental retardation, and autism (Findling et al, 2000; Buitelaar et al, 2001; Van Bellinghen and De Troch, 2001; Aman et al, 2002; RUPP Autism Network, 2002). About two thirds of the children randomized to risperidone showed clinically significant improvement as compared with only about 12% on placebo (RUPP Autism Network, 2002). These data indicate that the effect size of risperidone (i.e. the standardized difference versus placebo, used as a measure of efficacy) in decreasing aggression is large.

The usual starting dose is 0.5 mg/day given with a bid dosing (Table 10.3). A lower starting dose of 0.25 mg/day can be used in young children of 5–6 years of age. The effective dose can range from 0.5 to 3.5 mg/day, with an average around 2 mg/day, given in two separate doses. The therapeutic benefit tends to emerge early, usually within the first week of treatment, and persists in time. Upon discontinuation, however, about 75% of patients relapse (RUPP Autism Network, 2005).

Administration of risperidone can cause sedation, orthostatic hypotension, dizziness, appetite increase, and weight gain. It can also cause extrapyramidal effects (EPS), such as dystonia, muscle rigidity, and tremor, but these are not common if the dose is maintained low, below about 4 mg/day. As with all the antidopaminergic agents, the use of risperidone entails a risk for tardive dyskinesia and for the rare but potentially life-threatening neuroleptic malignant syndrome. Weight gain tends to occur in the first few months of treatment, with an average increase of about 3 kg over 2 months, as compared to about 1 kg on placebo. In an open-label, 12-month study during which risperidone was administered to children aged 5–12 years at a mean dose of 1.5 mg/day, the mean weight gain was 5.5 kg, of which half was attributable to normal development (Findling et al, 2004). Weight gain can be massive and problematic in some patients, as it has been associated with fatty liver, hyperlipidemia, impaired glucose tolerance, and type II diabetes.

No negative effects of risperidone on cognitive performance have emerged, but the impact of early or chronic treatment on cognitive development of children has not been systematically evaluated. Through dopamine-2 receptor inhibition, risperidone increases prolactin. The implications of hyperprolactinemia for children and adolescents are still not fully understood. Probably due to its alpha-adrenolytic effects, risperidone can cause priapism, an infrequent but potentially serious toxicity.

From the adverse effects profile, it follows that careful assessment and recording of weight, fasting glycemia, lipid profile, blood pressure, and pulse should occur before treatment is started, and periodically during treatment with risperidone. Monthly recording of weight, blood pressure, and pulse, and quarterly first, then semi-annual, assessment of glycemia, and plasma lipids allow the clinician to monitor effectively for possible adverse effects. In the presence of obesity or type II diabetes, alternative treatments should be considered. Drug discontinuation is often accompanied by the loss of at least part of the excessive weight gained during treatment.

Risperidone is rapidly absorbed after oral administration, with a plasma peak at about 1 hour after dosing. Food does not interfere with absorption. Risperidone is primarily oxidized by the hepatic CYP 2D6 isoenzyme into 9-hydroxyrisperidone, which is also pharmacologically active. CYP 2D6 is subject to genetic polymorphism that affects the rate and extent of risperidone metabolism. About 8% of the Caucasian population are "poor metabolizers," that is they metabolize the drug much more slowly than the rest of the population ("extensive metabolizers"). The elimination plasma half-life of risperidone is about 3 hours in adults who are extensive metabolizers, but 20 hours in poor metabolizers. Because, however, the main metabolite has pharmacologic activity, it has been found that the half-life of the active moiety is overall comparable in the two groups of metabolizers. Thus, the clinical relevance of the genetic polymorphism is unclear.

The plasma level of risperidone and its metabolite can also be altered during the concomitant use of other medications. For instance, certain drugs, such as fluoxetine, compete with risperidone for the CYP 2D6 isoenzyme, thus causing increased plasma levels of risperidone. Other drugs, such as phenytoin or carbamazepine, can induce the CYP 2D6 isoenzyme and cause a more rapid metabolism and decreased plasma levels.

In summary, risperidone is an effective agent in the treatment of children and adolescents with impulsive aggression. Its tolerability and safety profile includes a number of adverse effects and potential toxicities that require careful monitoring of the patient, especially during long-term treatment. If the dosage is titrated slowly and maintained below 4 mg/day, risperidone is well tolerated, at least for up to 6 months of treatment, and side-effects, although present, are seldom reason for discontinuation (RUPP Autism Network, 2002, 2005).

Other atypical antipsychotics   At this time, there are no controlled studies supporting the efficacy of other atypical antipsychotics in children with impulsive aggression. The following compounds, all marketed for the treatment of schizophrenia, are also used in children with aggression on the basis of uncontrolled studies and clinical anecdotal experience.

Olanzapine has the advantage of having few EPS, but the drug-induced weight gain can be problematic. During a 2-month treatment of 7–13-year-old children at an average dose of about 15 mg/day, a 6 kg mean weight gain was reported (Stephens et al, 2004). Olanzapine has been associated with decreased glucose tolerance and onset of type II diabetes. Its plasma elimination half-life ranges from 21 to 54 hours in adults.

Quetiapine and ziprasidone have been anecdotally used in adults and children with impulsive aggression, but very little is known about their potential efficacy and safety in pediatric patients. Ziprasidone can cause prolongation of the QTc interval of the ECG, thus theoretically increasing the risk for arrhythmias and requiring careful ECG monitoring during treatment.

Aripiprazole (5–15 mg/day) is a recently introduced atypical antipsychotic that has the advantage of not increasing the body weight or inducing ECG changes. Aripiprazole has a unique pharmacologic profile, as it functions as a partial agonist at the dopamine D2 and serotonin 5-HT$_{1A}$ receptors, in addition to being an antagonist to the serotonin 5-HT$_{2A}$ receptor. The daily dose ranges from 5 to 15 mg, given once a day (plasma half-life is about 2–3 days). This drug is metabolized in the liver primarily by CYP 2D6 and CYP 3A4. This drug

Table 10.3 Selected medications used in the treatment of impulsive aggression in children and adolescents

Medication	Starting dose mg/day	Usual therapeutic dose mg/day	Dosing	Evidence for efficacy[a]	Main safety concerns
Antipsychotics					
risperidone	0.25–0.5	0.5–3.5	bid	A	Weight gain, obesity, diabetes
haloperidol	0.25–0.5	0.5–6.0	Once a day	A	Dystonias, tardive dyskinesia
olanzapine	1.25–2.5	2.5–20	Once a day	C	Weight gain, obesity, diabetes
aripiprazole	5	5–15	Once a day	C	Nausea, sedation
Mood stabilizers					
lithium	300	900–2100	bid[b]	A (inpatients) C (outpatients)	Nausea, vomiting, cognitive impairment, hypothyroidism
valproate	125–250	500–1500	bid	B	Risk for liver toxicity
carbamazepine	200–400	400–1200	bid	C	Aplastic anemia, agranulocytosis
Stimulants					
methylphenidate	10	10–60	bid/tid Once a day	B	It can worsen psychosis and mania; It can be abused
Alpha-adrenergics					
clonidine	0.1–0.4	0.05–0.3	bid/tid	C	Sedation, hypotension
guanfacine	0.5–4	0.02–0.06	bid	C	Hypotension

[a]Level of evidence for efficacy as antiaggressive treatment; A: two or more controlled clinical trials; B: only one controlled clinical trial; C: only uncontrolled studies and/or anecdotal case reports.

[b]Gastrointestinal adverse events are less common with bid dosing as they are associated with the rate of rise in serum medication levels.

has an attractive pharmacologic profile and appears a good candidate for controlled studies of its potential antiaggressive activity.

Clozapine, the first introduced atypical antipsychotic, has antiaggressive properties, at least in adults, but also a problematic tolerability and safety profile that makes its use unwieldy in children. It can cause agranulocytosis, seizures, myocarditis, and syncope due to orthostatic hypotension. Its use requires periodic monitoring of white blood cells, on a weekly basis initially, then biweekly. Clozapine can also induce major weight gain and type II diabetes. The use of this drug is restricted to treatment-resistant psychosis.

Typical antipsychotics

Haloperidol   Haloperidol is a typical antipsychotic that is primarily marketed for the treatment of schizophrenia. It has also been found to be effective in placebo-controlled investigations at doses ranging from 1 to 6 mg/day (average 3 mg/day) given orally to children for aggressive conduct disorder (Campbell et al, 1984). Lower doses, between 0.5 and 4 mg/day, can be effective in children with aggression in the context of pervasive developmental disorders (Perry et al, 1989).

Administration of haloperidol is commonly associated with the emergence of dose-related adverse events, including acute dystonias, tremor, muscle rigidity, sedation, hyperprolactinemia, and withdrawal dyskinesia (Campbell et al, 1997). Less commonly, it can cause tardive dyskinesia, which is related to the cumulative dose received and can emerge after treatment for several months. Infrequently, it can cause neuroleptic malignant syndrome, which is characterized by hyperpyrexia, muscle rigidity, and confusion, and can lead to coma and death. The high incidence of acute EPS and withdrawal dyskinesia, and the risk for tardive dyskinesia and neuroleptic malignant syndrome that the use of haloperidol entails limit the usefulness of this medication, which is now seldom used as first-step treatment.

Other typical antipsychotics   Other typical antipsychotics, such as pimozide, have been used in the management of children with disruptive behavior. The scanty evidence for their efficacy, tolerability problems, and the presence of alternative treatments all contribute to limit the therapeutic value of these drugs in the management of children with impulsive aggression.

Stimulants

Methylphenidate

Methylphenidate is an effective antiaggressive agent in children with ADHD who also have symptoms of impulsive aggression. The dosage is the same as used in the treatment of ADHD (see Chapter 9). One controlled investigation also supports the efficacy of this drug in aggressive children who meet criteria for conduct disorder without ADHD (Klein et al, 1997).

The relative safety of methylphenidate makes this medication the first choice in the pharmacologic treatment of impulsive aggression occurring as part of disruptive behavior disorders, such as ADHD and conduct disorder. Methylphenidate is not, however, a suitable treatment for children with impulsive aggression in the context of psychosis or mania, because it can worsen the underlying condition. When given to children with autism or other pervasive developmental disorders, methylphenidate is less effective and less well tolerated than among typical children with ADHD (see Chapter 9). Finally, methylphenidate can be abused, and this consideration limits its use in adolescents with substance abuse.

Mood stabilizers

Mood stabilizers, including lithium, valproate, and carbamazepine, are used in the management of impulsive aggression in children. The evidence of their efficacy is, however, rather limited. The best evidence is for lithium in severe aggression among hospitalized children. Case reports, uncontrolled studies, and a small controlled study suggest that valproate may be effective. Only uncontrolled observations are available at this time for carbamazepine.

Lithium

Lithium, a basic metallic element that is marketed as a salt for the treatment of bipolar disorder, is also efficacious in decreasing aggressive behavior in hospitalized children with severe conduct disorder. Its efficacy has been demonstrated in two placebo-controlled trials, one in 5–12-year-old children (Campbell et al, 1984) and the other in 10–17-year-old children and adolescents (Malone et al, 2000). The dose ranged from 900 to 2100 mg/day and the serum lithium levels from 0.5 to 1.8 mEq/l in the first study, and 0.8–1.5 mEq/l in the second one. In general, there was little clinical advantage in exceeding the plasma level of 1.1 mEq/l. Lithium, however, has not been found better than placebo for the treatment of outpatients who suffer from less severe forms of aggression than inpatients.

Most common adverse events are nausea, vomiting, and frequent urination. Lithium can also induce a fine intentional tremor, motor incoordination, and dysarthria. These effects are dose related. Studies in adult subjects suggest that lithium may impair some components of learning (Stip et al, 2000). Chronic treatment can cause hypothyroidism and, rarely, impairment in renal function and kidney failure.

Lithium is not metabolized and is excreted unchanged by the kidney. Its elimination depends on renal clearance. Since children have a greater clearance than adults, they eliminate lithium faster, with a mean half-life of 18 hours as compared to 24 in adults (Vitiello et al, 1988).

Before lithium treatment is started, a series of laboratory tests and exams need to be completed. These include renal function tests (plasma creatinine, blood urea nitrogen, and urinalysis), serum electrolytes, plasma thyroid stimulating hormone (TSH), and ECG. Lithium can cause T-wave flattening or inversion, which is usually not indicative of toxicity, and, at toxic levels, S–T segment depression and QTc prolongation. Renal function tests, TSH, and ECG should be repeated after 6 months of treatment and then semiannually or annually.

For lithium titration, the conventional approach is:

1. start a low dose (150 mg in young children under 7 years of age, and 300 mg in older subjects) the first day;
2. increase it by 150 mg or 300 mg daily increments to 600 mg/day;
3. obtain a serum level after about 4 days of continuous treatment; and
4. adjust the dose, aiming to reach a serum level of around 0.8–1.2 mEq/l.

An alternative approach is to dose according to body weight (Weller et al, 1986), as follows:

- under 25 kg: 600 mg/day
- between 25 and 40 kg: 900 mg/day
- 40–50 kg: 1200 mg/day
- 50–60 kg: 1500 mg/day

The dose for individual subjects required to reach a lithium serum concentration in the therapeutic range can also be predicted using the single-point method (Cooper et al, 1973), which has also been applied to children (Malone et al, 2000). This method, which is particularly suitable for hospitalized patients consists of using a serum lithium measurement obtained 24 hours after a single oral administration of lithium carbonate 600 mg in order to predict, through a nomogram, the dose required for achieving therapeutic serum levels in individual patients.

Valproate

Valproate, usually formulated as divalproex, is marketed as an anticonvulsant and for the treatment of mania and migraine. There is limited support from uncontrolled studies and one small placebo-controlled study for the efficacy of divalproex (750–1500 mg/day) in decreasing the frequency and severity of recurrent impulsive aggression in youths age 10 to18 years (Donovan et al, 2000). Because of the risk of liver toxicity and thrombocytopenia, testing of blood cells and liver function before and during treatment is needed. Therapeutic plasma levels are estimated to be around 50–100 mg/l.

Valproate is metabolized by the liver and has an elimination plasma half-life of about 9–16 hours in subjects above 10 years of age, while younger children have a 50% faster clearance. Consequently, twice-a-day (bid) dosing is needed. An extended-release formulation has also been introduced that can be administered with once-a-day dosing, at least in children older than 7 years of age (Dutta et al, 2004). Treatment is started at a dose of 125–250 mg/day and increased by 125–250 mg daily increments to a dose of 500–750 mg, which is in the lower range of the possible effective dose. Further increases are implemented on the basis of clinical response, adverse events, and plasma levels.

Carbamazepine and oxcarbazepine

Carbamazepine is marketed as an anticonvulsant and is also prescribed for the treatment of impulsive aggression in children, despite the fact that there are no controlled studies that support this practice. Small clinical trials have been conducted, but no difference from placebo has emerged (Cueva et al, 1996).

The starting dose is 200 mg/day in children under 12 years and 400 mg/day in older subjects, given with bid dosing. The therapeutic dose ranges from 400 to 1200 mg/day (10–20 mg/kg per day), to reach serum levels between 4 and 12 µg/ml. Carbamazepine has a plasma elimination half-life of 12–60 hours. It is metabolized in the liver by CYP 3A4. The drug induces its own metabolism, so that plasma levels tend to decrease with chronic treatment and the dosage needs to be adjusted to maintain therapeutic levels.

Carbamazepine often causes leukopenia (white blood cell count below 4000 cells/mm³) and rarely aplastic anemia, agranulocytotosis, and thrombocytopenia, which are life-threatening conditions. Careful monitoring of blood cells is required weekly during dose titration and every 3–6 months afterwards.

Oxcarbazepine, a related compound which is also marketed for seizure control, is also used for management of impulsive aggression, although this use is not supported by any controlled studies. Based on data from epilepsy studies, the starting dose is 8–10 mg/kg per day (maximum daily dose 600 mg) given bid. The drug is then slowly titrated over 2 weeks up to 900–1800 mg/day, based on body weight, clinical response, and adverse effects. Sedation, nausea, vomiting, and abdominal pain are the most common side-effects that can occur in up to 20–30% of patients, but they are usually mild and transient.

Unlike carbamazepine, oxcarbazepine has not been linked with hematopoietic adverse effects, but can cause hyponatremia, and it is recommended that serum electrolytes be checked periodically during chronic treatment. More problematic are serious, potentially life-threatening dermatologic reactions, including Stevens–Johnson syndrome and toxic epidermal necrolysis, which have been reported in both children and adults treated with this drug. Oxcarbazepine undergoes extensive hepatic metabolism, yielding an active metabolite that is primarily responsible for the pharmacologic activity. The elimination plasma half-life is about 2 hours for oxcarbazepine and 9 hours for the active metabolite in children 8 years and older, and 30–40% shorter in younger children, who clear the drug faster.

Other medications

Clonidine and guanfacine are alpha-2 adrenergic medications used in the treatment of ADHD, especially when associated with Tourette's disorder (see Chapter 9). These medications are also used for the management of children with impulsive aggression (Table 10.2). This use is supported only by uncontrolled investigations.

The involvement of serotonin in the neurobiology of aggressive behavior (Stoff and Cairns, 1997) has spurred interest in the possible therapeutic benefit of serotonergic drugs, such as buspirone and selective serotonin re-uptake inhibitors (SSRIs), for patients with impulsive aggression. Fluoxetine was found to be effective in adults with impulsive aggression and personality disorder (Coccaro et al, 1997). Only open-label pilot data with citalopram 10–40 mg/day are available in children with impulsive aggression (Armenteros and Lewis, 2002). Caution and careful clinical monitoring are required if SSRI medications are used in children and adolescents, because some patients can become negatively activated by these drugs, with the possible emergence of irritability, anxiety, and suicidal or aggressive behavior (see Chapter 4 on the treatment of depression).

Beta-blockers have been proposed as possible antiaggressive agents based on uncontrolled studies in subjects with mental retardation, but controlled studies have either failed to support the efficacy or found a high rate of intolerable adverse events.

Sedative-hypnotics, such as benzodiazepines, are sometimes used in the management of acute episodes of aggression (e.g. lorazepam 0.5–1.0 mg intramuscularly), but do not have a demonstrated therapeutic benefit in the prevention of recurrent impulsive aggression. Acute outbursts of aggression are best managed with non-pharmacologic interventions and strategies.

References

Achenbach TM. *Manual for the Child Behavior Checklist/4-18 and 1991 Profile*. Department of Psychiatry, University of Vermont; Burlington, VT; 1991.

Aman MG, De Smedt G, Derivan A, Lyons B, Findling RL. Risperidone Disruptive Behavior Study Group: double-blind, placebo-controlled study of risperidone for the treatment of disruptive behaviors in children with subaverage intelligence. *Am J Psychiatry* 2002; **159**: 1337–46.

Armenteros JL, Lewis JE. Citalopram treatment for impulsive aggression in children and adolescents: an open pilot study. *J Am Acad Child Adolesc Psychiatry* 2002; **41**: 522–9.

Arnold LE, Vitiello B, McDougle C, et al. Parent-defined target symptoms respond to risperidone in RUPP autism study: customer approach to clinical trials. *J Am Acad Child Adolesc Psychiatry* 2003; **42**: 12443–50.

Buitelaar JK, van der Gaag RJ, Cohen-Kettenis P, Melman CTM. A randomized controlled trial of risperidone in the treatment of aggression in hospitalized adolescents with subaverage cognitive abilities. *J Clin Psychiatry* 2001; **62**: 239–48.

Campbell M, Anderson LT, Small AM, et al. The effects of haloperidol on learning and behavior in autistic children. *J Autism Dev Disord* 1982; **12**: 167–75.

Campbell M, Small AM, Green WH, et al. Behavioral efficacy of haloperidol and lithium carbonate. A comparison in hospitalized aggressive children with conduct disorder. *Arch Gen Psychiatry* 1984; **41**: 650–6.

Campbell M, Armenteros JL, Malone RP, et al. Neuroleptic-related dyskinesias in autistic children: a prospective, longitudinal study. *J Am Acad Child Adolesc Psychiatry* 1997; **36**: 835–43.

Coccaro EF, Kavoussi RJ. Fluoxetine and impulsive aggressive behavior in personality-disordered subjects. *Arch Gen Psychiatry* 1997; **54**: 1081–8.

Cooper TB, Bergner PE, Simpson GM. The 24-hour serum lithium level as a prognosticator of dosage requirements. *Am J Psychiatry* 1973; **130**: 601–3.

Cueva JE, Overall JE, Small AM, et al. Carbamazepine in aggressive children with conduct disorder: a double-blind and placebo-controlled study. *J Am Acad Child Psychiatry* 1996; **35**: 480–90.

Donovan SJ, Stewart JW, Nunes EV, et al. Divalproex treatment for youth with explosive temper and mood lability: a double-blind, placebo-controlled crossover design. *Am J Psychiatry* 2000; **157**: 818–20.

Dutta S, Zhang Y, Conway JM, et al. Divalproex-ER pharmacokinetics in older children and adolescents. *Pediatr Neurol* 2004; **30**: 330–7.

Findling RL, McNamara NK, Branicky LA, et al. A double-blind pilot study of risperidone in the treatment of conduct disorder. *J Am Acad Child Adolesc Psychiatry* 2000; **39**: 509–16.

Findling RL, Aman MG, Eerdekens M, Derivan A, Lyons B. Risperidone Disruptive Behavior Study Group: long-term, open-label study of risperidone in children with severe disruptive behaviors and below-average IQ. *Am J Psychiatry* 2004; **161**: 677–84.

Halperin JM, McKay KE, Newcorn JH. Development, reliability, and validity of the Children's Aggression Scale – Parent Version. *J Am Acad Child Adolesc Psychiatry* 2002; **41**: 245–52.

Jensen PS, Youngstrom E, Steiner H, et al. Consensus report: impulsive aggression as a symptom across diagnostic categories in child psychiatry – implications for medication development (under review).

Kafantaris V, Lee DO, Magee H, et al. Assessment of children with the overt aggression scale. *J Neuropsychiatry Clin Neurosci* 1996; **8**: 186–93.

Klein RG, Abikoff H, Klass E, et al. Clinical efficacy of methylphenidate in conduct disorder with and without attention deficit hyperactivity disorder. *Arch Gen Psychiatry* 1997; **54**: 1073–80.

Malone RP, Luebbert JF, Delaney MA, et al. Nonpharmacological response in hospitalized children with conduct disorder. *J Am Acad Child Adolesc Psychiatry* 1997; **36**: 242–7.

Malone RP, Delaney MA, Luebbert JF, Cater J, Campbell MA. A double-blind placebo-controlled study of lithium in hospitalized aggressive children and adolescents with conduct disorder. *Arch Gen Psychiatry* 2000; **57**: 649–54.

Pappadopulos E, MacIntyre JC, Crimson ML, et al. Treatment recommendations for the use of antipsychotics for aggressive youth (TRAAY). Part II. *J Am Acad Child Adolesc Psychiatry* 2003; **42**: 145–61.

Pelham WE, Gangy EM, Greiner AR. Behavioral versus behavioral and pharmacological treatment in ADHD children attending a summer treatment program. *J Abnorm Child Psychology* 2000; **28**: 507–25.

Perry R, Campbell M, Adams P, et al. Long-term efficacy of haloperidol in autistic children: continuous versus discontinuous drug administration. *J Am Acad Child Adolesc Psychiatry* 1989; **28**: 87–92.

Research Units on Pediatric Psychopharmacology (RUPP) Autism Network. Risperidone in children with autism and serious behavioral problems. *N Engl J Med* 2002; **347**: 314–21.

RUPP Autism Network. Risperidone treatment of autistic disorder: longer term benefits and blinded discontinuation after six months. *Am J Psychiatry* 2005; **163**: 1361–9.

Schur SB, Sikich L, Findling RL, et al. Treatment recommendations for the use of antipsychotics for aggressive youth (TRAAY). Part I: A review. *J Am Acad Child Adolesc Psychiatry* 2003; **42**: 132–44.

Silver JM, Yudofsky SC. The Overt Aggression Scale: overview and guiding principles. *J Neuropsychiatry Clin Neurosci* 1991; **3**: S22–S29.

Stephens RJ, Bassel C, Sandor P. Olanzapine in the treatment of aggression and tics in children with Tourette's syndrome – a pilot study. *J Child Adolesc Psychopharmacol* 2004; **14**: 255–66.

Stip E, Dufresne J, Lussier I, Yatham L. A double-blind, placebo-controlled study of the effects of lithium on cognition in healthy subjects: mild and selective effects on learning. *J Affect Disord* 2000; **60**: 147–57.

Stoff DM, Cairns RB, eds. *Aggression and violence: genetic, neurobiological, and biosocial perspectives*. Mahwah, NJ: Erlbaum; 1997.

Van Bellinghen M, De Troch C. Risperidone in the treatment of behavioral disturbances in children and adolescents with borderline intellectual functioning: a double-blind, placebo-controlled pilot trial. *J Child Adolesc Psychopharmacol* 2001; **11**: 5–13.

Vitiello B, Stoff DM. Subtypes of aggression and their relevance to child psychiatry. *J Am Acad Child Adolesc Psychiatry* 1997; **36**: 307–15.

Vitiello B, Behar D, Malone R, et al. Pharmacokinetics of lithium carbonate in children. *J Clin Psychopharmacol* 1988; **8**: 355–9.

Weller EB, Weller RA, Fristad MA. Lithium dosage guide for prepubertal children: a preliminary report. *J Am Acad Child Psychiatry* 1986; **25**: 92–5.

chapter 11

Pharmacotherapy of eating disorders in children and adolescents

Gabriele Masi

Introduction

Eating disorders are characterized by a severe disorder in eating behavior. They have been removed from the category of disorders first diagnosed in infancy, childhood and adolescence, where they were included in the previous versions of the DSM-IV (American Pyschiatric Association, 1994), and are now included in a specific diagnostic category. Anorexia nervosa (AN) is characterized by a refusal to mantain the body weight, associated with an extreme fear of becoming fat. Bulimia nervosa (BN) is characterized by repeated episodes of binge eating followed by compensatory behaviors such as self-induced vomiting, or the use of laxatives and diuretics, or excessive exercise. Binge-eating disorder (BED), previously included in the eating disorders not otherwise specified (NOS), has more recently been considered a specific psychiatric diagnosis. It is characterized by uncontrolled binge eating without compensatory behaviors, both in obese and, more rarely, in non-obese individuals. When an eating disorder fails to meet diagnostic criteria for AN, BN, or BED, an eating disorder NOS is diagnosed. Among the clinical situations included in this category are anorexic behavior without amenorrhea or severe weight loss, with the current weight still in the normal range, bulimic behavior, with a low frequency of episodes (fewer than two per week for at least 3 months), and the compensatory behaviors (vomiting, exercise, laxatives) after a small amount of food has been eaten.

Although AN is an exclusionary criterion for BN, at least one out of four patients with severe BN has a history of AN. Furthermore, analogies between these two disorders are more evident than discrepancies. Patients with AN do not have appetite suppression, but a resistence to feeding drive, and patients with BN do not have a primary tendence to overeat, but to restrain their food intake, with a fear of weight gain, their overeating is transitory, and usually preceded and followed by dieting behavior (Kaye and Walsh, 2002). Furthermore, episodes of binge eating are quite frequent in patients with AN. Finally, a disturbance in the perception of body shape is shared by both disorders.

Obesity is not included in the DSM-IV, as it is considered not invariably related to a specific emotional or behavioral syndrome. However, hyperphagia and obesity can be symptoms of different psychiatric disorders, including mood disorders, psychotic disorders, and personality disorders.

Eating disorders are not rare in the general population. The prevalence rate of AN with full diagnostic criteria is estimated at 0.5–1%, and subjects with a subthreshold form of the disorder are much more frequent. BN is even more frequent, with a prevalence of 1–2%. The male/female ratio is about 1:10 for both disorders. According to US community studies, more than 10% of girls attending secondary school have presented episodes of self-induced vomiting, or have taken laxatives, diuretics, or medication to reduce appetite, and 30–40% have serious concerns about their weight and body shape (Fisher et al, 1995). A minority of these conditions probably meets the criteria for eating disorder NOS (Killen et al, 1986).

Prepubertal onset is rare in AN, and the first peak is between 13 and 17 years, while the peak of BN is later, around 17 years. Disorders of feeding and eating, which primarily occur during infancy and early childhood, such as rumination disorder, will not be considered in this chapter, as they do not have pharmacologic implications. Eating problems during preschool years are more frequent in males than in females, while the opposite happens during adolescence, suggesting a discontinuity between these forms of eating disorders.

The management of child and adolescent eating disorders is typically multi-modal (Gowers and Bryant-Waugh, 2004). In the following paragraphs an overview of clinical and pharmacotherapeutic issues in eating disorders will be presented. Unfortunately, even though most of the cases have an onset during adolescence, most of the studies describe young adult samples, and the role of medication in adolescent patients is still relatively unexplored. There is still a need to define specific interventions for the younger patients, including preventive interventions for the most vulnerable, although still strictly non-symptomatic subjects, who are probably increasingly under the influence of the current models of beauty and "ideal" body shape (Steinhausen, 2002).

We have decided to include in this review the data from adult studies, assuming that a cautious approach may allow these findings to be generalized to adolescents. In effect, the clinical features of both AN and BN are consistent across ages, in terms of behaviors, psychopathology, and associated features (Gowers and Bryant-Waugh, 2004). An even more careful approach to pharmacotherapy is needed in these young patients, particularly when malnutrition or (semi)starvation increase their vulnerability to adverse effects.

Anorexia nervosa

Clinical picture

The main feature of AN is the refusal to maintain the body weight, associated with an extreme fear of gaining weight, and with a severe distortion of body image. In postpubertal girls, amenorrhea is usually co-occurring (at least three consecutive menses). Two main subtypes of AN are specified, according to the presence or absence of regular binge eating or purging. The restricting subtype is diagnosed when weight loss is achieved through dieting, fasting, or exercise, but without regular binge eating or purging. The binge-eating/purging subtype is characterized by a regular binge eating or purging, or both, usually with self-induced vomiting, laxatives, diuretics, or enemas. Patients with the binge-eating/purging subtype are usually more likely to present a history of behavioral dyscontrol and family conflicts, and to have a higher risk of substance abuse.

The weight is less than 85% of that considered normal, according to the norms for age, height, and gender. A more rigid criterion requires that the subjects have a body mass index (BMI) (that is weight in kg/height in m^2) below 17.5 kg/m^2. The weight loss is almost always associated with an intense fear of weight gain, which paradoxically increases as the weight continues to decrease, parallel to the distortion of the body perception. Amenorrhea is usually the consequence of the weight loss, even though, more rarely, it can precede the decrease in body weight.

Many symptoms of AN are related to starvation, such as constipation, abdominal pain, hypotension, hypothermia, cold intolerance, periods of lethargy (alternated with an excess of energy and hyperactivity), dry skin (some girls can develop a lanugo on the forearms), and peripheral edemas. Dental enamel erosion is progressively evident in vomiting patients. In the chronic forms, anemia, impaired renal and cardiovascular function, and osteoporosis can complicate the clinical picture and the prognosis.

Atypical eating behaviors during childhood are not rare in subjects who will develop an adolescent-onset AN. Furthermore, a true prepubertal onset of AN can also occur. The criterion of weight loss is less stringent in this age range, while the interference with the normal growth in weight and stature is more evident. In these very early forms the criterion of amenorrhea is absent, while a delayed onset of menses is frequent. The evidence of the dread of fatness and/or weight gain is affected by cognitive development, being less clear in the prepubertal age. Most frequent behaviors are refusal to eat, slowness of eating behavior, a tendency to hide food, or eating rituals before and during the meals. Therefore, developmentally adapted diagnostic criteria are warranted. Some studies suggest that prepubertal AN is more frequently associated with a heavier comorbidity, while most studies suggest a better prognosis, compared with the later-onset AN. The frequency of male cases seems to be higher (20–30% instead of the 10% in the adolescent-onset AN). These boys appear to present a more severe comorbidity and a poorer psychopathologic outcome, even though longitudinal studies are still insufficient.

It is possible that AN in males may be underdiagnosed, even though the clinical picture is similar to that of females. Earlier onset of the illness, atypical gender role behavior, more severe symptomatology, and poorer outcome have been reported (Carlat et al, 1997).

Comorbidity

Most of the data on comorbidity are derived from inpatient studies, which may have selected the most severe forms of the disorder, with the higher frequency of comorbidity. The most frequent comorbidity is depression, which is reported by 20% of the patients, with social withdrawal and low self-esteem, primarily related to body image, in both the prepubertal and adolescent AN. Depressive symptomatology may be partly affected by the starvation, and it seems to be more frequent in mixed forms, with combined anorexic and bulimic behavior.

Anxiety disorders co-occur in about 20–25% of the patients, and they can be associated with the depressive comorbidity. Their rate, as well as the nature of the comorbidity with the obsessive-compulsive disorder, is still under discussion, as an obsessive ideation about eating and body shape, and a compulsive behavior of dieting, even when the patient is emaciated, are core symptoms of AN. However, at least 1 out of 10 patients presents a real comorbid obsessive-compulsive disorder, and obsessive-compulsive traits are frequently reported before the onset of the eating disorder, such as highly restricted domains of interests, rigid thinking, and perfectionism.

Social phobic behavior, such as not eating in front of others, or a body dysmorphic disorder, such as not considering oneself thin, must be considered as part of the AN and not as comorbid conditions. However, they can become a real comorbidity when they are not restricted to the eating domain or to the fatness.

A personality disorder, usually of the avoidant type (whereas the borderline is more typical of the BN), is reported in about 15% of the patients. The binge-eating subtype of AN is more frequently associated with impulsivity, self-harm behaviors, and suicidality, which are more similar to those reported in bulimic patients (Casper et al, 1992; Herzog et al, 1992).

Diagnosis

AN is not usually a difficult diagnosis, and the most important differential diagnosis is with the appetite and weight loss related to another psychopathologic disorder, such as depression, or to general medical conditions. In these conditions, a disorder of the body image is usually absent, as well as the desire of weight loss.

Beliefs about body shape are so severe, and far from reality, that they can be erroneously interpreted as a delusion in the context of a psychotic disorder, even though they are usually restricted to body shape or to food, while the relationship with external reality is preserved. Compulsive behaviors, usually reported in AN, can be misinterpreted as an obsessive-compulsive disorder, at least in the first phases of the disorder, but they allow for a comorbid diagnosis only when the obsessions and/or compulsions are not limited to food.

When an eating disorder is suspected, a careful assessment, including history, development of the symptoms, comorbid conditions, and family functioning, is warranted, using a structured clinical interview with the patient and the parents, and rating scales for the follow-up. Interviews can explore the wide range of psychopathology (i.e. the Schedule for Affective Disorders and Schizophrenia for School-Age Children – Present and Lifetime Version (K-SADS-PL)) (Kaufman et al, 1997), as well as the area of the eating disorder, such as the Eating Disorder Examination (for both parents and patients) (Fairburn and Cooper, 1993; Bryant-Waugh et al, 1996), or the Structured Interview for Anorectic and Bulimic Disorders (Fichter et al, 1998), or self-reported questionnaires such as the Eating Disorders Inventory (Garner et al, 1983).

A behavioral assessment of eating behavior, including thought and attitudes towards eating, weight, and body image, should include the patients and informed others.

A careful examination of the clinical status is needed, including body weight and stature, in order to calculate the BMI, according to age. The following BMI values represent the 5th percentiles for females, aged 8 to 18 (Hammer et al, 1991).

- 8 years, 13.7
- 9 years, 14
- 10 years, 14.2
- 11 years, 14.6
- 12 years, 15.1
- 13 years, 15.6
- 14 years, 16.1
- 15 years, 16.6
- 16 years, 17.2
- 17 years, 17.7
- 18 years, 18.3

For subjects over 18 years, BMI values equivalent to those of subjects below 18 years are indicative of starvation (Kotler and Walsh, 2000).

Laboratory findings should consider blood urea nitrogen and liver function. Not infrequent findings in affected patients are hypercholesterolemia, hypophosphatemia, hypozincemia, and hyperamylasemia.

When the patients are vomiting, metabolic alkalosis (high serum levels of bicarbonate), hypochloremia, and hypokalemia can be relevant, while a metabolic acidosis is more frequent in patients with abuse of laxatives. Low thyroid function, hyperadrenocorticism, and low estrogen levels (low serum testosterone in males) are the most frequent endocrine abnormalities. An ECG can show sinus bradycardia and, more rarely, arrhythmias. In the more severe and chronic AN, an EEG can show diffuse abnormalities, resulting from fluid and electrolyte disturbances, and an increase of the ventricular–brain ratio can be evident on brain imaging.

Natural history

The premorbid condition is usually non-specific, with poor self-esteem, social sensitivity, rigid thinking, restricted interests, poor social contacts, and, in the older adolescents, infrequent sexual activity. The typical AN starts with a diet, with reduction of sweets and high-caloric foods, often induced by a family member or a schoolmate, due to a slight overweight. Several months pass before the parents notice the loss of control of dieting and the weight loss. Usually the patient is not aware of the pathologic condition. A disturbance of body image is already present, and often an inability to recognize internal states such as hunger or satiety is associated. Patients continue the diet restriction, as well as the attempt to further reduce weight, possibly with self-induced vomiting, or with excessive exercise, laxatives, and diuretics. Amenorrhea is usually present in this phase, although it can sometimes appear in the earlier period of reduction in food intake. Some patients start to binge eat, with the consumption of large amounts of food in a short time, with restrictive phases and guilty feelings in the following days.

Comorbid disorders may appear, namely major depression, obsessive-compulsive disorder, and anxiety disorders (see above). A low self-esteem is often associated, independently of comorbid conditions, and it is strongly related to body shape.

The physical status progressively deteriorates, in parallel with the weight loss, leading to the onset of bradycardia, hypotension, hypothermia, and, later, possible complications in every system, including a higher susceptibility to infections.

A review of more than 100 follow-up studies in the last 50 years (Steinhausen, 1999), 31 of them concerning children and adolescents shows that a normalization of weight and menses in about 60% of the patients and a normalization of eating behaviors in less than half of the patients. In summary, about one half of the patients recovers, one third improves, and one fifth is chronic. However, even in the group with a good outcome, many have persistent psychiatric symptoms, including dysthymia, obsessive-compulsive disorder, and social phobia. The mean mortality rate is about 5.5% in all the patients (range 0–21%), and 2.2% (range 0–11%) in children and adolescents (Sullivan, 1995). Suicide contributes to the mortality of AN, accounting for 20% of the mortality.

During the natural history, the comorbidity can strongly affect the clinical picture and the outcome. Affective disorders may also persist in the patients with the better outcome. About two thirds of the patients achieve normal education and employment; a minority of them have a normal intimate relationship or marriage.

Prognostic factors are still uncertain. Favorable prognostic factors are the earlier onset of the disorder, a short interval between onset of symptoms and intervention, and a higher social status or level of education. Vomiting, bulimic behaviors, chronicity or compulsiveness, and poor premorbid functioning are negative predictors of outcome.

Among the possible short- and long-term medical sequelae there are the effects of the low growth hormone on height, a hypothalamic hypogonadism, a hypoplasia of the bone marrow, structural abnormalities of the CNS (including a decreased volume of white matter), and cardiac and gastrointestinal diseases. Delayed statural development, delayed or arrested pubertal development, and ostepoenia-osteoporosis are the most worrying complications of the earliest form of AN.

Long-term studies of patients who have recovered from AN show the persistence of obsessional behaviors, inflexible thinking, increased perfectionism, restraint in emotional expression, high impulse control, and limited social spontaneity (Steinhausen et al, 1993; Eckert et al, 1995). Some of them continue to present overconcern about body image, thinness, and abnormal eating habits (Kaye and Walsh, 2002).

Treatment

When a careful clinical assessment has confirmed the diagnosis of AN, this severe and potentially lethal disorder requires a multi-modal and multi-disciplinary individual, familial, medical, and nutritional intervention. A physical management is of particular importance, given the risk of potentially irreversible effects on growth, particularly if the disorder occurs before fusion of the epiphyses, and impaired bone calcification and mass during the second decade of life, predisposing to osteoporosis and increased fracture risk (Kreipe et al, 1995). The medical management of endocrine effects on bone density should be an important part of the treatment, possibly with calcium, vitamin D, and endocrinologic treatments. Evidence supporting the efficacy of estrogen replacement to reduce the risk of osteoporosis is scarce. Regular monitoring of heart rate, vital signs, and serum electrolytes, namely phosphorus, magnesium, calcium, and potassium, is warranted, remembering that total body electrolytes may be depleted even in subjects with normal serum levels. In younger subjects, medical complications may occur before a severe weight loss.

When an early psychoeducational approach with the subject and his/her family have failed to rapidly improve the clinical picture, psychotherapy and possibly family therapy, and a careful monitoring of the physical condition should be performed by a multi-disciplinary team. In the context of this intervention, the role of possible hospitalization should be considered in the crisis phases. Only during this multi-modal treatment plan can pharmacotherapy have a possible role, as adjunctive intervention.

The knowledge about the neurobiology of symptoms in AN is not as advanced as to give a rationale for pharmacologic treatment based on etiology. Unfortunately, even the symptomatic approach to the core symptoms of AN is often disappointing. The restricted AN seems to be more treatment refractory than the binge-eating/purging subtype. Furthermore, a heavier comorbidity is usually a negative predictor of response.

Most of the studies are characterized by small sample sizes, brief duration of the trials, and often inadequate (low) doses of medications. Most of the studies have been conducted on inpatients, prevalently late adolescent or young adult women. Finally, medications were usually associated with other treatments, and therefore the specific effect of pharmacotherapy is still unclear. The most frequently used medications are antipsychotics and antidepressants, while mood stabilizers and medications that affect appetite and gastrointestinal kinetics are less frequently used and studied.

Antidepressants

A rationale for the use of an antidepressant in AN may be based on the frequency of comorbid affective disorders, which can further worsen the clinical picture and interfere with the compliance to other interventions, as well as on the antiobsessive properties of this medication.

Before the SSRIs, tricyclics were used, in the hope that they would increase appetite through their histaminergic activity. Results from a controlled study with amitriptyline were disappointing (Biederman et al, 1985). Clomipramine (50 mg daily) resulted in an increased appetite during the first phase of the treatment, but also in a reduced rate of weight gain, possibly because of increased activity, and marginal improvement was noted in more stable eating habits (Crisp et al, 1987). Moreover, tricyclics may be particularly dangerous in patients with AN, given their possible cardiotoxicity in malnourished patients.

More recently, SSRIs, which have a much more favorable side-effect profile, have been investigated in several studies, with conflicting results. Fluoxetine, which is a first-choice drug in BN, is the most frequently used SSRI in AN. Controlled studies have failed to support the efficacy of fluoxetine in AN patients during the acute phase (Attia et al, 1998; Strober et al, 1999), but have suggested a possible role in reducing relapse after weight restoration (Kaye et al, 2001), even though other studies did not find any effect of fluoxetine on a 24-month follow-up in treated and untreated patients (Strober et al, 1997).

Sertraline (Santonastaso et al, 2001) and citalopram (Fassino et al, 2002) resulted in an improvement in the associated affective symptoms, but not in the weight. A modest efficacy of SSRI treatment during the acute phase has been confirmed in a recent open-label study involving children and adolescents (Holtkamp et al, 2005).

In summary, empirical studies suggest that SSRIs may be useful when a depressive and/or anxious and/or obsessive symptomatology is prevalent, especially during the follow-up and after the acute phase. However, it has been suggested that malnourished patients may have a reduced synaptic serotonin concentration, which in turn strongly reduces the response to SSRIs. This may explain why fluoxetine is effective only when a weight restoration has occurred.

Older and newer antipsychotics

The use of antipsychotics can be based on a double rationale, that is the effect on appetite and weight gain and the effect on delusional perception of body image. Both typical and atypical antipsychotics have been used. Data on typical antipsychotics are based on adult samples. Pimozide (Vandereycken and Pierloot, 1982) and sulpiride (Vandereycken, 1984) have been explored by the same research group. Sulpiride did not appear to affect psychopathologic status and weight gain, while patients treated with pimozide presented a weight gain and a better attitude towards the treatment program (including behavioral therapy). More recently, Cassano and colleagues (2003) found a benefical effect of low-dose haloperidol as an adjunctive treatment in 13 patients with treatment-resistant AN-restricted subtype, according to specific questionnaires, CGI-I, and BMI.

Given the risk of side-effects during treatment with conventional antipsychotics, their use in children and adolescents cannot be considered as a first choice.

More recently, atypical antipsychotics have been increasingly used in clinical practice, even though controlled studies in patients with AN are lacking. Olanzapine treatment is supported by open trials, some of them including children and adolescents (Jensen and Mejlehde, 2000; La Via et al, 2000; Mehler et al, 2001; Powers et al, 2002; Boachie et al, 2003; Malina et al, 2003; Barbarich et al, 2004), showing a possible positive effect on both core symptoms and related affective and behavioral disorders. According to these studies, olanzapine was well tolerated. Much less evidence is available on risperidone, which has been effectively used in two adolescents (Newman-Toker, 2000).

Available evidence suggests that low- or medium-dose olanzapine may represent a possible effective treatment in patients with treatment-resistant AN, namely when a severe disturbance of body image and a strong refusal of concomitant non-pharmacologic interventions are associated.

Mood stabilizers

Lithium can increase appetite and induce weight gain. Its efficacy in anorexic patients has been explored only in a 4-week placebo-controlled study on 16 patients (Gross et al, 1981), with a mild effect on weight gain in the lithium group, compared to the placebo group, at weeks 3 and 4. Lithium plasma levels were 1 ± 0.1 mEq/l.

Appetite enhancers

Cyproheptadine is a serotonin antagonist with an antihistamine effect, which was noted to induce weight gain during treatment of allergic dermatologic illnesses. Efficacy of cyproheptadine in AN is based on early studies, and it is still controversial. One study supported efficacy in the more severe patients (Goldberg et al, 1979), and another showed a weight gain in the restrictive subtype and a weight loss in the binge-eating subtype (Halmi et al, 1986). Given the controversial findings and the mild modification during treatment, this medication has a secondary role in the pharmacotherapy of AN.

Prokinetic agents

Patients with AN often complain of gastric fullness or bloating. Cisapride, a prokinetic agent, has been proposed to improve these symptoms and, through this action, to decrease food rejection. However, both an open study (Stacher et al, 1993) and a controlled study (Szmukler et al, 1995) failed to show an effect of cisapride on gastric emptying time and weight gain. Furthermore, more recently, cisapride has been withdrawn from the market because of the risk of cardiotoxicity. The role of other prokinetic agents may be limited to the cases with clear evidence of a difficulty in gastric emptying.

Zinc

Based on the phenomenic similarities between zinc deficiency and AN (including reduced appetite, weight loss, and depressed mood), a putative role for zinc in the pathophysiology of AN has been proposed. An early open study seemed to support this hypothesis, with a significant weight gain after zinc supplementation in adolescent and young adult patients with AN (Safai-Kutti, 1990).

Two controlled studies (Katz et al, 1987; Birmingham et al, 1994) found a lower dietary zinc intake and a lower urinary zinc excretion, compared to controls, a trend to an improvement in depressive and anxiety symptoms, and a trend to a greater weight gain in subjects receiving zinc supplementation. A third controlled study (Lask and Bryant-Waugh, 1993) did not confirm these results. To date, the role of zinc supplementation is still controversial and it is not recommended in routine clinical practice.

Summary

According to the above literature review, the first step in treatment is to restore feeding and weight, and enhance the patient's cooperation in the context of a treatment plan, including educational and psychologic support to the patient and the family, nutritional support aimed at a target weight, and medical management of complications, as outpatient, or, when necessary, during hospitalization (American Psychiatric Association, 2000). Pharmacotherapy should not be used as the sole or primary treatment, and it should be reserved to the treatment-resistant cases, or those complicated by comorbid diagnoses (Gowers and Bryant-Waugh, 2004). Anxiety and depression can remit with weight gain, thus a decision on the use of medication should be considered after weight restoration, in view of the poor evidence for an efficacy of medication in weight gain. In patients with weight restoration and persisting obsessional or affective symptoms, or with difficulties in weight maintenance, a trial with fluoxetine is recommended.

In refractory patients with the least self-awareness and the most severe body distortion, a trial with olanzapine may improve anxiety during the refeeding. In both cases, the treatment should be continued for at least several months after the clinical and physiologic improvement.

Bulimia nervosa

Clinical picture

Bulimia nervosa (BN) is characterized by episodes of binge eating large amounts of food, during phases of clear loss of control and altered states of consciousness, associated with compensatory behaviors, for at least 3 months, at least twice a week. These episodes can last from some minutes to hours; they may be precipitated by anxiety, dysphoric mood, depression, or loneliness, and are usually followed by intense feelings of guilt or shame (usually binge episodes and vomiting occur in secrecy), and severe concerns about body shape. Sometimes vomiting becomes a goal in itself, and it occurs even after ingestion of a small amount of food. Constant preoccupations with weight, body size, and food are associated with both BN and AN. However, body weight is normal in most of the BN patients. Menstrual irregularities are common, but less frequent than in AN. However, a history of AN months or years before the onset of BN is not rare.

According to DSM-IV, two subtypes of BN are specified, the first with patients purging through self-induced vomiting, laxatives, or diuretics (purging type), the second with patients who do not purge, but control the weight gain through excessive exercise or fasting (non-purging type).

Beyond a purging and non-purging distinction, a clinically relevant differentiation is between a multi-impulsive subtype, when the bulimic behavior is associated with severe difficulties in self-regulation and emotional instability (including substance abuse and self-injurious behaviors), and a subtype with dependence on external rewards and excessive compliance.

In the (rare) prepubertal-onset BN, DSM-IV diagnostic criteria are more rarely met, as sometimes binge eating or purging is not present, or the frequency of the episodes is lower than two episodes for 3 months.

The frequency of BN is higher than AN (1–2%). Furthermore, a sizeable minority of teenagers in the community exhibits binge-eating and/or purging behaviors (Fisher et al, 1995). Age at onset is more variable than AN, it even peaks in mid- or late-adolescence. The male/female ratio is 1:10.

Males and females with BN have a similar symptomatology. A higher frequency of disturbances in psychosexual development and gender identity is reported in males; furthermore, sexual activity can be inhibited in heterosexual males with bulimia.

Comorbidity

About 25% of the patients with BN have an affective disorder, 15% an anxiety disorder, 15% substance abuse, and 5% a personality disorder. As in AN, in BN the most frequent comorbidity is with depression (major depressive disorder or dysthymia), which usually follows the eating disorder. Anxiety disorders are frequent as well, particularly social phobia. The multi-impulsive subtype presents a higher comorbidity with bipolar disorder type II and/or borderline personality disorder, with a high risk of substance or alcohol abuse (about 30% of the patients), antisocial behavior, hypersexuality, and suicide risk (Herzog et al, 1992). A relationship between BN and previous child abuse is more frequently reported in BN than in AN (Fallon et al, 1994; Schoemaker et al, 2002).

Natural history

Medical complications are often overlooked, but are usually less severe than in AN. However, fluid and electrolyte imbalance (namely hypokalemia, hyponatremia, and hypochloremia), metabolic acidosis, dehydration, lesions in the gastrointestinal tract, and blood pressure abnormalities may become so severe as to require hospitalization. The adverse dental effect of vomiting should be monitored, with specific guidance on oral hygiene (Gowers and Bryant-Waugh, 2004). Amenorrhea or menstrual irregularity may also occur. The mortality rate is about 0.7–1%.

The course of BN is usually oscillating, and influenced by comorbidities. Outcome analyses indicate that about half fully recovers, a quarter improves, and a quarter becomes chronic (Steinhausen, 1999). One third of the patients is still symptomatic 3 years after the index episode. Among those who recover, two thirds have a relapse within 18 months, and half of those who recovered from the second episode relapses again. Globally speaking, about 60% have a positive course, 30% have a partial improvement, 10% have a negative course, and 1% dies.

There are few predictors of outcome, based on the available literature (Herzog et al, 1993). A better prognosis is related to a younger age at onset, a shorter duration of illness, and a higher social class. The most severe BN cases have the worst prognosis. Personality disorders, suicide attempts, alcohol abuse, and low self-esteem are negative prognostic factors (Casper et al, 1992). Low self-esteem seems to be associated with a poor outcome. A persisting pressure to be thin has been found to predict the maintenance of bulimic symptoms, as well as caloric restriction.

Diagnosis

Diagnosis may be more difficult than in AN, as the weight loss is often absent. Many patients remain undiagnosed, and many are diagnosed by chance, during a routine medical assessment. Questionnaires and clinical interviews have been reported above in the section on AN. A differential diagnosis with affective disorders, both depression and bipolar disorder, can be difficult when binge and compensatory behaviors are not evident. A borderline personality disorder and substance abuse are frequently co-occurring, and they can mask the eating disorder.

Treatment

Even though the pharmacologic treatments are more effective in BN than in AN, they must be considered in the context of a multi-modal treatment, including educational, psychologic, familial, and medical interventions, and a nutritional management, including diary-keeping and self-monitoring. Cognitive-behavioral therapy has been proven to be effective in bulimic patients (Agras et al, 1992; Steinhausen, 1999), and it is probably more effective than a single course of an antidepressant medication (American Psychiatric Association, 2000). Family therapy can be useful as well (Dodge, 1995).

According to these findings psychotherapy can be considered a first-choice treatment. A summary of psychological interventions is available in Gowers and Bryant-Waugh (2004).

Pharmacologic treatment should be considered in the first phases of the disorder in the most severe patients, or when a comorbid depressive or bipolar symptomatology may worsen the clinical picture and reduce the efficacy of non-pharmacologic interventions.

The development of the pharmacotherapy of BN has been much less disappointing than in AN, since the 1980s. However, only antidepressants have received empirical support of established efficacy.

Antidepressants

Multiple studies have shown that antidepressants are significantly superior to placebo, including SSRIs, tricyclics (imipramine, desipramine, amitriptyline), MAOIs (phenelzine, isocarboxazide, brofaramine), trazadone, and bupropione (associated with an increased risk of seizure). SSRIs are currently the most frequently studied medications (Mitchell et al, 1993; Mayer and Walsh, 1998), and among them fluoxetine is the most frequently studied (Fluoxetine Bulimia Nervosa Collaborative Study Group, 1992; Goldstein et al, 1995), and approved by the US Food and Drug Administration. Support for fluvoxamine efficacy derives from a European study (Fichter et al, 1996), showing that fluvoxamine was superior to placebo (despite a high dropout rate) in reducing the re-emergence of bulimic behaviors after the completion of an inpatient treatment. No studies are available comparing the efficacy of different SSRIs.

Controlled trials have shown that high doses of fluoxetine (60 mg/day) but not low-medium doses (20 mg/day) were effective in controlling binge eating. When depression is comorbid, this co-occurrence does not predict the degree of improvement after antidepressant treatment, and this, as well as the need for higher doses of fluoxetine than in depression, suggests that the antibulimic mechanism is separate from the antidepressant mechanism, i.e. on the neural systems underlying the control of appetite (Kaye and Walsh, 2002). Romano et al (2002) have shown that continued fluoxetine treatment after an acute phase is associated with a significantly longer time to relapse.

A study involving ten adolescents (aged 12–18 years) explored the efficacy of an 8-week trial with fluoxetine (60 mg/day), showing a significant decrease of weekly binges and purges and an improvement in the CGI-I, with good tolerability and no dropouts (Kotler et al, 2003).

Fichter et al (1996) reported a placebo-controlled, 12-week study on fluvoxamine treatment in subjects who had completed an inpatient psychotherapy treatment. Fluvoxamine was significantly superior to placebo in reducing a relapse to binge-purge behavior, even though the dropout rate was higher in the active drug group than in the placebo group (38% versus 14%).

Several studies have compared cognitive-behavioral psychotherapy and pharmacotherapy. Fichter and colleagues (1991) blindly treated with fluoxetine or placebo, hospitalized patients with BN, intensively treated by behavioral psychotherapy. No significant differences were found between the two groups, suggesting a "ceiling effect" of the psychotherapy.

Walsh and colleagues (1997) compared two different types of psychotherapy (cognitive-behavioral therapy and supportive psychotherapy) and the effect of combining medication with psychotherapy (first desipramine, then fluoxetine, when the tricyclic was not tolerated or ineffective). Cognitive-behavioral therapy was superior to supportive psychotherapy, and the medication modestly but significantly augmented the effect of psychotherapy. The group of patients receiving medication only and the group with cognitive behavioral therapy plus placebo showed a similar outcome.

Mitchell and colleagues (2002) explored the efficacy of medication or interpersonal psychotherapy in patients who were unsuccessfully treated with cognitive-behavioral therapy. The response rate was similar in the two groups (medication and psychotherapy), and response rates were low.

In summary, most of these studies suggest that BN responds similarly to antidepressants and psychotherapy. In refractory cases, the combination of the two interventions can determine an additional but modest benefit, mainly in the short term. These three treatment strategies (psychotherapy, medication, both) can be effective, but it is not yet clear which patients to match with specific treatments (Mayer and Walsh, 1998). Predictors of response are still unclear. However, when the treatment is effective, the response is usually rapid irrespective of the treatment. For this reason, many experts believe that a first trial of psychotherapy is recommended, particularly in adolescents, and a medication can be added when this trial is ineffective (Wilson et al, 1999; Mitchell et al, 2001). However a first trial with medication may be needed when patients have to wait for access to psychotherapy, or when a trained psychotherapist is not available, or when the patient's compliance to psychotherapy is clearly absent. When pharmacologic treatment is effective, it should be continued in order to prevent relapses.

Topiramate

Topiramate has been shown to be superior to placebo in a 10-week, randomized, double-blind controlled study (Hedges et al, 2003; Hoopes et al, 2003). Topiramate was started at 25 mg/day, and increased by 25–50 mg/week, up to a maximum of 400 mg/day. The mean number of binge and/or purge days decreased by 44.8% in the topiramate group and by 10% in the placebo group. Other measures of binge and purge symptoms improved similarly in the topiramate group, compared with the placebo group. An improvement was reported also in behavioral measures, such as body dissatisfaction and drive for thinness. A significant improvement was found in anxiety, but not in depression.

Other medications

Kaplan and colleagues (1983) reported on an effective use of carbamazepine in six bulimic outpatients in a double-blind, cross-over study. Even if only one patient had a history suggestive of bipolar disorder, the authors hypothesize a possible link between bulimia and affective illness.

Lithium treatment has been tested in a randomized, double-blind, placebo-controlled study in an 8-week trial (Hsu et al, 1991). The 68 completers experienced a significant decrease in the bulimic episodes, as well as an improvement in depression and other psychopathologies.

However, at a relatively low plasma level, lithium was not more effective than placebo. The management of lithium may be problematic in bulimic patients, because the lithium levels may shift markedly with rapid volume changes.

Some experimental studies suggested that antagonism of endogenous opioids suppresses feeding behavior in human and infrahuman models. Mitchell and colleagues (1989) explored the efficacy of low-dose naltrexone (50–120 mg/day) in a double-blind, cross-over study in 16 bulimic outpatients. The active drug was not superior to placebo in reducing the binge-eating or vomiting episodes. Marrazzi et al (1995) treated with naltrexone (at higher doses than the previous study, that is 200–300 mg/day) or placebo 19 patients with BN or AN with binge eating, in a cross-over study. A reduction of the binge-purge symptomatology was evident during the naltrexone treatment in 18 out of 19 patients. The importance of the higher doses of the medication is unclear.

Summary

According to the available literature, antidepressants are effective as a component of a multi-modal treatment program. Antidepressants can reduce the frequency of abnormal eating behaviors, such as binge eating and vomiting, and can also improve depressive, anxiety, and obsessional symptoms, and, sometimes, impulse dyscontrol. SSRIs are the safest antidepressants, and among them fluoxetine is the best supported medication and should be considered as the first-line drug, especially in patients with symptoms of anxiety, depression, obsession, or impulse dyscontrol. High doses of fluoxetine (up to 60 mg/day) should be tested before considering the patient as a non-responder to treatment. A comorbid bipolar disorder should be investigated before starting an antidepressant medication, in order to avoid an acute worsening of the clinical picture.

When a mood stabilizer is needed, lithium and valproic acid can cause an undesirable increase in appetite and weight gain. Topiramate may be an alternative medication in non-responders to SSRIs, or when the clinical picture (particularly the impulse dyscontrol) has worsened after SSRI treatment, or when a bipolar disorder is comorbid. A slow titration of topiramate (starting dose 25 mg/day, with increases of 25 mg/day every week, up to the clinical response or 150–200 mg/day) can reduce the risk of side-effects, namely psychiatric side-effects, such as psychotic-like symptoms or impulsiveness, which are more frequent with a rapid titration and in long-term treatment.

The efficacy of alternative medications, such as opioid antagonists, is less supported by sufficient evidence, and they should not be used in the routine management of bulimic patients.

Binge eating

Clinical picture

Binge eating disorder (BED) is a psychiatric diagnosis of more recent origin. It is characterized by the occurrence of binge eating without inappropriate compensatory behaviors in obese and non-obese subjects. The most frequent clinical cluster is characterized by binge eating, obesity, body image distress, and psychopathology, namely depression (Devlin et al, 2003). Diagnostic criteria include the eating of an amount of food largely exceeding what most people would eat in a similar period of time, with a sense of lack of control. Furthermore, at least three of the following associated features are present:

- eating much more rapidly than normal
- eating until feeling unconfortably full
- eating when not feeling physically hungry
- eating alone because of being embarrassed by how much one is eating
- feeling disgusted with oneself, or depressed or guilty after overeating.

The binge eating occurs at least twice a week for 6 months, and determines marked distress. The specificity of BED is still being questioned, as obese persons with or without binge eating are not distinguishable, and the binge eating is often unstable, with possible remission during treatment or placebo (Devlin et al, 2003). The nosological status is also under discussion, whether BED is a distinct diagnostic entity, or a variant or subtype of BN, or a behavioral subtype of obesity (just like night eating, overeating all day, eating too much at the scheduled meals), or an associated feature emerging when primary disorders, such as obesity and depression, coexist.

However, despite these uncertainties, the patients with binge-eating behavior, particularly when they are obese, often need specialized treatment. About one third of the obese patients who attend a specialized clinic meet diagnostic criteria for BED. An effective treatment for this disorder is thus of clinical utility (Kaye and Walsh, 2002). This is particularly true for BED in children and adolescents (Marcus and Kalarchian, 2003). Even though the onset of BED is usually in late adolescence, two different patterns of onset can be identified, the first after the start of dieting behavior, similar to patients with BN, and the second before a dieting behavior, with an earlier age at onset (11–13 years) and more psychiatric disturbances, particularly depression and BN. Available studies suggest a continuity between childhood, adolescence, and adulthood BED.

The assessment of BED in overweight children and adolescents is of particular interest in clinical practice, given the increased risk of developing diabetes mellitus or hypertension. Loss of control over eating in overweight children is present in about one third of obese children aged 6–10 years, and 5.3% meet the diagnostic criteria for BED. These children report more anxiety, depression, negative moods, and body dissatisfaction (Morgan et al, 2002). A clinically significant binge eating was reported in 30% of a group of obese adolescent girls (14–16 years) (Berkowitz et al, 1993), a rate which is similar to that reported in adult obese patients. These data show that binge eating is a common problem in overweight children and adolescents. In order to properly identify those young patients, less stringent criteria may be needed to characterize binge-eating problems, even in prepubertal childhood (Marcus and Kalarchian, 2003). For example, a binge-eating episode may be characterized by food seeking in the absence of hunger and with a sense of lack of control, associated with at least one of the following features: food seeking in response to a negative affect, or as a reward, or sneaking or hiding food. These behaviors should persist for at least 3 months, without compensatory behaviors (Marcus and Kalarchian, 2003).

Treatment

Three categories of medication have been used in the treatment of BED: antidepressants, centrally acting appetite suppressants, and anticonvulsants (Carter et al, 2003). Controlled trials are needed to support the efficacy of pharmacotherapy, given that most of the treatments determine a short-term improvement, as a suggestion or placebo effect. However, the high placebo effect may obscure the efficacy of medication.

Antidepressants

A placebo-controlled trial in the early 1990s explored the efficacy of the tricyclic desipramine (100–300 mg/day) in non-purging BN, when diagnostic criteria for BED were still not available (McCann and Agras, 1990). Desipramine was superior to placebo in reducing binge frequency, but this effect was not associated with a weight loss in the short term.

SSRIs have been successfully used in BED, including fluvoxamine (50–300 mg/day) (Hudson et al, 1998), sertraline (50–200 mg/day) (McElroy et al, 2000), fluoxetine (20–80 mg/day) (Arnold et al, 2002), and citalopram (20–60 mg/day) (McElroy et al, 2003a). Grouping the effects of the above-mentioned four studies (Carter et al, 2003), the difference between medication and placebo according to the percentage of subjects presenting an improvement of at least 50% in the frequency of binges was 23, whereas the difference according to the percentage of subjects with cessation of binges was 20.2. Similar rates were found according to the CGI-I score 1 or 2. The mean placebo response in the four studies was 33.3%. These data support the efficacy of SSRIs in the treatment of BED. More recently, Grilo and colleagues (2005) randomized 108 patients with BED into one of the following 16-week treatment groups: cognitive-behavioral therapy, fluoxetine (60 mg/day), placebo, cognitive-behavioral therapy plus fluoxetine, and cognitive-behavioral therapy plus placebo. Remission rates were affected by cognitive-behavioral therapy, but not by fluoxetine. Furthermore, binge eating, but not weight loss, was affected by cognitive-behavioral therapy.

Centrally acting appetite suppressants

D-Fenfluramine was shown to be effective in reducing binges, but without a significant effect on body weight (Stunkard et al, 1996). However, fenfluramine has been withdrawn from the market because of the risk of causing heart valve defects.

Sibutramine was shown to be effective in 7 out of 10 patients with BED after a 12-week trial, according to both number of binges and weight reduction (Appolinario et al, 2002a). This finding has been confirmed in a placebo-controlled study (Appolinario et al, 2003), supporting the efficacy of sibutramine (15 mg/day) on binge eating, weight, and related depressive symptoms.

Topiramate

The role of the anticonvulsant topiramate in BED may be related to the effects of these medications on both mood and impulse control. Most of the available anticonvulsants, such as lithium and valproic acid, can increase appetite and weight gain, and therefore they are contraindicated in these patients. The most frequently studied medication is topiramate.

Several open trials (Shapira et al, 2000; Appolinario et al, 2002b) supported the efficacy of topiramate in reducing the frequency of binges and weight gain. A placebo-controlled trial (McElroy et al, 2003b) confirmed these findings, as 64% of the topiramate-treated patients, compared with 30% of the placebo-treated patients, significantly improved in terms of frequency of binges and weight, with a mean weight loss of 5.9 kg in the topiramate group and 1.2 kg in the placebo group. McElroy and colleagues (2004) have reported on long-term (42-week) treatment with topiramate (starting dose 25 mg/day, maximum dose 600 mg/day) in patients with BED and obesity, with an enduring improvement in both binge frequency and body weight, but with a high rate of discontinuation for adverse events.

Summary

A multi-modal treatment should be considered in patients with BED, particularly in overweight subjects, including behavioral weight loss methods, psychologic treatments, and pharmacotherapy. The aim of the treatment of BED is to reduce the eating binges, and in the obese patients to reduce the body weight and to normalize the eating behavior and the daily caloric intake. The goals should be realistic, in order to prevent a fall in motivation after the first enthusiasm. Management of the associated features, such as shame about eating, should be addressed as well. Finally, the psychopathologic symptoms or disorders, such as depression or impulse dyscontrol, may be the target of the treatment. However, even though abnormal eating behavior, overweight, and symptoms of anxiety and depression are closely related, a common clinical experience is that treatments can be effective on binge eating and on anxiety depression, but they more rarely determine a change in weight. In contrast, the binge eating can be rapidly responsive to non-specific interventions, included placebo, even though the effect of all the interventions, included pharmacotherapy, can fade once the intervention has been discontinued (Kaye and Walsh, 2002).

Pharmacotherapy should be considered in patients who are refractory to other treatments, or in patients with associated psychopathologies, or in the most severe obesity.

The first-line medication are the SSRIs, at the adequate doses (upper end range used in other indications), and for an adequate duration of time (at least 4–6 weeks), according to the literature indications. When successful, the treatment should be maintained for at least 6–12 months.

When the patients are clearly overweight and unresponsive to SSRIs, or when a bipolar disorder is comorbid, topiramate should be considered, following the guidelines reported above (see BN).

The scant experience with sibutramine currently limits the use of this medication, at least in young patients.

References

Agras WS, Rossiter E, Arnow B. Pharmacologic and cognitive-behavioral treatment for bulimia nervosa: a controlled comparison. *Am J Psychiatry* 1992; **149**: 82–7.

American Psychiatric Association. *Diagnostic and statistical manual of mental disorders*, 4th edn. Washington, DC: American Psychiatric Assocation; 2000.

American Psychiatric Association. Practice guideline for the treatment of patients with eating disorders (revision). *Am J Psychiatry* 2000; **157**: 1–39.

Appolinario JC, Godoy-Matos A, Fontenelle LF, et al. An open label trial of sibutramine in obese patients with binge eating disorder. *J Clin Psychiatry* 2002a; **63**: 28–30.

Appolinario JC, Fontenelle LF, Papelbaum M, et al. Topiramate use in obese patients with binge eating disorder: an open study. *Can J Psychiatry* 2002b; **47**: 271–3.

Appolinario JC, Bacaltchuk J, Sichieri R, et al. A randomized, double-blind, placebo-controlled study of sibutramine in the treatment of binge-eating disorder. *Arch Gen Psychiatry* 2003; **60**: 1109–16.

Arnold LM, McElroy SL, Hudson JI, et al. A placebo-controlled randomized trial of fluoxetine in the treatment of binge-eating disorder. *J Clin Psychiatry* 2002; **63**: 1028–33.

Attia E, Haiman C, Walsh BT, Flater SR. Does fluoxetine augment the inpatient treatment of anorexia nervosa? *Am J Psychiatry* 1998; **155**: 548–51.

Barbarich NC, McConaha CW, Gaskill J, et al. An open trial of olanzapine in anorexia nervosa. *J Clin Psychiatry* 2004; **65**: 1480–2.

Berkowitz R, Stunkard AJ, Stallings VA, et al. Binge-eating disorder in obese adolescent girls. *Ann NY Acad Science* 1993; **699**: 200–6.

Biederman J, Herzog DB, Rivinus TM, et al. Amitriptyline in the treatment of anorexia nervosa: a double-blind, placebo-controlled study. *J Clin Psychopharmacol* 1985; **5**: 10–16.

Birmingham CL, Goldner EM, Bakan R. Controlled trial of zinc supplementation in anorexia nervosa. *Int J Eat Disord* 1994; **15**: 251–5.

Boachie A, Goldfield GS, Spettigue W. Olanzapine use as an adjunctive treatment for hospitalized children with anorexia nervosa: case reports. *Int J Eat Dis* 2003; **33**: 98–103.

Bryant-Waugh RJ, Cooper PJ, Taylor CL, Lask BD. The use of the eating disorder examination with children: a pilot study. *Int J Eat Dis* 1996; **19**: 391–7.

Carlat DJ, Camargo CA, Herzog DB. Eating disorders in males: a report of 135 patients. *Am J Psychiatry* 1997; **54**: 1127–32.

Carter WP, Hudson JI, Lalonde JK, et al. Pharmacologic treatment of binge eating disorder. *Int J Eat Disord* 2003; **34**: S74–S88.

Casper R, Hedecker D, McClough J, et al. Personality dimensions in eating disorders and their relevance for subtyping. *J Am Acad Child Adolesc Psychiatry* 1992; **31**: 830–40.

Cassano GB, Miniati M, Pini S, et al. Six-month open trial of haloperidol as an adjunctive treatment for anorexia nervosa: a preliminary report. *Int J Eat Disord* 2003; **33**: 172–7.

Crisp AH, Lacey JH, Ctutchfield M. Clomipramine and "drive" in people with anorexia nervosa: an in-patient study. *Br J Psychiatry* 1987; **150**: 355–8.

Devlin MJ, Goldfein JA, Dobrow I. What is this thing called BED? Current status of binge eating disorder nosology. *Int J Eat Disord* 2003; **34**: S2–S18.

Dodge E. Family therapy for bulimia nervosa in adolescents: an exploratory study. *J Fam Ther* 1995; **17**: 59–77.

Eckert ED, Halmi KA, Marchi P, Grove W, Crosby R. Ten-year follow-up of anorexia nervosa: clinical course and outcome. *Psychol Med* 1995; **25**: 143–56.

Fairburn CG, Cooper Z. The eating disorder examination. In: Fairburn CT, Wilson GT, eds. *Binge-eating: nature, assessment and treatment.* New York: Guilford Press; 1993; 317–60.

Fallon BA, Sadik C, Saoud JB, Garfinkel RS. Childhood abuse, family environment, and outcome of bulimia nervosa. *J Clin Psychiatry* 1994; **55**: 424–8.

Fassino S, Leombruni P, Daga G, et al. Efficacy of citalopram in anorexia nervosa: a pilot study. *Eur Neuropsychopharmacol* 2002; **12**: 453–9.

Fichter MM, Leibl K, Rief W, et al. Fluoxetine versus placebo: a double-blind study with bulimic inpatients undergoing intensive psychotherapy. *Pharmacopsychiatry* 1991; **24**: 1–7.

Fichter MM, Kruger R, Rief W, Holland R, Dohne J. Fluvoxamine in prevention of relapse in bulimia nervosa: effects on eating specific psychopathology. *J Clin Psychopharmacol* 1996; **16**: 9–18.

Fichter MM, Herpertz S, Quadflieg N, Herpertz-Dahlmann B. Structured interview for anorectic and bulimic disorders for DSM IV and ICD 10: updated (third) revision. *Int J Eat Dis* 1998; **24**: 400–6.

Fisher M, Golden NH, Katzman DK, et al. Eating disorders in adolescents: a background paper. *J Adolesc Health Care* 1995; **16**: 420–37.

Fluoxetine Bulimia Nervosa Collaborative Study Group. Fluoxetine in the treatment of bulimia nervosa: a multicenter, placebo-controlled, double-blind trial. *Arch Gen Psychiatry* 1992; **49**: 139–47.

Garner DM, Olmsted MP, Polivy J. Development and validation of a multidimensional eating disorder inventory for anorexia nervosa and bulimia. *Int J Eat Dis* 1983; **2**: 15–34.

Goldberg SC, Halmi KA, Eckert ED, et al. Cyproheptadine in anorexia. *Br J Psychiatry* 1979; **134**: 67–70.

Goldstein DJ, Wilson MG, Thomson VL, et al. Fluoxetine Bulimia Nervosa Collaborative Study Group. Long-term fluoxetine treatment of bulimia nervosa. *Br J Psychiatry* 1995; **1666**: 660–6.

Gowers S, Bryant-Waugh R. Management of child and adolescent eating disorders: the current evidence base and future directions. *J Child Psychol Psychiatry* 2004; **45**: 63–83.

Grilo CM, Masheb RM, Wilson GT. Efficacy of cognitive behavioral therapy and fluoxetine for the treatment of binge eating disorder: a randomized double blind placebo controlled comparison. *Biol Psychiatry* 2005; **57**: 301–9.

Gross HA, Ebert MH, Faden VB, et al. A double-blind controlled trial of lithium carbonate in primary anorexia nervosa. *J Clin Psychopharmacol* 1981; **1**: 376–81.

Halmi KA, Eckert E, La Dru TJ, Cohen J. Anorexia nervosa. Treatment efficacy of cyproheptadine and amytriptiline. *Arch Gen Psychiatry* 1986; **43**: 177–81.

Hammer LD, Kraemer HC, Wilson DM, Ritter PL, Dornbusch SM. Standardized percentile curves of body-mass index for children and adolescents. *Am J Dis Child* 1991; **145**: 259–63.

Hedges D, Reimherr F, Hoopes S, et al. Part II. Treatment with topiramate is associated with improvements in psychiatric measures of bulimia nervosa: a randomized, double-blind, placebo-controlled trial. *J Clin Psychiatry* 2003; **64**: 1449–54.

Herzog DB, Keller MB, Lavori PW. The prevalence of personality disorders in 210 women with eating disorders. *J Clin Psychiatry* 1992; **53**: 147–52.

Herzog DB, Sacks NR, Keller MB, et al. Patterns and predictors of recovery in anorexia nervosa and bulimia nervosa. *J Am Acad Child Adolesc Psychiatry* 1993; **32**: 835–42.

Holtkamp K, Konrad K, Kaiser N, et al. A retrospective study of SSRI treatment in adolescent anorexia nervosa: insufficient evidence for efficacy. *J Psychiatr Res* 2005; **39**: 303–10.

Hoopes S, Reimherr F, Hedges H, et al. Part I. Topiramate in the treatment of bulimia nervosa: a randomized, double blind, placebo-controlled trial. *J Clin Psychiatry* 2003; **64**: 1335–41.

Hsu LKG, Clement L, Santhouse R, Ju ESY. Treatment of bulimia nervosa with lithium carbonate: a controlled study. *J Nerv Ment Dis* 1991; **179**: 351–5.

Hudson JI, McElroy SL, Raymond NC, et al. Fluvoxamine in the treatment of binge-eating disorder: a multicenter placebo-controlled, double-blind trial. *Am J Psychiatry* 1998; **155**: 1756–62.

Jensen VS, Meylehde A. Anorexia nervosa: treatment with olanzapine. Br J Psychiatry 2000; **177**: 87.

Kaplan AS, Garfinkel PE, Darby PL, Garner DM. Carbamazepine in the treatment of bulimia. *Am J Psychiatry* 1983; **140**: 1225–6.

Katz RL, Keen CL, Litt IF, et al. Zinc deficiency in anorexia nervosa. *J Adolesc Health Care* 1987; **8**: 400–6.

Kaufman J, Birmaher B, Brent D, et al. Schedule for Affective Disorders and Schizophrenia for School-Age Children – Present and Lifetime version (K-SADS-PL): initial reliability and validity data. *J Am Acad Child Adolesc Psychiatry* 1997; **36**: 980–8.

Kaye WH, Walsh BT. Psychopharmacology of eating disorders. In: Davis KL, Charney D, Coyle JT, Nemeroff C, eds. *Neuropsychopharmacology: the fifth generation of progress*. Philadelphia: Lippincott Williams Wilkins; 2002: 1677–83.

Kaye WH, Nagata T, Weltzin TE, et al. Double-blind placebo-controlled administration of fluoxetine in restricting and restricting-purging-type anorexia nervosa. *Biol Psychiatry* 2001; **49**: 644–52.

Killen JD, Taylor CB, Telch MJ, et al. Self-induced vomiting and laxative and diuretic use among teenagers: precursor of binge-purge syndrome? *JAMA* 1986; **255**: 1447–9.

Kotler LA, Walsh BT. Eating disorders in children and adolescents: pharmacological therapies. *Eur Child Adolesc Psychiatry* 2000; **9**: 108–16.

Kotler LA, Devlin MJ, Davies M, Walsh BT. An open trial of fluoxetine for adolescents with bulimia nervosa. *J Child Adolesc Psychopharmacol* 2003; **13**: 329–35.

Kreipe RE, Golden NH, Katzman DK, et al. Eating disorders in adolescence. A position of the Society of Adolescent Medicine. *J Adolesc Health* 1995; **16**: 476–9.

La Via MC, Grey N, Kaye WH, et al. Case reports of olanzapine treatment of anorexia nervosa. *Int J Eat Disord* 2000; **27**: 363–6.

Lask B, Bryant-Waugh R. Zinc deficiency and childhood-onset anorexia nervosa. *J Clin Psychiatry* 1993; **54**: 63–6.

McCann UD, Agras WS. Successful treatment of nonpurging bulimia nervosa with desipramine: a double-blind, placebo-controlled study. *Am J Psychiatry* 1990; **148**: 1097–8.

McElroy SL, Arnold LM, Shapira NA, et al. Placebo-controlled trial of sertraline in the treatment of binge-eating disorder. *Am J Psychiatry* 2000; **157**: 1004–6.

McElroy SL, Hudson JI, Malhotra S, et al. Citalopram in the treatment of binge-eating disorder. *J Clin Psychiatry* 2003a; **64**: 807–13.

McElroy SL, Arnold LM, Shapira NA, et al. Topiramate in the treatment of binge-eating disorder associated with obesity: a randomized placebo controlled trial. *Am J Psychiatry* 2003b; **160**: 255–61.

McElroy SL, Shapira NA, Arnold LM, et al. Topiramate in the long-term treatment of binge-eating disorder associated with obesity. *J Clin Psychiatry* 2004; **65**: 1463–9.

Malina A. Gaskill J, McConaha C, et al. Olanzapine treatment of anorexia nervosa: a retrospective study. *Int J Eat Disord* 2003; **33**: 234–7.

Marazzi MA, Bacon JP, Kinzie J, Luby ED. Naltrexone use in the treatment of anorexia nervosa and bulimia nervosa. *Int Clin Psychopharmacol* 1995; **10**: 163–720.

Marcus MD, Kalarchian MA. Binge eating in children and adolescents. *Int J Eat Disord* 2003; **34**: S47–S57.

Mayer LES, Walsh T. The use of selective serotonin reuptake inhibitors in eating disorders. *J Clin Psychiatry* 1998; **59**: 28–34.

Mehler C, Wewetzer C, Schulze U, et al. Olanzapine in children and adolescents with chronic anorexia nervosa. A study of five cases. *Eur Child Adolesc Psychiatry* 2001; **10**: 151–7.

Mitchell JE, Christenson G, Jennings J, et al. A placebo controlled, double-blind crossover study of naltrexone hydrocloride in outpatients with normal weight bulimia. *J Clin Psychopharmacol* 1989; **9**: 94–7.

Mitchell JE, Raymond N, Specker S. A review of the controlled trials of pharmacotherapy and psychotherapy in the treatment of bulimia nervosa. *Int J Eating Dis* 1993; **14**: 229–47.

Mitchell JE, Peterson CB, Myers T, Wonderlich S. Combining pharmacotherapy and psychotherapy in the treatment of patients with eating disorders. *Psychiatr Clin North Am* 2001; **24**: 315–23.

Mitchell JE, Halmi K, Wilson GT, et al. A randomized secondary treatment study of women with bulimia nervosa who fail to respond to CBT. *Int J Eat Disord* 2002; **32**: 271–81.

Morgan CM, Yanovsky FZ, Nguyen TT, et al. Loss of control over eating, adiposity, and psychopathology in overweight children. *Int J Eat Disord* 2002; **31**: 430–41.

Newman-Toker J. Risperidone in anorexia nervosa. *J Am Acad Child Adolesc Psychiatry* 2000; **39**: 941–2.

Powers PS, Santana CA, Bannon YS. Olanzapine in the treatment of anorexia nervosa: an open label trial. *Int J Eat Dis* 2002; **32**: 146–54.

Romano S, Halmi K, Sarkar N, et al. A placebo-controlled study of fluoxetine in continued treatment of bulimia after successful acute fluoxetine treatment. *Am J Psychiatry* 2002; **159**: 96–102.

Safai-Kutti S. Oral zinc supplementation in anorexia nervosa. *Acta Psychiatr Scand* 1990; **361**: S14–S17.

Santonastaso P, Friederici S, Favaro A. Sertraline in the treatment of restricting anorexia nervosa: an open controlled trial. *J Child Adolesc Psychopharmacol* 2001; **11**: 143–50.

Schoemaker C, Smit F, Bijl RV, Vollebergh WA. Bulimia nervosa following psychological and multiple child abuse: support for the self-medication hypothesis in a population-based cohort study. *Int J Eat Disord* 2002; **32**: 381–8.

Shapira NA, Goldsmith TD, McElroy SL. Treatment of binge-eating disorder with topiramate: a clinical case series. *J Clin Psychiatry* 2000; **61**: 368–72.

Stacher G, Abatzi TA, Wiesnagrotzki S, et al. Gastric emptying, body weight and symptoms in primary anorexia nervosa: long term effects of cisapride. *Br J Psychiatry* 1993; **162**: 398–402.

Steinhausen HC. Eating disorders. In: Steinhausen HC, Verhulst F, eds. *Risks and outcomes in developmental psychopathology*. Oxford: Oxford University Press; 1999: 210–30.

Steinhausen HC. Anorexia and bulimia nervosa. In: Rutter M, Taylor E, eds. *Child and adolescent psychiatry*. Oxford: Blackwell Publishing; 2002: 555–70.

Steinhausen HC, Rauss-Mason C, Seidel R. Follow-up studies of anorexia nervosa: a review of four decades of outcome research. *Psychol Med* 1993; **21**: 447–54.

Strober M, Freeman R, DeAntonio M, et al. Does adjunctive fluoxetine influence the post-hospital course of anorexia nervosa?: a 24-month prospective, longitudinal follow-up and comparison with historical control. *Psychopharmacol Bull* 1997; **33**: 425–31.

Strober M, Pataki C, Freeman R, DeAntonio M. No effect of adjunctive fluoxetine on eating behavior or weight phobia during the inpatient treatment of anorexia nervosa: an historical case-control study. *J Child Adolesc Psychopharmacol* 1999; **9**: 195–201.

Stunkard A, Berkowitz R, Tanrikut C, et al. D-Fenfluramine treatment of binge eating disorder. *Am J Psychiatry* 1996; **153**: 1455–9.

Sullivan PF. Mortality in anorexia nervosa. *Am J Psychiatry* 1995; **152**: 1073–4.

Szmukler G, Young GP, Miller G, et al. A controlled trial of cisapride in anorexia nervosa. *Int J Eat Dis* 1995; **17**: 347–57.

Vandereycken W. Neuroleptics in the short-treatment of anorexia nervosa: a double-blind placebo-controlled study with sulpiride. *Br J Psychiatry* 1984; **144**: 288–92.

Vandereycken W, Pierloot R. Pimozide combined with behavior therapy in the short term treatment of anorexia nervosa. *Acta Psychiatr Scand* 1982; **66**: 445–50.

Walsh BT, Wilson GT, Loeb KL, et al. Medications and pyschotherapy in the treatment of bulimia nervosa. *Am J Psychiatry* 1997; **154**: 523–31.

Wilson GT, Loeb KL, Walsh BT, et al. Psychological versus pharmacological treatments of bulimia nervosa: predictors and process of change. *J Consult Clin Psychol* 1999; **67**: 451–9.

chapter 12

Pharmacotherapy of pervasive developmental disorders in children and adolescents

Gabriele Masi

Introduction

Pervasive developmental disorders (PDDs) are severe psychiatric disorders, with onset in the first 3 years of life, which typically determine marked impairments in reciprocal social interaction, communication, and cognitive development. Stereotyped behavior, interests, and activities are shared, in different ways and intensities, by the five subtypes of PDDs, that is autistic disorder, the prototypical disorder, Asperger syndrome, Rett syndrome, childhood disintegrative disorder, and PDD not otherwise specified (PDDNOS) (American Psychiatric Association, 2000).

The treatment of PDDs is comprehensive and largely based on educational techniques, behavioral management principles, and family counseling. Speech and/or psychomotor therapy and occupational therapy are often helpful. However, sometimes behavioral symptoms, particularly hyperactivity, aggression, self-injurious behaviors, ritualized or stereotyped behaviors, are so severe as to reduce the effectiveness of these interventions. The appropriate use of medications can improve some maladaptive behaviors and increase the person's ability to benefit from non-pharmacologic interventions. Furthermore, pharmacotherapy may be considered in the presence of comorbid conditions, such as anxiety disorders, mood disorders, or ADHD. Unfortunately, the clinical picture of PDDs is often so severe that other comorbid disorders are usually unrecognized and left untreated.

However, when pharmacotherapy is started, it should always be part of a multi-modal treatment plan, including psychologic and psychosocial interventions. Furthermore, appropriate targets of the pharmacologic treatment should be selected, and specifically monitored with adequate instruments, along with possible side-effects.

Several neurochemical systems are believed to be of particular relevance to the pathophysiology and drug treatment of the syndrome (Anderson and Hoshino, 1997). Investigations have principally included subjects suffering from autistic disorder, Asperger's disorder, and PDDNOS. Because most biologic research in the pathophysiology of autism to date has implicated serotonin (5HT) and, to some extent, dopamine (DA) neuronal dysfunction, drugs acting on these systems have been more frquently used and they will be the principal focus of this review. However, to date, given that the neurochemical basis of PDD is largely unknown, there is no room for a pharmacotherapy based on a pathogenic core deficit. Other drugs which have been studied in PDD populations will be briefly analyzed. This chapter will address the available literature on children and adolescents with PDDs. Data on adults will be considered only when included in samples with children and/or adolescents, and when the mean age of the participants in the studies is less than 18 years.

Subtypes of pervasive developmental disorders

Five subtypes of PDD are listed in the DSM-IV-TR: autistic disorder, Rett's syndrome, childhood disintegrative disorder, Asperger's syndrome, and PDD not otherwise specified (PDDNOS). Clinical features of these disorders will be briefly summarized. However, most of the available treatment studies do not consider specific subtypes of PDDs, and they have included mixed samples of subjects with autistic disorder, Asperger's disorder, and PDDNOS. Studies addressing the pharmacotherapy of Rett's disorder and childhood disintegrative disorder are extremely rare.

Autistic disorder

The essential feature of autistic disorder is a markedly abnormal or impaired development in social interaction and communication, and a markedly restricted repertoire of activity and interests. The impaired social interaction includes the restricted use of multiple non-verbal behaviors (eye-to-eye gaze, facial expression, body postures, and gestures), the failure to develop peer relationships appropriate to the developmental level (ranging from a lack of interest in establishing friendships to a lack of understanding of the conventions of social interaction), and the lack of spontaneous seeking to share emotions, feelings, or interests with other people. The impaired communication includes spoken language, which may be absent, or grossly atypical, stereotyped, and repetitive (e.g. repeating jingles or commercials), echolalic, idiosyncratic, or abnormal in terms of intonation, rate, and rhythm. When speech is adequate, it is characterized by a gross inability to initiate or to sustain a conversation with others. Symbolic and imaginative play or social imitation play is also markedly impaired.

The restricted pattern of behavior, interests, and activities includes an abnormal (in terms of intensity and focus) preoccupation with one or a few stereotyped and restricted patterns of interests, an inflexible adherence to non-functional routines, stereotyped body movements or mannerisms, including the hands (clapping, finger flicking) or the whole body (rocking, swaying, walking on tiptoe), or a persistent fascination with parts of objects (buttons, wheels of toys), or movements (electric fan or other rapidly revolving objects). The subjects often insist on sameness, and they show a marked distress after apparently trivial changes. The impairment in social interaction, and/or language, and/or symbolic and imaginative play must be manifest prior to age 3 years, usually without a clear period of normal development. In approximately 75% of the cases there is an associated diagnosis of mental retardation, although sometimes specific areas of functioning (e.g. memory) may be abnormally developed. Severe behavioral disorders may be associated, including impulsivity, aggressiveness, self-injurious behaviors, as well as abnormalities of mood and affects, or of eating and sleeping.

Autistic disorder is considered a rare disorder, with a suggested prevalence rate of 2–5 cases per 10 000 individuals, with numbers expanding to 10–20 per 10 000 when broader definitions are considered. It is four to five times more frequent in males.

Rett's syndrome

The essential feature of Rett's syndrome is the development of multiple specific deficits following a period of normal development in the prenatal and perinatal period and in the first 5 months of life. Between the ages of 5 and 48 months the head circumference, which was normal at birth, begins to decrease its growth. A progressive, massive loss of previously acquired hand skills is evident, often associated with stereotyped hand movements resembling hand-wringing or hand-washing, and with gross problems in the coordination of gait and trunk movements. Interest in the social environment rapidly decreases during the first years of life, both expressive and receptive language are severely impaired, and typically a severe or profound mental retardation is associated. There is an increased frequency of EEG abnormalities and seizures. The course of the disorder is lifelong, and the loss of skills persistent and progressive.

Rett's disorder is considered much less common than the autistic disorder, and has been reported only in females. A mutation in the gene encoding X-linked methyl-CpG-binding protein 2 (MECP2) has been identified as the cause of some cases of Rett's disorder.

Childhood disintegrative disorder

The characteristic feature of the childhood disintegrative disorder is an insidious or abrupt regression in multiple areas of functioning after a period of at least 2 years of normal development, in terms of verbal and non-verbal communication, social relationships, play, and adaptive behavior. After the first 2 years of life (but before age 10 years) a significant loss of previously acquired skills in at least two of the following areas is evident: expressive or receptive language, social skills or adaptive behavior, bowel or bladder control, play or motor skills. Social and communicative deficits are similar to those observed in autistic disorder. A mental retardation is usually associated, as well as various non-specific neurologic signs, and only a limited improvement may occur. When the disorder is associated with a progressive neurologic condition, the loss of skills is progressive. Suggested prevalence rates are much lower than in autistic disorder, and more common among males.

Asperger's syndrome

The essential features of Asperger's syndrome, a severe and sustained impairment in social interaction, and the development of restricted, repetitive patterns of behavior, interests, and activities, are similar to those of the autistic disorder. In contrast to autistic disorder, no significant delays are evident in language, in cognitive development, in age-appropriate self-help skills, and in adaptive behavior, other than in social interaction.

Usually Asperger's syndrome is recognized later than autistic disorder. Motor delays or clumsiness are often noted in the preschool years, as well as an early language development, with sophisticated, adult-like words, and atypicalities and oddities in the tone of voice or rate or rhythm of the speech. Idiosyncratic or circumscribed interests typically appear or are recognized during the school years. As adolescents and adults, these subjects have persisting problems with empathy and modulation of social interaction.

No clear data about the prevalence of Asperger's syndrome are available.

Pervasive developmental disorders not otherwise specified (PDDNOS)

PDDNOS shoud be diagnosed when impairments of social interaction and of verbal and non-verbal communication, stereotyped interests, and behaviors are present, but the criteria for a specific PDD are not met. This category includes forms which can be considered atypical in terms of age at onset, and/or symptomatology, and/or subthreshold severity.

Medications in pervasive developmental disorders

Drugs acting on the serotonin system

Elevated levels of 5HT in the whole blood of autistic subjects compared to normal controls have been found in several studies (Anderson et al, 1987; Minderaa et al, 1989; Cook et al, 1990). Elevated levels of 5HT are found in about one third of the subjects, with a 25% increase with respect to normal subjects. Increased activity of the serotonin transporter of platelets and decreased binding to the 5HT2 receptor have been reported (Cook and Leventhal, 1996). However, the specificity of this finding is questionable. McBride et al (1998) reported that diagnosis, race, and pubertal status are important variables in assessing hyperserotonemia. Furthermore, high levels of 5HT were reported in non-autistic, mentally retarded individuals (Partington et al, 1973).

Further data suggest that 5HT function may be reduced in the central nervous system (CNS) of autistic patients, and the peripheral hyperserotonemia may be compensatory. Antibodies against human brain 5HT receptors were identified in the blood and cerebrospinal fluid (CSF) of a child with autism (Todd and Ciaranello, 1985), even though other studies reported inconsistent data (Yuwiler et al, 1992; Cook et al, 1993). Blunted neuroendocrine responses to pharmacologic probes of the 5-HT system have been identified in autistic children, using 5-hydroxytryptophan (Hoshino et al, 1984), and in adults, employing fenfluramine (McBride et al, 1989), compared with normal subjects, suggesting a low central tone of 5HT. Acute dietary depletion of the 5HT precursor tryptophan was associated with a worsening of aberrant behaviors in drug-free, autistic adults (McDougle et al, 1996b).

Preliminary evidence suggests that 5HT re-uptake inhibitors (SRIs), including the non-selective SRI tricyclic clomipramine and the selective SRIs (SSRIs) fluoxetine, paroxetine, sertraline, fluvoxamine, and citalopram, may be useful for reducing interfering repetitive behavior and aggression, and possibly for improving aspects of social relatedness, in some children and adolescents with autism and other PDDs. SSRIs do not affect cardiac function significantly, have a lower effect on seizure threshold than tricyclics, and are increasingly used in young PDD patients. However, definite conclusions cannot be drawn from these studies, because the great majority are uncontrolled, and the similarity of repetitive thoughts and behaviors in PDDs and in patients with obsessive-compulsive disorder is questionable (McDougle et al, 1995).

Conventional antipsychotics

Scarce evidence from neurobiologic studies suggests that DA function may be dysregulated in some patients with autism. Gillberg et al (1983) found that mean basal cerebral spinal fluid concentrations of homovanillic acid (HVA), the primary metabolite of brain DA, were elevated in 13 medication-free autistic children compared with matched controls, but other studies did not confirm this finding (Anderson and Hoshino, 1997). To date, a possible role for DA in the pathophysiology of autism is prevalently supported by findings from treatment studies with DA antagonists. These studies have supported the use of neuroleptics, particularly haloperidol, in young autistic patients.

Atypical antipsychotics

A common feature of the atypical antipsychotics is the ability to produce an antipsychotic effect with a lower incidence of acute or sub-acute extrapyramidal side-effects, both in clinical and preclinical studies (little or no ability to induce catalepsy in animal models). Other (possible) clinical features include a low incidence of tardive dyskinesias with prolonged treatment, little effect on prolactin levels, superior efficacy on the negative symptoms of schizophrenia, and reduced cognitive toxicity. Whether these features are better accounted for by a relatively high ratio of 5HT2A/D2 receptor antagonism (Meltzer et al, 1989), or by a looser binding with the D2 receptor, with a transient occupation and rapid dissociation (Kapur and Seeman, 2001), or by both these mechanisms, is still a matter of debate.

It has been suggested that the negative symptoms of schizophrenia are comparable to some of the core symptoms of PDDs, mainly emotional and social withdrawal, lack of interest in social relationships, stereotyped thinking, blunted affect, lack of spontaneity, and conversation (Fisman and Steele, 1996). All these features may be ameliorated by atypical antipsychotics. To date, reports have appeared principally with risperidone and, to a lesser degree, with olanzapine, clozapine, quetiapine, and ziprasidone.

Other medications

Exogenous opioids have been found to induce socio-emotional blindness and absence of separation distress in animal models, and these phenomena were reversed by opioid receptor blockage (Panksepp, 1979). Furthermore, autistic subjects have a heightened pain threshold and frequent self-injurious behaviors, which can be found in animals in which an opioid dependence has been induced (Leboyer et al, 1992). These features have suggested that an excess of opioid system activity in the brain may contribute to the genesis of autistic symptoms (Leboyer et al, 1992). Gillberg (1995) reviewed evidence supporting high levels of beta-endorphin in autistic subjects, compared to normal controls. These findings need further support, since there is contradictory evidence of lower levels of beta-endorphin in autistic subjects (Sandman et al, 1991). The use of naloxone and naltrexone has been explored in autistic children on the basis of these considerations.

Based on the hypothesis of a glutamatergic component in the physiopathology of autism (Carlsson, 1998), interest in the efficacy of glutamatergic compounds like lamotrigine and amantadine in the treatment of autism has led to specific studies.

Treatment with vitamins and other nutritional agents has been repeatedly used during the past decades. As early as 1978, Rimland and colleagues treated 16 children with autistic symptoms with vitamin B6, and even though several methodologic flaws were present in their study, further research on megavitamin therapy for autism was encouraged, without significant empirical support.

Some anecdotal evidence suggested the efficacy of secretin, a poly-peptide hormone secreted by endocrine cells in the upper small intestine and involved in the control of pancreatic exocrine function, in the social functioning of some autistic children treated for gastrointestinal problems. However, several controlled studies did not support these early findings. To date, even if research on the psychotropic effects of gastrointestinal hormones is a promising research field, findings do not support the use of secretin in the treatment of autistic symptoms.

Other medications have been used in PDDs on the basis of clinical considerations. Symptoms of attention deficit hyperactivity disorder (ADHD) are frequently reported in children with PDDs, and this has prompted the use of psychostimulants, namely methylphenidate and the alpha-adrenergics clonidine and guanfacine. Impulsivity and mood instability have also been frequently reported in PDD children and adolescents, and this has suggested the use of mood stabilizers, such as lithium and, more frequently, valproic acid. Anxiety disorders are also frequently reported, and this clinical consideration has prompted the use of buspirone, that is less disinhibiting than benzodiazepines. Niaprazine, an antagonist of histaminic H1 receptors, characterized by its sedative properties, has been found to improve sleep disorders, without the risks of behavioral activation related to the use of benzodiazepines. In the following paragraphs opiate antagonists and beta-blockers will be more deeply described. The other medications above mentioned have been considered in other chapters of this handbook; antidepressants in Chapters 3 and 4, mood stabilizers in Chapter 5 and antipsychotics in Chapter 8.

Opiate antagonists

Morphine-like substances are normally present in the CNS, and they are released principally during pain, stress, and fatigue, accounting for post-traumatic analgesia and euphoria after intense fatigue. They act through the interaction with specific receptors. Opiate antagonists block the effect of exogenous opiate (such as morphine and heroin) and endogenous opiate, such as endorphins and enkephalins. Naloxone and other parenteral opiate antagonists have long been used in the management of exogenous opiate toxicity, but some animal studies suggest that these medications may be of interest in some other mental disorders, such as hyperphagia and obesity, aggression, and emotional numbing in post-traumatic stress disorder. They have become a focus of clinical research in child psychiatry since an increased opiate activity has been proposed to underlie social and behavioral abnormalities in autism, namely self-injurious behaviors.

Two forms of opiate antagonists are used in psychiatry, parenteral naloxone and oral naltrexone, and only the latter is of interest in child psychiatry. It is variably absorbed, and it reaches its peak concentration in one hour. The mean half-life is 4 hours in adults, but it has not been well established in children.

Naltrexone is not approved for use in patients under 18 years. After a single test dose of 0.25 mg/kg per day, the starting dose should be 0.5 mg/kg per day, with a 0.5 mg/kg per day increase every week. The effective dose 1.5 mg/kg per day and the maximum dose is 2.0 mg/kg per day. Naltrexone liver toxicity has been reported in adult patients with a history of drug and alcohol abuse. However, even though liver abnormalities have not been found in autistic children taking naltrexone (Campbell et al, 1993) monitoring of liver function is recommended in these patients, and pre-existing hepatic disease should be a contraindication. For the same reason, baseline procedures should include liver function tests. Side-effects are drowsiness, anorexia, and vomiting.

Clonidine

Clonidine is an alpha-2 adrenergic agonist, which activates the presynaptic receptors, and through a negative feed-back action, results in a post-synaptic inhibition of central noradrenergic neurons, reducing hyperarousal states, with hyperactivity, impulsivity, and aggressiveness. It has been utilized in Tourette syndrome, ADHD and in behavioral symptoms of autistic and/or mentally retarded children and adolescents.

The starting dose is 0.05 mg at bedtime, with a slow increase of 0.05 mg every 3–7 days, and an optimal dose of 3–5 µg/kg/day, 3 or 4 times per day, with meals and at bedtime. It is important that clonidine be withdrawn gradually. After a treatment of at least 4 weeks, clonidine should be reduced by 0.05 mg every 3–7 days. Parents must be informed that an abrupt withdrawal is dangerous. Contraindications to clonidine use are depression in the subject or in the family history, cardiovascular disorders, and renal disease (clonidine is partly metabolized by the kidney).

Side-effects most frequently reported are sedation, mainly during the first 3–4 weeks of treatment (usually manageable decreasing the rapidity of titration), which can persist in a minority of patients, hypotension (10% decrease of systolic pressure), headache and dizziness (mainly when the titration is too fast), and gastrointestinal symptoms (in the first days of treatment).

Clonidine increases the effect of antipsychotic and anticholinergic medications. Nonsteroidal anti-inflammatory analgesics decrease the effect of clonidine. Baseline procedures are blood pressure and pulse measurements; CBC and differential, electrolytes, BUN, creatinine, liver function tests, thyroid function tests, ECG, and fasting blood glucose. Blood pressure and pulse measurement every week during the titration, and every 2 months when the dose is stabilized. Overdose with clonidine can be life-threatening.

Beta-blockers

The beta-blockers antagonize the actions of epinephrine and norepinephrine at the beta-adrenergic receptors. Two types of beta-adrenergic receptors, beta-1 and beta-2, are known, and they are largely found both in the CNS and peripherally. In the CNS, beta-1 receptors are predominant, while beta-2 receptors are prevalently found in the glia. Peripherally, beta-1 receptors stimulate heart activity (both chronotropically and inotropically), while beta-2 receptors are prevalently located in the lung and in the blood vessels, and they determine broncodilatation and vasodilatation.

The use of beta-blockers in child and adolescent psychiatry is limited to impulsive and aggressive behavior dyscontrol, while the indication in anxiety disorders is very limited, even though central and peripheral mechanisms of psychiatric effects, as well as the roles of beta-1 and beta-2 receptors, are not fully understood. Atenolol, which has a specific beta-1 activity with minimal central activity, has shown antianxiety and antiaggressive properties, while specific beta-2 agents do not have these psychiatric effects. These observations suggest that the peripheral sympatholytic activity of propranolol (e.g. on somatic effects of anxiety) may have a stronger antianxiety and antiaggressive effect, compared to the central effect. It has also been suggested that the antianxiety and antiaggressive effects may be prevalently accounted for by beta-1 receptors rather than by beta-2 receptors.

Beta-blockers differ according to receptor affinity, lipophilicity (affecting prevalent central or peripheral activity), half-life, and elimination. Propranolol and nadolol beta-bockers are non-selective, as they act on both beta-1 and beta-2 receptors, whereas atenolol and metoprolol are selective for beta-1 receptors. Propranolol and metoprolol have both central and peripheral effects, whereas atenolol and nadolol have scarce central action. Propranolol and metoprolol have a hepatic metabolism, whereas atenolol and nadolol have a mainly renal metabolism.

Little is known about the pharmacokinetics of beta-blockers in children and adolescents. Propranolol, a non-specific beta-1 and beta-2 antagonist in the brain and peripherally, is the most frequently used and investigated beta-blocker, and will be considered in this chapter. It has been used in aggressive patients with mental retardation and/or brain damage, PTSD, and somatic symptoms of anxiety disorders.

The most frequent side-effects of propranolol are a reduction of the pulse, fatigue, depression, and bronchoconstriction. Propranolol is contraindicated in patients with diabetes mellitus (beta-blockers may interfere with the normal response to hypoglycemia), asthma, cardiovascular disorders, hyperthyroidism, and depression.

Overdose with propranolol is a medical emergency, with bradycardia, hypotension, cardiac arrest, gastrointestinal symptoms, psychotic symptoms, and seizures. Propranolol is not dialyzable, so an immediate gastric evacuation is necessary. Atropine is needed for bradycardia; digitalization and diuretics can be used for cardiac failure, vasopressors (epinephrine) for hypotension, and isoproterenol and aminophylline for bronchospasm.

Interactions of propranolol are of clinical interest. Propranolol increases the effects of antipsychotics, clonidine, epinephrine, and thyroxine. Propranolol decreases the effects of insulin and oral hypoglycemia. Carbamazepine, estrogens, and non-steroidal anti-inflammatory analgesics decrease the effect of propranolol.

After documentation of cardiovascular function and baseline vital signs, the clinical use of propranolol can be started with a low dose of 10 mg/day for children, with 10 mg increments every 4 days, and 10 mg twice a day for adolescents, with 10–20 mg increments every 4 days. The therapeutic range is 10–120 mg/day for children and 20–300 mg/day for adolescents, in three doses. Monitoring of cardiovascular functioning is warranted. Gradual withdrawal is needed after a chronic treatment, reducing by 10–20 mg every 4 days, with monitoring of vital signs because of the risk of hypertension, tachycardia, and arrythmias after abrupt discontinuation.

Medications in pervasive developmental disorders: available evidence

Serotonergic medications (Table 12.1)

Clomipramine

Gordon and colleagues found clomipramine (mean dose 152 mg daily) superior to placebo and noradrenergic tricyclic desipramine in reducing some core symptoms of autism, obsessive-compulsive behaviors, and anger/uncooperativeness, assessed with the Child Psychiatric Rating Scale (CPRS) and the Clinical Global Impression (CGI) scale in a 10-week, double-blind, crossover study of 24 children and adolescents with autistic disorder (Gordon et al, 1993). Clomipramine and desipramine were similar in reducing hyperactivity. Adverse effects were a prolongation of the QT interval on the ECG, tachycardia, and grand mal seizures. Some studies suggest that children may tolerate clomipramine less well than adults, being more prone to cardiac side-effects (Biederman et al, 1993). Furthermore, two studies suggest that children with PDDs are less responsive to clomipramine than adults, and show an increased risk of seizure and exacerbation of agitation and aggressiveness (Brasic et al, 1994; Sanchez et al, 1996). Finally, a direct comparison of clomipramine–haloperidol (main dose 128 mg/day and 1.3 mg/day, respectively) and placebo in a double-blind, cross-over study in 36 autistic patients, prevalently adolescents (age range 10–36 years, mean 16.3 years), showed that the efficacy of clomipramine was similar to haloperidol in autistic symptoms, assessed with the Children Autism Rating Scale (CARS), and not better tolerated (only 37.5% of the patients receiving clomipramine completed the trial, due to adverse effects, lack of efficacy, and behavioral activation) (Remington et al, 2001). Because of this side-effect and efficacy profile, clomipramine is not currently a first-line medication in the pediatric population with PDDs.

Fluoxetine

Fluoxetine (10–80 mg/day) was given openly to 23 autistic subjects (age range 7–28 years, mean age 15.9 years) and was effective in 15 patients, based on the Clinical Global Impression – Improvement (CGI-I) score 1 or 2 (very much or much improved), with moderate side-effects (behavioral activation in 6 of 23 subjects) (Cook et al, 1992). Fatemi et al (1998) reported significant improvement of irritability, lethargy, and stereotypy, assessed with the Aberrant Behavior Checklist (ABC), in seven autistic adolescents (age range 9–20 years, mean age 16 years) after fluoxetine treatment (mean dose 37 mg/day, range 20–80 mg/day) over a mean duration of 18 months (range 1.3–32 months). More recently, DeLong and coworkers have treated 37 autistic children (ages 2.25 to 7.75 years) with fluoxetine (0.2–1.4 mg/kg per day), with excellent response in 11 subjects and good response in the other 11, mainly in behavioral, cognitive, and affective areas (DeLong et al, 1998). Hyperactivity, aggression, and agitation were the most frequent reasons for discontinuation. Interestingly, the main predictor of good response was a familial history of affective disorders. These findings have been confirmed by the same research group in an extension of the previous study, involving 129 autistic children (aged 2 to 8 years) (DeLong et al, 2002). Fluoxetine (0.15–0.5 mg/kg) was given for 5–76 months (mean 32 to 36 months), with excellent response in 22 subjects (17%), good response in 67 (52%), and fair/poor response in 40 (31%). Treatment response highly correlated with familial major affective disorder (mainly bipolar disorder) and unusual intellectual achievement (defined as exceptional abilities and achievements requiring systematic organization of large amounts of information that is emotionally neutral, mostly in scientific fields) and, in the affected children, with hyperlexia. Five children (treated for more than 3 years) developed a bipolar disorder during the treatment.

Citalopram

Two studies describe the efficacy and tolerability of citalopram in PDDs. Couturier and Nicolson (2002) retrospectively assessed efficacy of treatment with citalopram (5–40 mg, mean dose 19.7±7 mg) in 17 patients (4–15 years, mean age 9.4±2.9 years). Ten patients (59%) were considered responders according to the CGI-I, in behavioral and anxiety symptoms, even though social relatedness did not improve significantly. Namerow and colleagues (2003) reviewed the medical charts of 15 subjects (aged 6–16 years) with PDDs treated with citalopram (16.9±12.1 mg) for 218±167 days. Eleven subjects were improved on the last-visit CGI, with greater improvements in anxiety and mood symptoms, and good tolerability.

Sertraline

A decrease in anxiety symptoms, irritability, and need for sameness has been reported in a case series of nine autistic children treated for 2–8 weeks with a low dose of sertraline (25–50 mg daily) (Steingard et al, 1997). However, three of the eight responders had a recurrence of symptoms after 3–7 months. Two patients showed behavioral activation when sertraline dosage was increased to 75 mg/day, suggesting a possible dose effect.

Fluvoxamine

Promising results from a placebo-controlled study in autistic adults treated with fluvoxamine (McDougle et al, 1996a) were not confirmed in a 12-week, double-blind, placebo-controlled study in 34 PDD children and adolescents from the same research group; the medication was poorly effective (only one of the 18 treated patients was significantly improved) and many subjects had significant side-effects (insomnia, hyperactivity, agitation, aggression) (McDougle et al, 2000). Developmental differences in the 5-HT system across the life-span, as well as specific features of serotonergic function in autistic patients, may affect efficacy and tolerability of SSRIs in younger patients. According to the findings of Chugani et al (1999), humans show a period of high brain serotonin synthesis capacity during childhood (more than 200% of adult values until the age of 5 years, then declining to adult levels), but this process is disrupted in autistic children.

Escitalopram

Escitalopram is the pure S-enantiomer of citalopram and shares similar pharmacological activity with the racemic parent compound, but at half the dose of citalopram. An open trial assessed the efficacy of escitalopram (up to 20mg/day) in 28 subject with PDD (mean age 10 years) (Owley et al, 2005). A significant improvement in the subscales of the Aberrant Behavior Checklist – Community Version (including the irritability subscale) and in the Clinical Global Impression – Severity score. A wide variability of dose was found, and 25% of the participants did not tolerate a 10 mg/day dose.

Paroxetine

Two case reports describe the effects of paroxetine in children and adolescents with autism. A 15-year high-functioning autistic adolescent improved his self-injurious behaviors after treatment with paroxetine (20 mg/day) (Snead et al, 1994). A 7-year-old autistic boy was treated with paroxetine (10 mg/day) and an improvement in irritability and temper tantrums was seen, but an attempt to increase the dosage lead to the emergence of aggression and agitation (Posey et al, 1999a).

Newer antidepressants with dual serotonergic-noradrenergic action

More recently, newer antidepressants with a dual action, on both serotonin and norepinephrine, but without the cholinergic, histaminergic, and alpha-adrenergic effects of tricyclics, have been marketed. The noradrenergic action may improve hyperactive and inattentive symptoms, which are frequently associated with the core PDD symptomatology. Venlafaxine and mirtazapine share these serotonergic and noradrenergic properties, with different mechanisms of action (inhibition of monoamine reuptake for venlafaxine, blockade of serotonergic and noradrenergic autoreceptors for mirtazapine). Hollander and colleagues (2000) treated 10 consecutive PDD patients (age range 3–21 years, mean age 10.46 years) with venlafaxine (starting dose 12.5 mg/day, with flexible increases). Six subjects were considered responders at low dosages of medication (mean 24.37 mg/day, range 6.25–50 mg), based on the CGI-I score 1 or 2 (very much or much improved). As well as a decrease in repetitive behaviors and restricted interests, social and communication deficits (also reported in treatment with SSRIs), hyperactivity and inattention improved as well. Side-effects included mild behavioral activation.

Posey and colleagues (2001b) explored the efficacy and tolerability of mirtazapine (mean dose 30.3 mg/day, range 7.5–45 mg) in 26 subjects with PDDs (age range 3.8–23.5 years, mean age 10.1 years), 17 of whom were taking other psychotropic medications. Nine subjects (34.6%) showed a good clinical response, assessed with the CGI-I, with a significant improvement in aggression, self-injury, irritability, hyperactivity, anxiety, and depression. Core symptoms of social and communication impairment were not affected by the treatment. Increased appetite, mild transient sedation, and irritability were the most frequently reported side-effects.

Conventional antipsychotics

The high-potency antipsychotic haloperidol, with a DA (D2) receptor antagonism, has been extensively studied in controlled trials in children with autism. A seminal placebo-controlled, randomized study by Campbell et al (1978) showed the efficacy of haloperidol to a maximum of 4 mg/day (mean optimal dose was 1.65 mg/day) in a 12-week study in 40 hospitalized autistic children, aged 2.6 to 7.2 years (mean 4.5 years). Haloperidol treatment was associated with an improvement in stereotypies and withdrawal, but 12 children experienced dose-dependent sedation and two had acute dystonic reactions. In another study from the same research group, Anderson et al (1984) found that haloperidol (maximum dose 4.0 mg/day, optimal dose 1.1 mg/day) improved withdrawal, stereotypies, hyperactivity, abnormal object relationships, negativism, angry affect, and lability of mood, together with discrimination learning in a structured laboratory setting. Acute dystonic reactions occurred in 11 children. A third controlled investigation with lower doses of haloperidol (mean optimal dose 0.8 mg/day) in 45 autistic children showed a significant decrease in hyperactivity, temper tantrums, withdrawal, and stereotypies, and an increase in social relatedness, with fewer side-effects (Anderson et al, 1989).

Because long-term medication is often needed in severely affected autistic children, Perry et al (1998) studied the effects of haloperidol

(0.5 to 4.0 mg/day, mean optimal dose 1.23 mg/day) given for 6 months in 60 children with autism. A positive response to treatment was seen in 71.5% of the children, 20% showing no improvement, and 8.5% worsening. Twelve children developed haloperidol-related dyskinesias, three during administration and nine upon discontinuation.

A prospective, longitudinal study specifically addressed the occurrence of drug-related dyskinesias in 118 PDD patients during treatment with haloperidol (mean daily dose 1.75 mg) (Campbell et al, 1997). The mean duration of treatment was 708.4 days (range 25 to 3610 days). Forty children (33.9%) developed withdrawal dyskinesias, and nine developed tardive dyskinesia.

Pimozide, another DA receptor antagonist, was investigated in a multi-center, double-blind, cross-over study with haloperidol and placebo in children with behavior disorder aged from 3 to 16 years, including 34 autistic children (Naruse et al, 1982). At doses ranging from 1 to 9 mg/day, pimozide treatment improved aggression against persons and objects, but not self-injurious behaviors.

In summary, controlled and open-label studies show that haloperidol can significantly improve maladaptive behaviors in children and adolescents with autism. However, given the frequency of acute and withdrawal-related dyskinesias, as well as of cognitive toxicity, safer agents, such as the new atypical antipsychotics (clozapine, risperidone, olanzapine, quetiapine, and ziprasidone) have been studied in individuals with autism and other PDDs.

Atypical antipsychotics

Risperidone

Risperidone is currently the atypical antipsychotic most frequently used in PDD patients. Two controlled studies of risperidone have been published in individuals with autism and related PDDs, one in adult patients (McDougle et al, 1998), the other in children and adolescents (Research Unit on Pediatric Psychopharmacology, 2002). In the latter multi-site, double-blind, placebo-controlled study, 101 children and adolescents (age range 5–17 years, mean age 8.8 years) were randomized to receive risperidone (dose range 0.5 to 3.5 mg/daily) or placebo for 8 weeks. Based on the CGI-I and the Aberrant Behavior Checklist (ABC) Irritability score, 69% of the patients in the risperidone group and 12% in the placebo group were responders at week 8. At the sixth month, the rate of responders decreased to 47%. Irritability, hyperactivity, and stereotypies were more sensitive to treatment than social withdrawal and inappropriate speech. Increased appetite and weight gain (2.7±2.9 kg), fatigue, and drowsiness were the most commonly reported side-effects. In the expansions of this study (Research Units on Pediatric Psychopharmacology Autism Network, 2005; McDougle et al, 2005) risperidone was given openly for 4 months to 63 children at a mean dose of 1.96 mg/day, with a persistent efficacy and good tolerability (5 patients discontinued for loss of efficacy and one for adverse effects). Improvement was evident not only in the primary measures (Aberrant Behavior Checklist, irritability subscale, and CGI-Improvement score), but also in Ritvo-Freeman Real Life Rating Scale, in the Vineland Adaptive Behavior Scale, and in the Children's Yale-Brown Obsessive Compulsive Scale. However, no statistical significance was found in the social relatedness and language subscales of the Ritvo-Freeman Scale, suggesting that the social and communicative dimensions are more resistant to this pharmacological treatment. In 36 patients risperidone was blindly withdrawn, and replaced with placebo. The relapse rates were 62.5% with placebo and 12.5% with risperidone.

Multiple open-label reports of risperidone in PDD children and adolescents are available (Fisman and Steele, 1996; Hardan et al, 1996; Perry et al, 1997; Findling et al, 1997; McDougle et al, 1997; Nicolson et al, 1998; Zuddas et al, 2000; Malone et al, 2002), and some of the studies with larger samples will be presented in this review. In a case series of 14 young patients with PDD, 13 improved according to the Children's Global Assessment Scale (CGAS). Improvement was seen in aggression, agitation, social relatedness, concentration, anxiety, and obsessive symptoms (Fisman and Steele, 1996). Risperidone dosages ranged from 0.75 to 1.5 mg/day. Medication was well tolerated, and 10 of 14 patients maintained on risperidone monotherapy.

McDougle et al (1997) described a 12-week, prospective, open-label trial of risperidone (mean dose 1.8 mg/day) in 18 children and adolescents with autism and other PDDs (mean age 10.2±3.7 years). Based on the CGI-I score 1 or 2, 12/18 patients were considered responders. Significant improvement was seen in repetitive behavior, aggression, impulsivity, and in some aspects of social relatedness. The most significant side-effect (12/18 patients) was weight gain (range 3.7 to 13 kg; mean±SD: 6.6/2.8 kg).

Nicolson et al (1998) reported a 12-week, open-label trial of risperidone in 10 autistic children, aged 4.5 to 10.8 years. The mean final dose of risperidone was 1.3 mg/day, with a range of 1–2.5 mg/day. On the basis of the CGI-I, 8 out of 10 children were considered responders. Transient sedation was common, and the children gained an average of 3.5 kg.

Two studies consider the longer-term efficacy and safety of risperidone treatment. Zuddas and colleagues (2000) investigated the 6-month effect of risperidone treatment (dose range 1–6 mg/day) in 11 PDD patients (mean age 12.3±3.8 years). One patient worsened after 4 weeks (repetitive phenomena and fidgetiness) and dropped out. All the remaining 10 subjects were responders at the sixth month ("much improved" on the CGI-I), even though the core symptoms of social relatedness were less sensitive to change than hyperactivity and uncooperativeness. In the seven subjects who continued risperidone treatment for a further 6-month period, the benefit was maintained at 12 months. Three patients who discontinued at the sixth month worsened significantly. Weight gain was observed in six subjects, with an average gain of 7.2 kg at the sixth month.

Malone and colleagues (2002) treated 22 autistic outpatients (range 2.9–16.3 years, mean age 7.1 years) with risperidone (mean dosage 1.2 mg/day, range 0.5 to 2.5 mg/daily) for one month. Seventeen subjects (77.3%) were responders. (CGI-I 1 or 2). Eleven of these subjects completed a 6-month risperidone treatment, and 10 of them were much or very much improved on the CGI-I. Increased appetite occurred in 31.8% of participants, and persisted in the long term, and the weight gain was 2.7±1.4 kg. Thereafter, medication was discontinued, and the need for further drug treatment was reassessed. All the subjects had a worsening of their symptoms within 2 weeks of stopping risperidone. Two subjects developed withdrawal dyskinesia at drug discontinuation.

Although PDDs begin in the first 3 years of life, and a timely effective treatment (both psychosocial and pharmacologic) may help improve prognosis, only sparse data are available on pharmacologic treatments in preschool children. Psychopharmacology of preschool patients is increasingly considered a major topic of current research, even though several specific questions are largely unmet, including the paucity of information about the pharmacodynamic effect of drugs on the developing brain (Vitiello, 1998; Greenhill et al, 2003). Casaer et al (1994) reported a preliminary investigation on pharmacokinetics and safety (but not efficacy) of risperidone in six young autistic children (mean age 4.7), who received a single oral dose of the drug at 0.015 mg/kg daily (three subjects) or 0.030 mg/kg daily (three subjects). The medication was well tolerated, although five children had dose-related somnolence (Caesar et al, 1994). Other sparse data on preschoolers are available in the literature (Demb, 1996; Findling et al, 1997; McDougle et al, 1997; Nicolson et al, 1998; Schwamm et al, 1998; Posey et al, 1999b; Masi et al, 2001). The younger autistic patients treated with risperidone have been described by Posey et al (1999b). Two autistic children aged 29 and 23 months showed a significant behavioral improvement after risperidone (0.25 mg twice daily, one subject slowly increased to 1.25 during the following year).

Masi et al (2001) described the efficacy and tolerability of risperidone treatment in 24 children aged 3.6–6.6 years (mean 4.6 years) in a 16-week, open-label trial. Maximum risperidone dosage was 0.04 mg/kg daily. Two subjects did not complete the study due to side-effects (tachycardia in one subject, sedation and reduced appetite in the other). According to both a 25% improvement in the CPRS and a CGI-I score of 1 or 2, eight subjects (36.4%) were responders. Hyperactivity and lability of affect were more sensitive to treatment than social interaction. Risperidone was well tolerated; 13 subjects (54.1%) did not show any side-effect, and only three patients had a weight gain of more than 10%. Masi and colleagues have recently reported on the expansion of the previous study, describing systematic data from a 3-year naturalistic study on 53 PDD preschool children (age range 3.5 to 6.6 years, mean 4.6 years) (Masi et al, 2003). The patients received risperidone (maximum dose 1 mg/day) for a period ranging from 1 to 32 months (mean 7.9±6.8 months). Twenty-five patients (47.1%) are still receiving risperidone, while 28 (52.9%) discontinued, due to side-effects (22.6%), parents' choice (18.8%), lack of efficacy (5.6%), or decision of the treating psychiatrist (5.6%). Based on both an improvement of 25% at CPRS and a score of 1 or 2 in the CGI-I, 46.8% of the subjects were considered responders. Behavioral disorders and affect dysregulation were more sensitive to treatment than interpersonal functioning. Responders received higher doses of medication, for a longer period, and had a greater weight gain than non-responders. Increased prolactin levels without clinical signs and increased appetite were the most frequent side-effects.

Olanzapine

Three open-label studies (Potenza et al, 1999; Malone et al, 2001; Kemner et al, 2002) and several anecdotal case reports (Horrigan et al, 1997; Rubin 1997; Malek-Ahmadi et al, 1998) have described the clinical effects of the atypical antipsychotic olanzapine in patients with PDDs. The three studies will be described in more detail. A pilot study examined the efficacy and safety of olanzapine treatment in eight patients (age range 5 to 42 years) with autism and other PDDs (Potenza et al, 1999). Seven patients completed a 12-week open-label study, and six were responders based upon the CGI-I, with a mean dose of 7.8 ± 4.7 mg/day (range 5–20 mg/day). Social relatedness, lability of affect, language usage, self-injurious behavior, hyperactivity, and aggression significantly improved, as well as anxiety and depression. Improvement in repetitive behaviors did not occur. All four children and adolescents in the sample improved in core and associated symptoms of PDD, but two of them discontinued olanzapine due to weight gain.

Subsequently, Malone and colleagues (2001) compared olanzapine and haloperidol, openly randomizing 12 autistic children (mean age 7.8 ± 2.1 years) for 6 weeks into two treatment groups (final dosage of olanzapine 7.9 ± 2.5 mg/day, final dosage of haloperidol 1.4 ± 0.7 mg/day). Patients from both groups improved in their symptomatology; five out of six in the olanzapine group, and three out of six in the haloperidol group were responders according to the CGI-I score. Weight gain was significantly higher in the olanzapine group.

Finally, Kemner et al (2002) openly explored the efficacy and tolerability of olanzapine (final mean dose 10.7 mg/day) in 25 children and adolescents (age range 6 to 16 years). Twenty-three subjects completed the study and showed a significant improvement in irritability, hyperactivity, excessive speech, and in some autistic symptoms, assessed by the Aberrant Behavior Checklist. However, only three subjects were responders according to CGI-I scores. Increased appetite and weight gain were the most frequent side-effects, and three subjects showed extrapyramidal symptoms, which disappeared after the dosage was reduced.

Quetiapine

Quetiapine is an atypical antipsychotic with a clozapine-like neurochemical profile and a lower risk for seizures and no need for blood monitoring. Four reports of quetiapine in the treatment of children with PDDs are available. Six subjects with autism and mental retardation (mean age 10.9 ± 3.3 years) participated in a 16-week, open-label study of quetiapine (mean daily dose 225 ± 108 mg, range 100–350 mg/day), but only two subjects completed the trial and were considered responders, based on the CGI-I, and only one continued to benefit from long-term treatment (Martin et al, 1999). There was no statistically significant improvement during the study for the group on various rating scales. Sedation, behavioral activation, increased appetite, and weight gain (range 0.9 to 8.2 kg) were reported, and one subject had a possible seizure. The small sample size limits definite conclusions.

Corson et al (2004) examined efficacy and safety of quetiapine (mean dose 248.7 ± 198.4 mg/day, range 25–600 mg/day) for aggressiveness, hyperactivity, and self-injurious behaviors of 20 patients (age range 5–28 years, mean 12.1 ± 6.7 years). Eight patients (40%) were considered responders, but the mean CGI-I score was 3.0 ± 1.1 (minimally improved) suggesting a modest effect on maladaptive behaviors. Three subjects (15%) discontinued for side effects.

Findling et al (2004) examined the effectiveness of quetiapine (300 mg/day) in 9 autistic adolescents in a 12-week, open-label study. One two patients met the criteria for responders (much or very much improved) and continued the treatment after the end of the study.

Harden et al (2005) assessed efficacy and tolerability of quetiapine (477 ± 212 mg) in 12 young patients (12 ± 5.1 years) with PDD. Six patients were considered responders based on impression from chart review and Conners Parent Scale (conduct, inattention, and hyperactivity subscales). Mild sedation was the most frequent side-effect.

Ziprasidone

McDougle and coworkers (2002) reported a preliminary evaluation on efficacy and tolerability of ziprasidone in 12 patients with PDDs (age range 8–20 years, mean age 11.6 ± 4.4 years). The mean duration of treatment was 14.2 weeks (range 6–30 weeks) and the final dosage was 59.2 mg/day (range 20–120 mg). Six (50%) of the patients were considered responders according to the CGI-I. Mild sedation was the most frequent side-effect. No significant weight gain and cardiovascular effects were observed during the treatment.

Aripiprazole

Preliminary data on efficacy of aripiprazole in children with PDD are reported by Stigler et al (2004). Five youths (mean age 12 years) received aripiprazole (mean 12 mg/day, range 10–15 mg/day) for at least 8 weeks. All the patients were considered responders according to a CGI-I score 1 or 2. Mild somnolence and weight loss (probably due to discontinuation of atypical antipsychotics) were the most frequent side-effects.

Clozapine

Only a few reports on the use of clozapine in children and adolescents with autism are available in the literature. The first described three children (8–12 years) with marked hyperactivity, fidgetiness, or aggression who did not benefit from typical antipsychotics (Zuddas et al, 1996). Children's Psychiatric Rating Scale (CPRS) scores improved by 19, 35, and 39%, respectively, after 3 months' treatment at dosages up to 200 mg/day, but one patient returned to pretreatment values after 5 months with higher dosages of clozapine (up to 450 mg/day). The second report describes the case of a 17-year-old adolescent with autism and mental retardation, who showed a significant reduction in aggression, hyperactivity, and repetitive motions after clozapine treatment (275 mg/day) (Chen et al, 2001). The risk of agranulocytosis and seizures, as well as the frequent blood draws, accounts for the scarcity of reports in children with PDDs.

Other medications

Opioid antagonists

On the basis of the above mentioned findings, the opioid antagonist naltrexone has been investigated as a potential treatment for self-injurious behavior, social deficits, and aggressiveness. Controlled studies failed to confirm efficacy (Willemsen-Swinkles et al, 1996), or reported transient and moderate results on hyperactivity, and even though the medication is usually well tolerated, in some subjects there was a worsening of behavioral symptomatology and stereotypies (Campbell et al, 1993; Kolmen et al, 1995).

Percy et al (1994) have found that naltrexone was associated with a more rapid decline in motor function and a more rapid progression of the disorder in 10 patients with Rett syndrome. Thus naltrexone is contraindicated in this disorder.

Clonidine and guanfacine

The alpha-adrenergic medication clonidine, usually used in subjects with hyperactivity and impulsivity, has been used in a small double-blind, placebo-controlled, cross-over study in eight autistic children, with mixed results (efficacy according to teachers' and parents' ratings with the Conners scales, but not according to clinicians' ratings of videotaped observations) (Jaselskis et al, 1992). Transdermal clonidine was effective in a double-blind, placebo-controlled, cross-over study in nine autistic subjects (5 to 33 years, mean age 12.9 years), improving hyperactivity, anxiety, and global functioning (Ritvo–Freeman Real Life Rating Scale and CGI-I) (Fankhauser et al, 1992). Hypotension, fatigue, and sedation are frequent side-effects. Furthermore, many patients tend to develop tolerance to the positive effects of clonidine during the first months of treatment.

The efficacy of guanfacine in 80 PDD children and adolescents (age range 3–18 years, mean 7.7 years) has been retrospectively assessed by Posey and coworkers (Posey et al, 2001a). At a mean dose of 2.6 mg/day (range 0.25–9 mg) 19 subjects (23.8%) were responders according to the CGI score, with significant improvement in hyperactivity, inattention, insomnia, and tics. Subjects with Asperger's syndrome or PDDNOS demonstrated greater improvement.

Psychostimulants

Symptoms of ADHD are frequently reported in children with PDDs. Methylphenidate (dose 10 or 20 mg bid for 2 weeks) has been used in a double-blind, placebo-controlled, cross-over study of 10 autistic children (age range 7–11 years, mean 8.5 years) resulting in a significant reduction in hyperactivity and irritability, according to the Conners' Teacher Questionnaire (Quintana et al, 1995). Frequent side-effects, mainly agitation, irritability, aggressiveness, and sleep disorders, were more often reported in subjects with severe mental retardation (Aman et al, 1991).

More recently, 13 children with autism and symptoms of ADHD participated in a double-blind, placebo-controlled, cross-over study of methylphenidate (0.3 and 0.6 mg/kg dose) (Handen et al, 2000). Eight patients were considered responders, based on a reduction of at least 50% of the Conners Hyperactivity Index. However, scores on the Childhood Autism Rating Scales, which assess severity in global autistic symptoms, did not change. Furthermore, significant side-effects occurred during the treatment, mainly at 0.6 mg/kg dose, including irritability and social withdrawal. More recently, Di Martino and colleagues (2004) investigated the effects of methylphenidate in 13 subjects with PDD. Five patients showed increased hyperactivity, stereotypies, and dysphoria one hour after the first dose and did not receive further methylphenidate. Eight subjects received a 12-week open trial. Two of them remained unchanged, and discontinued the treatment after one week of the maximally tolerated doses. The other eight patients significantly improved behavioral measures of hyperactivity and impulsivity, without significant changes in autistic features. No significant adverse effects were observed in the subjects who completed the study.

Mood stabilizers

An emerging literature documents the co-occurrence of mania in children with PDDs, suggesting that up to 21% of PDD children may also meet criteria for mania (Wozniak et al, 1997). Identification of this comorbidity may have important therapeutic and theoretic implications, at least for a subgroup of autistic disorder related to bipolar disorder, in terms of occurrence of manic symptoms, extreme hyperactivity non-responsive to stimulants, cyclic component of symptomatic behaviors, and/or family history of bipolar disorder. Lithium carbonate has been seldom used in subjects with co-occurrence of autistic and manic symptoms (Kerbeshian et al, 1987; Steingard et al, 1987). More recently, a lithium augmentation of fluvoxamine in a patient with autistic disorder determined a significant improvement in aggression and impulsivity (Epperson et al, 1994).

Hollander and colleagues openly assessed the efficacy of divalproex sodium (mean dose 768 mg/day, range 125–2500 mg, mean blood level 75.8 µg/ml) in 14 PDD patients (age range 5–40, mean 17.9 years) (Hollander et al, 2001). Ten patients (71%) resulted responders, according to the CGI-I score. Core symptoms of autism, as well as impulsivity and aggression, improved during treatment.

Uvebrant and Bauziene (1994) treated with the anticonvulsant, lamotrigine, 13 young patients with autism and treatment-refractory epilepsy. Eight of these patients significantly improved their autistic symptoms. This finding has not been confirmed in a more recent double-blind study with lamotrigine (Belsito et al, 2001). Fourteen autistic children (age range 3–11 years, mean 5.8 years) received lamotrigine (5 mg/kg per day) for 4 weeks, without any significant difference from a placebo group, according to the Autism Behavior Checklist, ABC, Vineland scales, and CARS.

Buspirone

Buspirone is a serotonergic 5-HT1A partial agonist, with affinity for dopaminergic receptors, which is currently used in the treatment of anxiety disorders. Given its positive side-effect profile, it has been used, at dosages of 15–45 mg/day, as an adjuvant in the treatment of anxiety disorders in 22 subjects (6 to 17 years) with mental retardation and PDD (Buitelaar et al, 1998). Nine subjects had a marked improvement and seven a moderate response in the CGI-I after 6–8 weeks of treatment. Positive effects have been reported as a reduction in affective lability and decrease in anxieties and sleeping problems.

Glutamatergic compounds

Based on the hypothesis of a glutamatergic component in the physio-pathology of autism (Carlsson et al, 1998), interest in the efficacy of glutamatergic compounds like lamotrigine and amantadine in the treatment of autism has led to specific studies. Data on lamotrigine are discussed in the section on mood stabilizers (see above). The efficacy of amantadine has been assessed in a double-blind, placebo-controlled study in 39 autistic children and adolescents (age range 5–19 years, mean 7 years) (King et al, 2001). After a 1-week trial of placebo, patients were randomized to placebo or amantadine (2.5 mg/kg per day) in one daily dose for one week, then placebo or amantadine (5 mg/kg daily) in two daily doses for 3 weeks. A significant improvement in hyperactivity and inappropriate speech was found, according to the clinician-rated Aberrant Behavior Checklist – Community Version, even though the corresponding parent-rated measure failed to show any clinical effect. Amantadine was well tolerated.

Niaprazine

Niaprazine, an antagonist of histaminic H1 receptors, characterized by sedative properties, has been found to improve sleep disorders, as well as hyperactivity and behavior disorders, in 52% of 25 autistic patients, at a dose of 1 mg/kg per day for 60 days (Giovanardi Rossi et al, 1999).

Vitamins

As early as 1978, Rimland and colleagues treated with vitamin B6, 16 children with autistic symptoms (Rimland et al, 1978), and even though several methodologic flaws were present in their study, further research on megavitamin therapy for autism was encouraged. Another 12 significant papers were published up to 1995 (six of them with double-blind, placebo-controlled design), combining vitamin B6 and magnesium, and they were critically analyzed by Pfeiffer and colleagues (Pfeiffer et al, 1995). Two hundred and forty-eight subjects participated in these studies. The period of treatment ranged from 2 weeks to 8 months, the dosage of vitamin B6 was 600–1125 mg/day or 30 mg/kg per day, and the dosage of magnesium 400–500 mg or 10–15 mg/kg per day. Ten of the 12 studies reported a degree of behavioral improvement ranging from moderate to marked and two reported a significant decrease in autistic behavior, even though the outcome measures had questionable reliability and validity. Furthermore, none of the studies reported evidence beyond group data on the statistical improvement of the tests, and the rates of reponders were not available. Findling and colleagues conducted a 10-week, double-blind, placebo-controlled trial in 12 autistic children (mean age 6.6 years) with vitamin B6 (average dose 638.9mg/day) and magnesium (mean dose 216.3 mg/day) (Findling et al, 1997). Autistic behaviors, assessed by the CPRS, the CGI-I, and the NIMH Global Obsessive-Compulsive Scale, did not improve after the treatment.

Secretin

After some anecdotal reports, the first study randomized 56 children into two groups (secretin and placebo), and secretin was not superior to placebo in any of the standardized measures (Sandler et al, 1999). The second study first treated openly 56 children (mean age 6.4 years), with modest results after 3–6 weeks. The 17 best responder subjects were randomized to secretin or placebo, with a cross-over after 4 weeks (Chez et al, 2000). Differences between secretin and placebo were not significant. Dunn-Geier et al (2000) did not find significant differences in language performance and autistic behavior in 95 autistic children placed for 3 weeks in a secretin group or a placebo group. Owley and colleagues randomized 56 subjects with autistic disorder to receive secretin or placebo, and they did not find significant differences between groups according to the Autism Diagnostic Observation Schedule (ADOS) social-communication total score and other developmental measures (Owley et al, 2001). Coniglio et al (2001) assigned 60 autistic children to secretin or placebo, without significant differences in language skills and parents' behavioral assessment. Severity of autistic symptoms did not differ between groups at 6 weeks after treatment. Finally, Roberts and coworkers failed to find superiority of repeated doses of secretin (two doses, 6 weeks apart) in 64 children with autism randomly assigned to secretin or placebo (Roberts et al, 2001). Any significant therapeutic effect of secretin was found by subgrouping the patients according to intelligence level, presence or absence of diarrhea, and history of regression.

Treatment strategy

On the basis of the above literature review, some clinical guidelines can be proposed. There is no pharmacotherapy of PDDs, but a pharmacotherapy of some symptoms is possible. Thus, pharmacotherapy should be considered only when the severity of symptoms hampers other psychosocial, rehabilitative, and psychoeducational treatment programs.

Given the symptomatic nature of the pharmacologic intervention, it is not surprising that there is no consensus on the first-choice medication in PDDs, the choice being determined by the target symptoms. However, a symptom-targeted approach may be misleading, inducing a polypharmacy or an excessively changing strategy, given that autistic children often present many maladaptive symptoms. A possible strategy is to define broad symptomatologic domains which can orient a first pharmacologic approach, and at the same time to prefer medications with the broadest range of effects.

According to the first issue, four possible symptomatologic domains can be defined: impulsivity, aggression against self and others; repetitive phenomena; mood swings, temper tantrums; severe isolation with stereotypies.

According to the second issue, data from the literature suggest that atypical antipsychotics, SSRIs, and mood stabilizers present the broader spectrum of clinical effects.

According to both these criteria, when aggression or self-injurious behaviours are the target symptom, a trial with an atypical anti-psychotic (risperidone) can be started, at low doses. When repetitive phenomena are prevalent, an SSRI (fluoxetine) can be considered. When mood swings and temper tantrums are more evident, a mood stabilizer (valproic acid) can be the first choice. The pharmacologic management of severe isolation with stereotypies is more complex, this symptomatologic domain being particularly resistant to any kind of intervention, including medication. However, a trial with a low-dose atypical antipsychotic may reduce the severity of isolation and increase the effectiveness of co-administered non-pharmacologic treatments.

A careful psychiatric assessment may reveal possible comorbid con-ditions, often masked by the autistic symptomatology. These comor-bidities (anxiety, depression, bipolar disorder, ADHD) may be the target of pharmacologic treatment, according to the guiding principles exposed in the other chapters of this book.

When a treatment with an atypical antipsychotic is considered, the available evidence suggests risperidone (0.5–2 mg in children, up to 4–6 mg in adolescents) as the first choice, and olanzapine (2.5–5 mg in children, up to 20 mg in adolescents) as a possible alternative when the first trial has failed. Titration should be slow, with a lower target dose in children with severe isolation, and higher doses in children aggressive against self and others. Quetiapine should be given when risperidone or olanzapine were not effective or tolerated (especially increased appetite and weight gain).

When an SSRI is considered, fluoxetine (5–10 mg in children, up to 20–40 mg in adolescents), which is more activating, may be the first-line medication in children with lower activity, while sertraline or fluvoxamine (50–100 mg in children, up to 200 mg in adolescents) or citalopram (20 mg in children, up to 40 mg in adolescents) may be pre-ferred in patients with higher levels of agitation and restlessness. After an unsatisfying trial with an SSRI, a trial with another SSRI is possible. Alternatively, mirtazapine presents calming properties and improves sleep, while venlafaxine may be indicated when a behavioral activation is needed.

When a mood stabilizer is considered for agitation related to mood swings and anxiety, valproic acid can be considered as a first choice. Very few data are available on lithium and carbamazepine in PDDs, and the efficacy of the newer anti-epileptics, namely lamotrigine and topiramate, needs further research.

Severe sleep disorders may be managed using niaprazine, or mirtazapine or trazodone, especially when other anxiety disorders are comorbid. Benzodiazepines may determine a behavioral activation in younger patients.

When a combination of symptomatologic domains is present, only the most impairing domain should be considered with a monotherapy. Only when a trial with a single medication has been performed, with a partially positive but unsatisfying response, may an association with another medication be carefully started, monitoring possible emerging side-effects. It is important to remember that fluvoxamine, more than other SSRIs, when added to an antipsychotic, can elevate the serum levels of the antipsychotic.

The efficacy of all these treatments should be monitored after 6–8 weeks, using standardized measures. At the end of this period, a proper evaluation of risks and benefits of one or more medications used at appropriate doses for a sufficient length of time will be possible.

Practical guidelines for the management of atypical antipsychotics, SSRIs, and mood stabilizers have been described elsewhere in this book. Principal concerns are related to the use of atypical antipsychotics in children and younger adolescents. For this reason, specific recommendations on the tolerability of these medications in younger patients will follow. The principal concern with SSRIs in PDDs is the behavioral activation, which may occur during the first 1 or 2 weeks, or, more rarely, after some months. The possibility of a pharmacologic hypomania shoud be carefully considered (e.g. considering the familial history of affective disorders). In this case the medications should be rapidly discontinued.

Unfortunately, treatment non-response is not rare. After unsatisfying trials according to the above mentioned principles, alternative options, less supported by empirical evidence, can be considered. Methylphenidate and clonidine/guanfacine in ADHD-like symptoms, propranolol in explosive behavior disorders, and naltrexone in self-injurious behavior can be used as alternative or adjunctive medications, when these symptoms did not improve after treatment with the previously reported medications. This is particularly true in the case of self-injurious behavior, an extremely treatment-resistant symptom in autistic and/or mentally retarded children, which always requires a multi-modal intervention, including behavioral techniques and parental support.

When methylphenidate is used in children with PDDs, a higher rate of side-effects, including a worsening of agitation, isolation, repetitive phenomena, and stereotypies, has been reported, and this possibility should be actively monitored.

Naltrexone treatment should start with 12.5 mg twice a day for children, and 25 mg twice a day for adolescents, with possible titration after 2 weeks, up to 25 mg twice a day for children, and 50 mg twice a day for adolescents, even in association with other medications. Naltrexone is usually well tolerated.

Clonidine is contraindicated when a comorbidity with a depressive disorder is suspected, on the basis of the clinical picture and the familial history. The starting dose is 0.05 mg at bedtime, with an increase by 0.05 mg every 3–7 days, up to an optimal dose of 3–4 µg/kg per day, three or four times a day, after meals and at bedtime. Many of the patients tend to develop a tolerance to clonidine after 6–12 months. It is essential that clonidine be withdrawn gradually, especially after a chronic use, reducing by 0.05 mg every 3–7 days.

Propranolol treatment is contraindicated in patients with asthma, diabetes mellitus, cardiovascular diseases, and hypothyroidism, and a fasting blood glucose and an ECG should be performed before the treatment. A starting dose in children is 10 mg three times a day, with an increase every 3–4 days, up to 40 mg three times a day. Further increments may be considered after at least one month of treatment.

Atypical antipsychotics: data on safety

Given the increasing use of atypical antipsychotics in PDD, more information will be provided on the available data on side-effects in children and adolescents treated with these medications. Other side-effects of antipsychotics during treatment of psychotic disorders can be found in the Chapter 8.

Weight gain

Weight gain is the the most significant side-effect in all the studies on risperidone, olanzapine, and clozapine, in PDDs as well as in other psychiatric disorders. Increased appetite and weight gain are frequently reported in the subjects treated with risperidone (McDougle et al, 1997; Nicolson et al, 1998; Zuddas et al, 2000; Malone et al, 2002; Research Unit of Pediatric Psychopharmacology, 2002; Masi et al, 2003), with a mean increase in weight of 2.7 ± 2.9 kg in the double-blind study on risperidone in children and adolescents (Research Unit on Pediatric Psychopharmacology, 2002), to 7.2 kg (mean) in the long-term study (McDougle et al, 1997). Increased appetite and weight gain occurred during treatment with olanzapine in the studies by Potenza et al (1999) (about 8 kg), Malone et al (2001) (mean 3.3 kg) and Kemner et al (2002) (mean 4.7 kg).

Quetiapine and ziprasidone are reported to have a lower incidence of weight gain. However, increased appetite and body weight increase (0.9 to 8.2 kg) has been reported during quetiapine treatment in autistic children (Martin et al, 1999). In contrast, in the ziprasidone study, patients did not report increased body weight, and the change was –2.2 kg (range –13 to +2.2 kg) (McDougle et al, 2002).

This side-effect cannot be disregarded, given the increased morbidity and mortality in subjects with obesity. Furthermore, the difficult management of food craving in patients with PDDs adds further conflict in the families, reducing the compliance to treatment. Dietary recommendations and psychoeducational counseling are needed at the beginning of the treatment. A careful monitoring of weight gain, parallel to monitoring of liver functioning and glycemia, is highly recommended in all these patients. At present there is no standardized pharmacologic treatment for antipsychotic-induced weight gain (Baptista et al, 2002). Trials with amantadine, orlistat, metformin, nizatidine, and topiramate are reported in the literature on adult patients, but only topiramate has been tested anecdotally in children and adolescents (Lessig et al, 2001; Pavuluri et al, 2002).

Hyperprolactinemia

Although hyperprolactinemia is a common side-effect of antipsychotics in adult patients, scarce information is available in children and adolescents. Wudarski et al (1999) reported on prolactin levels in 35 children and adolescents with psychotic disorder (age range 9 to 19 years, mean age 14.1 years), during treatment with clozapine, olanzapine, and haloperidol. Prolactin levels did increase, but were within the normal range in all the subjects under clozapine treatment. All the patients under haloperidol treatment had an increase in prolactin above the upper limit of normal, while seven patients out of ten under olanzapine treatment showed a moderate hyperprolactinemia.

Risperidone appears to elevate prolactin levels to a greater extent than any other atypical antipsychotic. Frazier et al (1999) reported elevated prolactin levels (average level double the upper end of the normal range) in 9 of 11 patients with bipolar disorder (mean age 10.4 years) during risperidone treatment (mean dosage 1.7 ± 1.3 mg/day), but no baseline prolactin levels were available for comparison. Galactorrhea and amenorrhea, and delayed ejaculation were reported by two adolescent patients. A study specifically addressed prolactin levels during treatment with risperidone (dosage range 0.25 to 0.75 mg/day, mean dosage 0.50 mg/day) in 25 young autistic children (mean age 4.10 years) (Masi et al, 2001). Serum prolactin was 9.77 ± 3.94 ng/ml at baseline, and 25.92 ± 13.9 ng/ml at the 10th week of treatment ($P < 0.001$). Eight children (28%) had a prolactin level higher than double the upper limit (30 ng/ml). The level of prolactin did not show significant correlations with age, weight, risperidone dosage, or clinical outcome. Dose reduction of risperidone resulted in a decrease in prolactin levels. None of the children showed clinical signs of hyperprolactinemia. In the more recent 3-year naturalistic study from the same research group, data were available on 37 subjects (Masi et al, 2003). The mean prolactin level at baseline was 13.3 ± 7.8 ng/ml and the mean prolactin level at the last observation was 28.38 ± 22.45 ng/ml ($P < 0.0001$). Thirteen patients (35%) showed normal levels of prolactin (below 15 ng/ml), five (14%) had prolactin increases to between 30 and 50 ng/ml, and six (16%) had prolactin levels over 50 ng/ml. Subjects with the highest and the lowest prolactin levels did not differ according to age, drug dosage, severity scores at baseline, or weight gain. In some patients, when risperidone was newly introduced after a discontinuation due to high levels of prolactin, prolactin levels rose to a lesser degree.

The clinical implications of asymptomatic antipsychotic-induced hyperprolactinemia in young children are not clear. Data from children with prolactinomas suggest that growth arrest, osteopenia, and delayed pubertal development may be determined by enduring high levels of prolactin (Colao et al, 1998; Galli-Tsinopoulou et al, 2000). These data should be considered cautiously because prolactin levels in these patients are much higher than those normally found in children treated with antipsychotics (mean 688 ng/ml, SD 907 ng/ml in the 26 young patients described by Colao et al, 1998); furthermore, symptoms may be affected by the effect of a prolactinoma on pituitary function. Due to the lack of clear guidelines, monitoring of serum prolactin levels during treatment with risperidone is warranted. In the case of high levels of prolactin associated with a good efficacy of the treatment, a careful consideration of the risk–benefit ratio should include the switch to another atypical antipsychotic.

Extrapyramidal side-effects

Acute extrapyramidal side-effects (EPS) have been primarily observed in pediatric patients treated with risperidone, prevalently due to a higher starting dose and faster rate of dosage escalation (Mandoki, 1995). More recently, a more prudent approach to risperidone treatment, in terms of maximum dose and titration, has reduced this risk. Data from the above mentioned studies suggest that risperidone is associated with significantly milder and more transient EPS than typical antipsychotics, such as haloperidol. For example, acute dystonic reactions did not occur in the 49 patients taking risperidone in the placebo-controlled study (RUPP Autism Network, 2002), and only one of the 53 children in the 3-year naturalistic study showed dystonic movements during the first month of treatment, causing discontinuation of medication, while another had only mild and transient tremors (Masi et al, 2003). Data from the long-term studies report two cases of facial dystonia after 6 months of treatment (Zuddas et al, 2000) and two cases of withdrawal dyskinesia (Malone et al, 2002). No withdrawal diskinesias are reported in the study of Masi et al (2003).

The occurrence of EPS has been more rarely reported during treatment with olanzapine and quetiapine. However, in the study of Kemner et al (2002), three children showed mild EPS (rigidity and tremor), which disappeared after dosage reduction. Given the possibility of acute or tardive extrapyramidal phenomena, a close monitoring of abnormal motor movements is warranted.

Seizures

Even though atypical antipsychotics produce EEG abnormalities, the higher risk of dose-dependent epileptic seizures is associated with clozapine treatment, while the risk is milder with risperidone and quetiapine (Centorrino et al, 2002). This risk is particularly significant in autistic patients, who are particularly predisposed to developing seizures (Volkmar and Nelson, 1990).

Agranulocytosis

The higher risk of agranulocytosis is associated with clozapine treatment, and mandatory monitoring of white blood cells is recommended in the guidelines of the drug (Alvir et al, 1993). However, agranulocytosis and granulocytopenia are seldom reported during treatment with olanzapine (Kodesh et al, 2001) or quetiapine (Ruhe et al, 2001). A blood cell count is warranted when clinical indices of leukopenia are suspected (i.e. recurrent infections).

Hyperglycemia and hyperlipidemia

Atypical antipsychotics, particularly clozapine and olanzapine, are associated with higher levels of glucose and lipid levels (Hedenmalm et al, 2002; Wirshing et al, 2002), while for risperidone the risk is lower (Koller et al, 2003). Specific data on children and adolescents are scarce. Bloch and colleagues reported on five adolescents who developed overt diabetes (two subjects) or glucose dysregulation (three subjects) during olanzapine treatment (Bloch et al, 2003). A regular metabolic follow-up including fasting blood glucose is recommended in healthy adolescents receiving olanzapine and clozapine treatment.

Hepatotoxicity

Risperidone-induced hepatotoxicity, which may, in part, be related to weight gain in long-term use of this drug, has also been reported (Kumra et al, 1997). Two boys with psychotic disorder treated with risperidone (4 and 6mg/day) showed obesity and liver enzyme abnormalities (elevated serum aminotransferase levels), and abdominal ultrasound revealed fatty infiltration of the liver in both boys. In each case, liver damage was reversed after discontinuation of risperidone and/or weight loss. In the open-label risperidone study by Perry et al (1997), two children with PDD also developed possible hepatotoxicity associated with weight gain. The other studies on risperidone treatment in PDDs did not report specific concerns about this side-effect.

Liver function abnormalities during treatment with olanzapine are more frequently reported in children and adolescents than in adults (Woods et al, 2002). However, no significant changes in liver function were reported in the above mentioned studies on olanzapine in young patients with PDDs (Potenza et al, 1999; Malone et al, 2001; Kemner et al, 2002). Liver function should be monitored in children who are taking atypical antipsychotics, particularly in obese children or in those with rapid weight gain.

Cardiovascular effects

Cardiac symptoms in young children during risperidone treatment should be considered. A transient increase in heart rate was reported in two of the six preschool autistic patients in treatment with risperidone described by Casaer et al (1994), who considered these episodes as transitory and benign. Posey et al (1999b) reported tachicardia and QTc interval prolongation in the ECG in a very young autistic patient, which resolved when the risperidone dosage was reduced. In the study by Masi et al (2001a), one preschool child showed tachycardia and flushes one hour after drug intake. Tachycardia has been reported in 12% of the children in the placebo-controlled study (RUPP Autism Network, 2002). An ECG at baseline and as part of routine monitoring is recommended in younger patients.

Conclusions

Pharmacologic treatment can be considered a symptomatic intervention in children and adolescents with behavioral disorders associated with the autistic core symptomatology. Hyperactivity, aggression, lability of mood, and repetitive phenomena are the most sensitive target symptoms, while the social impairment is more resistant to pharmacologic interventions.

Further research is warranted, mainly considering the efficacy and safety of medications, for specific subtypes of patients, according to age and clinical profile. Long-term data are needed, given the paucity of information about the pharmacodynamic effect on the developing brain of drugs administered for extended periods of time during the first years of life, when dramatic developmental changes in neurotransmitters and receptors occur. Some animal data suggest a permanent up- or downregulation of receptor systems as a function of exposure to psychotropic drugs in the developing mammalian brain (Vitiello and Jensen, 1995). The greater immaturity of biologic systems may modify not only drug response (in terms of pharmacokinetics and/or pharmacodynamics), but also sensitivity to specific therapeutic or untoward effects. These considerations are non-specific to psycho-tropic medications, but they are common to pediatric pharmacology as a whole. Long-term, well-designed controlled studies on large samples of affected young children should expand the current knowledge on these issues.

Although the randomized, placebo-controlled clinical trials can be considered the gold standard when data on safety and efficacy are lacking, and/or when there is uncertainty regarding whether a med-ication is a valid alternative, an interesting issue is how far the results of controlled studies on very selected populations, intensively studied for short periods, can apply to everyday care. Systematic naturalistic observations of long-term outcome in routine care can yield their spe-cific kind of essential information needed to practice evidence-based health care (Masi et al, 2003). Long-term naturalistic prospective stud-ies might represent an important source of information regarding the effectiveness of a treatment over extended periods of time under routine clinical conditions.

References

Alvir JM, Lieberman JA, Safferman AZ, et al. Clozapine-induced agranulocytosis. Incidence and risk factors in the United States. *N Engl J Med* 1993; **329**: 162–7.

Aman MG, Marks RE, Turbott SH, et al. Clinical effects of methylphenidate and thiori-dazine in intellectually subaverage children. *J Am Acad Child Adolesc Psychiatry* 1991; **30**: 246–56.

American Psychiatric Association. *Diagnostic and statistical manual of mental disorders*, 4th edn. Washington, DC: American Psychiatric Association; 2000.

Anderson GM, Hoshino Y. Neurochemical studies of autism. In: Cohen DJ, Volkmar FR, eds. *Handbook of autism and pervasive developmental disorders*. New York: John Wiley & Sons; 1997: 325–43.

Anderson L, Campbell M, Grega D, et al. Haloperidol in the treatment of infantile autism: effects on learning and behavioral symptoms. *Am J Psychiatry* 1984; **141**: 1195–202.

Anderson GM, Freedman DX, Cohen DJ, et al. Whole blood serotonin in autistic and normal subjects. *J Child Psychol Psychiatry* 1987; **28**: 885–900.

Anderson L, Campbell M, Adams P, et al. The effects of haloperidol on discrimination learning and behavioral symptoms in autistic children. *J Autism Dev Disord* 1989; **19**: 227–39.

Baptista T, Kin NM, Beaulieu S, deBaptista EA. Obesity and related metabolic abnor-malities during antipsychotic drug administration: mechanism, management and research perspectives. *Pharmacopsychiatry* 2002; **35**: 205–19.

Belsito KM, Law PA, Kirk KS, et al. Lamotrigine therapy for autistic disorder: a random-ized, double-blind, placebo-controlled trial. *J Autism Dev Disord* 2001; **31**: 175–81.

Biederman J, Baldessarini R, Goldblatt A, et al. A naturalistic study of 24-hour electrocardiographic recordings in children and adolescents treated with desipramine. *J Am Acad Child Adolesc Psychiatry* 1993; **32**: 805–13.

Bloch Y, Vardi O, Mendlovic S, et al. Hyperglycemia from olanzapine treatment in adolescents. *J Child Adolesc Psychopharmacol* 2003; **13**: 97–102.

Brasic JR, Barnett JY, Kaplan D, et al. Clomipramine ameliorates adventitious movements and compulsions in prepubertal boys with autistic disorder and severe mental retardation. *Neurology* 1994; **44**: 1309–12.

Buitelaar JK, van der Gaag RJ, van der Hoeven J. Buspirone in the management of anxiety and irritability in children with pervasive developmental disorder: results of an open label study. *J Clin Psychiatry* 1998; **59**: 56–9.

Campbell M, Anderson L, Meier M, et al. A comparison of haloperidol and behavior therapy and their interaction in autistic children. *J Am Acad Child Psychiatry* 1978; **17**: 640–55.

Campbell M, Anderson LT, Small AM, et al. Naltrexone in autistic children: behavioral symptoms and attentional learning. *J Am Acad Child Adolesc Psychiatry* 1993; **32**: 1283–91.

Campbell M, Armenteros JL, Malone RP, et al. Neuroleptic-related dyskinesias in autistic children: a prospective, longitudinal study. *J Am Acad Child Adolesc Psychiatry* 1997; **36**: 835–43.

Carlsson ML. Hypothesis: is infantile autism a hypoglutamatergic disorder? Relevance of glutamate–serotonin interactions for pharmacotherapy. *J Neural Transm* 1998; **105**: 525–35.

Casaer P, Walleghem D, Vandenbussche I, et al. Pharmacokinetics and safety of risperidone in autistic children. *Ped Neurol* 1994; **11**: 89.

Centorrino F, Price BH, Tuttle M, et al. EEG abnormalities during treatment with typical and atypical antipsychotics. *Am J Psychiatry* 2002; **159**: 109–15.

Chen NC, Bedair HS, McKay B, et al. Clozapine in the treatment of aggression in an adolescent with autistic disorder. *J Clin Psychiatry* 2001; **62**: 479–80.

Chez MG, Buchanan CP, Bagan BT, et al. Secretin and autism: a two-part clinical investigation. *J Autism Dev Disord* 2000; **30**: 87–94.

Chugani DC, Muzik O, Behen M, et al. Developmental changes in brain serotonin synthesis capacity in autistic and nonautistic children. *Ann Neurol* 1999; **45**: 287–95.

Colao A, Loche S, Cappa M, et al. Prolactinomas in children and adolescents. Clinical presentation and long term follow-up. *J Clin Endocrinol Metab* 1998; **83**: 2777–80.

Coniglio SJ, Lewis JD, Lang C, et al. A randomized, double-blind, placebo-controlled trial of single-dose intravenous secretin treatment for children with autism. *J Pediatr* 2001; **138**: 649–55.

Cook EH Jr, Leventhal BL. The serotonin system in autism. *Curr Opin Pediatr* 1996; **8**: 348–54.

Cook EH Jr, Leventhal BL, Heller W, et al. Autistic children and their relatives: relationships between serotonin and norepinephrine levels and intelligence. *J Neuropsychiatry Clin Neurosci* 1990; **2**: 268–74.

Cook EH, Rowlett R, Jaselskis C, et al. Fluoxetine treatment of children and adults with autistic disorder and mental retardation. *J Am Acad Child Adolesc Psychiatry* 1992; **31**: 739–45.

Cook EH Jr, Perry BD, Dawson G, et al. Receptor inhibition by immunoglobulins: specific inhibition by autistic children, their relatives, and control subjects. *J Autism Dev Disord* 1993; **23**: 67–78.

Corson AM, Barkenbus JE, Posey DJ, et al. A retrospective analysis of quetiapine in the treatment of pervasive developmental disorders. *J Clin Psychiatry* 2004; **65**: 1531–6.

Couturier JL, Nicolson R. A retrospective assessment of citalopram in children and adolescents with pervasive developmental disorders. *J Child Adolesc Psychopharmacol* 2002; **12**: 243–8.

DeLong GR, Teague LA, Kamran MM. Effects of fluoxetine treatment in young children with idiopathic autism. *Dev Med Child Neurol* 1998; **40**: 551–62.

DeLong GR, Ritch CR, Burch S. Fluoxetine response in children with autistic spectrum disorder: correlation with familial major affective disorder and intellectual achievement. *Dev Med Child Neurol* 2002; **44**: 652–9.

Demb HB. Risperidone in young children with pervasive developmental disorders and other developmental disabilities. *J Child Adolesc Psychopharmacol* 1996; **6**: 79–80.

Di Martino A, Melis G, Cianchetti C, Zuddas A. Methylphenidate for pervasive developmental disorders: safety and efficacy of acute single dose and ongoing therapy: an open-pilot study. *J Child Adolesc Psychopharmacol* 2004; **14**: 207–18.

Dunn-Geier J, Ho HH, Auersperg E, et al. Effect of secretin on children with autism: a randomized controlled trial. *Dev Med Child Neurol* 2000; **42**: 796–802.

Epperson CN, McDougle CJ, Anand A, et al. Lithium augmentation of fluvoxamine in autistic disorder: a case report. *J Child Adolesc Psychopharmacol* 1994; **4**: 201–7.

Fankhauser MP, Karumanchi VC, German ML, et al. A double-blind, placebo-controlled study of the efficacy of transdermal clonidine in autism. *J Clin Psychiatry* 1992; **53**: 77–82.

Fatemi SH, Realmuto GM, Khan L, Thuras P. Fluoxetine in the treatment of adolescent patients with autism: a longitudinal open trial. *J Autism Dev Disord* 1998; **29**: 303–7.

Findling RL, Maxwell K, Scotese-Wojtila L, et al. High-dose pyridoxine and magnesium administration in children with autistic disorder: an absence of salutary effects in a double-blind, placebo-controlled study. *J Autism Dev Disord* 1997a; **27**: 467–78.

Findling RL, Maxwell K, Wiznitzer M. An open clinical trial of risperidone monotherapy in young children with autistic disorder. *Psychopharmacol Bull* 1997b; **33**: 155–9.

Findling RL, McNamara NK, Gracious BL, et al. Quetiapine in nine youths with autistic disorder. *J Child Adolesc Psychopharmacol* 2004; **14**: 287–94.

Fisman S, Steele M. Use of risperidone in pervasive developmental disorders: a case series. *J Child Adolesc Psychopharmacol* 1996; **6**: 177–90.

Frazier JA, Meyer MC, Biederman J, et al. Risperidone treatment for juvenile bipolar disorder: a retrospective chart review. *J Am Acad Child Adolesc Psychiatry* 1999; **38**: 960–5.

Galli-Tsinopoulou A, Nousia-Arvanitakis S, Mitsiakos G et al. Osteopenia in children and adolescents with hyperprolactinemia. *J Pediatr Endocrinol Metabol* 2000; **13**: 439–41.

Gillberg C. Endogenous opioid and opiate antagonists in autism: brief review of empirical findings and implications for clinicians. *Dev Med Child Neurol* 1995; **37**: 239–45.

Gillberg C, Svennerholm L, Hamilton-Hellberg C. Childhood psychosis and monoamine metabolites in spinal fluid. *J Autism Dev Disord* 1983; **13**: 383–96.

Giovanardi Rossi P, Posar A, Parmeggiani A, et al. Niaprazine in the treatment of autistic disorder. *J Child Neurol* 1999; **14**: 547–50.

Gordon CT, State RC, Nelson JE, et al. A double-blind comparison of clomipramine, desipramine, and placebo in the treatment of autistic disorder. *Arch Gen Psychiatry* 1993; **50**: 441–7.

Greenhill LL, Jensen PS, Abikoff H, et al. Developing strategies for psychopharmacological studies in preschool children. *J Am Acad Child Adolesc Psychiatry* 2003; **42**: 406–14.

Handen BL, Johnson CR, Lubetsky M. Efficacy of methylphenidate among children with autism and symptoms of attention-deficit hyperactivity disorder. *J Autism Dev Disord* 2000; **30**: 245–55.

Hardan A, Johnson K, Johnson C, et al. Risperidone treatment of children and adolescents with developmental disorders. *J Am Acad Child Adolesc Psychiatry* 1996; **35**: 1551–6.

Hardan AY, Jou RJ, Harden BL. Retrospective study of quetiapine in children and adolescents with pervasive developmental disorder. *J Autism Dev Disord* 2005; **35**: 387–91.

Hedenmalm K, Hagg S, Stahl M, et al. Glucose intolerance with atypical antipsychotics. *Drug Saf* 2002; **25**: 1107–16.

Hollander E, Kaplan A, Cartwright C, Reichman D. Venlafaxine in children, adolescents and adults with autism spectrum disorder: an open retrospective clinical report. *J Child Neurol* 2000; **15**: 132–5.

Hollander E, Dolgoff-Kaspar R, Cartwright C, et al. An open-trial of divalproex sodium in autism spectrum disorders. *J Clin Psychiatry* 2001; **62**: 530–4.

Horrigan JP, Barnhill LJ, Courvoisie HE. Olanzapine in PDD. *J Am Acad Child Adolesc Psychiatry* 1997; **36**: 1166–7.

Hoshino Y, Yamamoto T, Kanelo M, et al. Blood serotonin and free tryptophan concentration in autistic children. *Neuropsychobiology* 1984; **11**: 22–7.

Jaselskis CA, Cook EH Jr, Fletcher KE, et al. Clonidine treatment of hyperactive and impulsive children with autistic disorder. *J Clin Psychopharmacol* 1992; **12**: 322–7.

Kapur S, Seeman P. Does fast dissociation from the dopamine D(2) receptor explain the action of atypical antipsychotics? A new hypothesis. *Am J Psychiatry* 2001; **158**: 360–9.

Kemner C, Willemsen-Swinkels S, DeJonge M, et al. Open-label study of olanzapine in children with pervasive developmental disorders. *J Clin Psychopharmacol* 2002; **22**: 455–60.

Kerbeshian J, Burd L, Fisher W. Lithium carbonate in the treatment of two patients with infantile autism and atypical bipolar disorder. *J Clin Psychopharmacol* 1987; **7**: 401–5.

King BH, Wright DM, Habden J, et al. Double-blind, placebo-controlled study of amantadine hydrochloride in the treatment of children with autistic disorder. *J Am Acad Child Adolesc Psychiatry* 2001; **40**: 658–65.

Kodesh A, Finkel B, Lerner AG, et al. Dose-dependent olanzapine-associated leukopenia: three case reports. *Int Clin Psychopharmacol* 2001; **16**: 117–19.

Koller EA, Cross JT, Doraiswamy PM, Schneider BS. Risperidone-associated diabetes mellitus: a pharmacovigilance study. *Pharmacotherapy* 2003; **23**: 735–44.

Kolmen BK, Feldman HM, Handen BL, et al. Naltrexone in young autistic children: a double blind, placebo-controlled, cross-over study. *J Am Acad Child Adolesc Psychiatry* 1995; **34**: 223–31.

Kumra S, Herion D, Jacobsen LK, et al. Case study: risperidone-induced hepatotoxicity in pediatric patients. *J Am Acad Child Adolesc Psychiatry* 1997; **36**: 701–5.

Leboyer M, Bouvard MP, Launay JM, et al. A double-blind study of naltrexone in infantile autism. *J Autism Dev Disord* 1992; **22**: 309–19.

Lessig MC, Shapira NA, Murphy TK. Topiramate for reversing atypical antipsychotic weight gain. *J Am Acad Child Adolesc Psychiatry* 2001; **40**: 1364.

McBride PA, Anderson GM, Hertzig ME et al. Serotonergic responsivity in male young adults with autistic disorder: results of a pilot study. *Arch Gen Psychiatry* 1989; **46**: 213–21.

McBride PA, Anderson GM, Hertzig ME, et al. Effects of diagnosis, race, and puberty on platelet serotonin levels in autism and mental retardation. *J Am Acad Child Adolesc Psychiatry* 1998; **37**: 767–76.

McDougle CJ, Kresch LE, Goodman WK, et al. A case-controlled study of repetitive thoughts and behavior in adults with autistic disorder and obsessive-compulsive disorder. *Am J Psychiatry* 1995; **152**: 772–7.

McDougle CJ, Naylor ST, Cohen DJ, et al. A double-blind, placebo-controlled study of fluvoxamine in adults with autistic disorder. *Arch Gen Psychiatry* 1996a; **53**: 1001–8.

McDougle CJ, Naylor ST, Cohen DJ, et al. Effects of tryptophan depletion in drug-free adults with autistic disorder. *Arch Gen Psychiatry* 1996b; **53**: 993–1000.

McDougle CJ, Holmes JP, Bronson MR, et al. Risperidone treatment of children and adolescents with pervasive developmental disorders: a prospective open-label study. *J Am Acad Child Adolesc Psychiatry* 1997; **36**: 685–93.

McDougle CJ, Holmes JP, Carlson DC, et al. A double-blind, placebo-controlled study of risperidone in adults with autistic disorder and other pervasive developmental disorders. *Arch Gen Psychiatry* 1998; **55**: 633–41.

McDougle CJ, Scahill L, McCracken JT, et al. Research Units on Pediatric Psychopharmacology – Autism Network. Background and rationale for an initial controlled study of risperidone. *Child Adolesc Psychiatr Clin N Am* 2000; **9**: 201–24.

McDougle CJ, Kem DL, Posey DJ. Case series: use of ziprasidone for maladaptive symptoms in youths with autism. *J Am Acad Child Adolesc Psychiatry* 2002; **41**(8): 921–7.

McDougle CJ, Scahill L, Aman MG, et al. Risperidone for the core symptom domains of autism: results from the study by the autism network of the research units of pediatric psychopharmacology. *Am J Psychiatry* 2005; **162**: 1142–80.

Malek-Ahmadi P, Simonds JF. Olanzapine for autistic disorder with hyperactivity. *J Am Acad Child Adolesc Psychiatry* 1998; **37**: 902.

Malone RP, Cater J, Sheikh RM, et al. Olanzapine versus haloperidol in children with autistic disorder: an open pilot study. *J Am Acad Child Adolesc Psychiatry* 2001; **40**: 887–94.

Malone RP, Maislin G, Choudhury MS, et al. Risperidone treatment in children and adolescents with autism: short- and long-term safety and effectiveness. *J Am Acad Child Adolesc Psychiatry* 2002; **41**: 140–7.

Mandoki MW. Risperidone treatment of children and adolescents: increased risk of extrapyramidal side-effects? *J Child Adolesc Psychopharmacol* 1995; **5**: 49–67.

Martin A, Scahill L, Keonig K, et al. An open-label trial of quetiapine in children and adolescents with autistic disorder. *J Child Adolesc Psychopharmacol* 1999; **9**: 99–107.

Masi G, Cosenza A, Mucci M, De Vito G. Risperidone monotherapy in preschool children with pervasive developmental disorders: an open label study. *J Child Neurol* 2001; **16**: 395–400.

Masi G, Cosenza A, Mucci M. Open trial of risperidone in 24 young children with pervasive developmental disorders. *J Am Acad Child Adolesc Psychiatry* 2001a; **40**: 1206–14.

Masi G, Cosenza A, Mucci M. Prolactin levels in preschool autistic children during risperidone treatment. *J Child Adolesc Psychopharmacol* 2001b; **11**: 389–94.

Masi G, Cosenza A, Brovedani P, Mucci M. A three-year naturalistic study of 53 preschool children with pervasive developmental disorder treated with risperidone. *J Clin Psychiatry* 2003; **64**: 1039–47.

Meltzer HY, Matsubara S, Lee J-C. Classification of typical and atypical antipsychotic drugs on the basis of dopamine D1, D2 and serotonin 2 pKi values. *J Pharmacol Exp Ther* 1989; **251**(1): 238–46.

Minderaa RB, Anderson GM, Volkmar FR, et al. Whole blood serotonin and tryptophan in autism: temporal stability and the effects of medication. *J Autism Dev Disord* 1989; **19**: 129–36.

Namerow LB, Thomas P, Bostic JQ, et al. Use of citalopram in pervasive developmental disorders. *J Dev Behav Pediatr* 2003; **24**: 104–8.

Naruse H, Nagahata M, Nakane Y. A multi-center double-blind trial of pimozide (Orap), haloperidol and placebo in children with behavior disorders, using cross-over design. *Acta Paedopsychiatrica* 1982; **48**: 173–84.

Nicolson R, Awad G, Sloman L. An open trial of risperidone in young autistic children. *J Am Acad Child Adolesc Psychiatry* 1998; **37**: 372–6.

Owley T, McMahon W, Cook EH, et al. Multisite, double-blind, placebo-controlled trial of porcine secretin in autism. *J Am Acad Child Adolesc Psychiatry* 2001; **40**: 1293–9.

Owley T, Walton L, Salt J, et al. An open-label trial of escitalopram in pervasive developmental disorders. *J Am Acad Child Adolesc Psychiatry* 2005; **44**: 343–8.

Panksepp J. A neurochemical theory of autism. *Trends Neurosci* 1979; **2**: 174–7.

Partington MW, Tu JB, Wonf CY. Blood serotonin levels in severe mental retardation. *Dev Med Child Neurol* 1973; **15**: 616–27.

Pavuluri MN, Janicak PG, Carbray J. Topiramate plus risperidone for controlling weight gain and symptoms in preschool mania. *J Child Adolesc Psychopharmacol* 2002; **12**: 271–3.

Percy AK, Glaze DG, Schultz RJ, et al. Rett syndrome: controlled study of an oral opiate antagonist, naltrexone. *Ann Neurol* 1994; **35**: 464–70.

Perry R, Pataki C, Munoz-Silva DM, et al. Risperidone in children and adolescents with pervasive developmental disorder: pilot trial and follow-up. *J Child Adolesc Psychopharmacol* 1997; **7**: 167–79.

Perry R, Campbell M, Adams P, et al. Long-term efficacy of haloperidol in autistic children: continuous versus discontinuous drug administration. *J Am Acad Child Adolesc Psychiatry* 1998; **28**: 87–92.

Pfeiffer SI, Norton J, Nelson L, Shott S. Efficacy of vitamin B6 and magnesium in the treatment of autism: a methodology review and summary of outcomes. *J Autism Dev Disord* 1995; **25**: 481–93.

Posey DJ, Litwiller M, Koburn A, McDougle CJ. Paroxetine in autism. *J Am Acad Child Adolesc Psychiatry* 1999a; **38**: 111–12.

Posey DJ, Walsh KH, Wilson GA, et al. Risperidone in the treatment of two very young children with autism. *J Child Adolesc Psychopharmacol* 1999b; **9**: 273–6.

Posey DJ, Decker J, Sasher TM, et al. A retrospective analysis of guanfacine in the treatment of autism. *Proc Am Psychiatr Assoc* 2001a, New Research Abstract 816.

Posey DJ, Guenin KD, Kohn AE, et al. A naturalistic open-label study of mirtazapine in autistic and other pervasive developmental disorders. *J Child Adolesc Psychopharmacol* 2001b; **11**: 267–77.

Potenza MN, Holmes JP, Kanes SJ, et al. Olanzapine treatment of children, adolescents, and adults with pervasive developmental disorders: an open-label pilot study. *J Clin Psychopharmacol* 1999; **19**: 37–44.

Quintana H, Birmaher B, Stedge D, et al. Use of methylphenidate in the treatment of children with autistic disorder. *J Autism Dev Disord* 1995; **25**: 283–94.

Remington G, Sloman L, Konstantareas M, Parker K, Gow R. Clomipramine versus haloperidol in the treatment of autistic disorder: a double-blind, placebo controlled, crossover study. *J Clin Psychopharmacol* 2001; **21**: 440–4.

Research Unit on Pediatric Psychopharmacology (RUPP) Autism Network. Risperidone in childen with autism and serious behavioral problems. *N Engl J Med* 2002; **347**: 314–21.

Research Unit on Pediatric Psychopharmacology (RUPP) Autism Network. Risperidone treatment of autistic disorder: longer-term benefits and blinded discontinuation after 6 months. *Am J Psychiatry* 2005; **162**: 1361–9.

Rimland B, Callaway E, Dreyfus P. The effect of high doses of vitamin B6 on autistic children. *Am J Psychiatry* 1978; **135**: 472–5.

Roberts W, Weaver L, Brian J, et al. Repeated doses of porcine secretin in the treatment of autism: a randomized, placebo-controlled trial. *Pediatrics* 2001; **107**: E71.

Rubin M. Use of atypical antipsychotics in children with mental retardation, autism and other developmental disabilities. *Psychiatr Ann* 1997; **27**: 19–221.

Ruhe HG, Becker HE, Jessum P, et al. Agranulocytosis and granulocytopenia associated with quetiapine. *Acta Psychiatr Scand* 2001; **104**: 311–13.

Sanchez LE, Campbell M, Small AM, et al. A pilot study of clomipramine in young autistic children. *J Am Acad Child Adolesc Psychiatry* 1996; **35**: 537–44.

Sandler AD, Sutton KA, DeWeese J, et al. Lack of benefit of a single dose of synthetic human secretin in the treatment autism and pervasive developmental disorders. *N Engl J Med* 1999; **341**: 1801–6.

Sandman CA, Barron JL, Chicz-DeMet A, et al. Brief report: plasma beta-endorphin and cortisol levels in autistic patients. *J Autism Dev Disord* 1991; **21**: 83–8.

Schwamm JS, Klass E, Alonso C, Perry R. Risperidone and refusal to eat. *J Am Acad Child Adolesc Psychiatry* 1998; **37**: 572–3.

Snead RW, Boon F, Presberg J. Paroxetine for self-injurious behavior. *J Am Acad Child Adolesc Psychiatry* 1994; **33**: 909–10.

Steingard R, Biederman J. Lithium-responsive manic-like symptoms in two individuals with autism and mental retardation. *J Am Acad Child Adolesc Psychiatry* 1987; **26**: 932–5.

Steingard RJ, Zimnitzky B, De Maso DR, et al. Sertraline treatment of transition-associated anxiety and agitation in children with autistic disorder. *J Child Adolesc Psychopharmacol* 1997; **7**: 9–15.

Stigler KA, Posey DJ, McDougle CJ. Aripiprazole for maladaptive behavior in pervasive developmental disorders. *J Child Adolesc Psychopharmacol* 2004; **14**: 455–63.

Todd RD, Ciaranello RD. Demonstration of inter- and intraspecies differences in serotonin binding sites by antibodies from an autistic child. *Proc Natl Acad Sci USA* 1985; **82**: 612–16.

Uvebrant P, Bauziene R. Intractable epilepsy in children: the efficacy of lamotrigine treatment, included non-seizure-related benefits. *Neuropediatrics* 1994; **25**: 284–9.

Vitiello B. Pediatric psychopharmacology and the interaction between drugs and the developing brain. *Can J Psychiatry* 1998; **43**: 582–4.

Volkmar FR, Nelson DS. Seizure disorders in autism. *J Am Acad Child Adolesc Psychiatry* 1990; **29**: 127–9.

Willemsen-Swinkels SHN, Buitelaar JK, van Engeland H. The effects of chronic naltrexone treatment in young autistic children: a double-blind placebo-controlled crossover study. *Biol Psychiatry* 1996; **39**: 1023–31.

Wirshing DA, Boyd JA, Meng LR, et al. The effects of novel antipsychotics on glucose and lipid levels. *J Clin Psychiatry* 2002; **63**: 856–65.

Woods SW, Martin A, Spector SG, McGlashan TH. Effects of development on olanzapine-associated adverse events. *J Am Acad Child Adolesc Psychiatry* 2002; **26**: 1409–11.

Wozniak J, Biederman J, Faraone SV, et al. Mania in children with pervasive developmental disorders revisited. *J Am Acad Child Adolesc Psychiatry* 1997; **36**: 1552–9.

Wudarski M, Nicolson R, Hamburger SD, et al. Elevated prolactin in pediatric patients on typical and atypical antipsycotics. *J Child Adolesc Psychopharmacol* 1999; **9**: 239–45.

Yuwiler A, Shih JC, Chen CH, et al. Hyperserotoninemia and antiserotonin antibodies in autism and other disorders. *J Autism Dev Disord* 1992; **22**: 33–45.

Zuddas A, Ledda MG, Fratta A, et al. Clinical effects of clozapine on autistic disorder. *Am J Psychiatry* 1996; **153**: 738.

Zuddas A, Di Martino A, Muglia P, Cianchetti C. Long-term risperidone for pervasive developmental disorder: efficacy, tolerability, and discontinuation. *J Child Adolesc Psychopharmacol* 2000; **10**: 79–90.

Index

Page numbers in *italics* represent tables, those in **bold** represent figures.